SMOKING AND LUNG CANCER

SMOKING AND LUNG CANCER

EVELYN N. POWERS
AND
JASMINA B. CABBOT
EDITORS

Nova Science Publishers, Inc.
New York

For permission to use material from this book please contact us:
Telephone 631-231-7269; Fax 631-231-8175
Web Site: http://www.novapublishers.com

Library of Congress Cataloging-in-Publication Data

Smoking and lung cancer / [edited by] Evelyn N. Powers and Jasmina B. Cabbot.
p. ; cm.
Includes bibliographical references and index.
ISBN 978-1-60692-367-2 (hardcover)
1. Lungs--Cancer--Etiology. 2. Smoking--Health aspects. I. Powers, Evelyn N. II. Cabbot, Jasmina B.
[DNLM: 1. Lung Neoplasms--etiology. 2. Smoking--adverse effects. WF 658 S666 2009]
RC280.L8S648 2009
616.99'424--dc22

2008041721

Published by Nova Science Publishers, Inc. ✦ New York

Contents

Preface

Smoking is responsible for 90% of cancer deaths. Incidence of lung cancer is rising. Lung cancer is responsible for more cancer deaths than colorectal cancer, breast cancer, and prostate cancer combined. Lung cancer primarily strikes people over age 45. By the time that an individual develops symptoms, spread has usually occurred. Lung cancer is directly related to smoking. Over 40 carcinogens have been identified in cigarette smoke. The risk of developing lung cancer is directly related to the number of cigarettes smoked. The change in consumption from unfiltered high tar cigarettes to filtered low tar cigarettes parallels the change in incidence from squamous cell carcinoma to adenocarcinoma. There is a long interval between quitting smoking and elimination of lung cancer risk. Up to 40% of newly diagnosed lung cancer occurs in former smokers (median abstinence duration 9 years). This new book presents the latest research in the field from around the world.

Expert Commentary - Lung cancer exhibits symptoms only after the disease has made cure unlikely. Because early-stage disease can be successfully treated, a screening technique that can detect lung cancer before it has spread might be useful in decreasing lung cancer mortality. In this chapter, the authors review the evidence on the benefit and harm on the early detection of lung cancer, with a focus on three technologies: chest x-ray (CXR), sputum cytology, and low-dose CT (LDCT) scanning and offer recommendations regarding its usefulness for asymptomatic patients with no history of cancer. Studies of lung cancer screening with chest radiograph and sputum cytology have failed to demonstrate that screening lowers lung cancer mortality rates. Published studies of newer screening technologies such as low-dose CT and "biomarker" screening report primarily on lung cancer detection rates and do not present sufficient data to determine whether the newer technologies will benefit or harm. Although researchers are conducting randomized trials of low-dose CT, results will not be available for several years. In the meantime, cost-effectiveness analyses and studies of nodule growth are considering practical questions but producing inconsistent findings. Studies of symptomatic patients suggest that surgery causes morbidity and mortality. Overall, mortality rates range from 1.3% to 11.6% and morbidity rates from 8.8% to 44% and these figures might be higher among asymptomatic patients. Another potential harm of screening is false-negative findings with possible false reassurance. In current practice, the best estimate of the rate of false-negative results from chest x-rays comes from the CT studies, where false-negative rates as high as 75% were shown. In conclusion, for high-risk populations, no screening modality has been shown to alter mortality outcomes. Individuals undergo screening only when it is administered as a component of a well-designed clinical trial with appropriate protection for human subjects. Current smokers should be clearly informed that the most immediate preventive health priority is the elimination of tobacco use altogether, because smoking cessation offers the surest route at this time for reducing the risk of premature death from lung cancer.

Chapter I - Tobacco smoke is the single most important etiologic factor in the development of lung cancer, accounting for approximately 90% of all lung cancer deaths in men and approximately 60% in women, although a great deal of variation was present between countries. This review provides a current understanding of the epidemiologic evidence on lung cancer. The major objectives of this article were 3-fold: 1) to review the updated risk estimates associated with smoking for lung cancer by histologic type, 2) to summarize the relationship between passive smoking and lung cancer risk, 3) to describe the effect of smoking reduction and cessation on lung cancer risk. Lung cancer in never smokers is seventh leading cause of cancer deaths in the world. Epidemiological studies of lung cancer in never smokers have identified significant gender and geopraphic variations. This review also summarizes the epidemiological features of lung cancer in never smokers. Cigarette smoking plays a part in the development of Chronic Obstructive Pulmonary Disease (COPD) in only a proportion of smokers. The association of susceptibility to COPD and the prognostic outcome of smokers with early-stage lung cancer were also reviewed. In the present article, the authors also provide a summary of current understanding about the computed tomography screening for lung cancer and lung cancer outcomes.

Chapter II - An estimated 85% of the lung cancer cases worldwide in men, and 47% in women, are attributable to tobacco smoking. In other words, smoking is an important risk factor for developing lung cancer. On the other hand, the impact of smoking status on survival after the diagnosis of lung cancer, especially in the surgical setting, has long been controversial, although numerous relevant studies have been conducted. Recently, we reported that the preoperative smoking history is an important clinical postoperative prognostic factor in patients with primary resected non-small cell lung cancer (NSCLC), and since then, several studies have reported identical findings. Furthermore, smoking cessation even after the diagnosis is associated with improved survival in early-stage NSCLC patients. In addition, the longer the time has been since the cessation of smoking, the better the survival outcome. Interestingly, a possible association between exposure to passive smoking prior to diagnosis of early-stage NSCLC and survival after treatment has also been reported. Here, the authors review several studies investigating the relationship between smoking and prognosis of non-small cell lung cancer in surgical settings.

Chapter III - Background: Cigarette smoking-induced lung damage is one of the most important factors predisposing to lung cancer with aggressive clinical features. However, the relationship between lung damage and the clinical features of lung cancer is still unclear.

Methods: The subjects of this study were a consecutive series of 72 smokers who underwent complete resection of pathological stage I non-small-cell lung cancer. Pulmonary emphysema and airflow limitation was diagnosed based on the findings of quantitative computed tomography and spirometry, respectively. The authors compared the clinicopathological features of smokers with, and smokers without lung damage.

Results: Pulmonary emphysema and airflow limitation were diagnosed in 39 and 30 patients, respectively. Pulmonary emphysema was associated with higher risks of death and recurrence, whereas airflow limitation was not. Male gender and poorly differentiated type were more common in patients with emphysema than in those without emphysema. However, according to a multivariate analysis, emphysema, tumor size, and microvessel invasion were the independent predictors of survival and recurrence.

Conclusion: Although smoking-induced lung dysfunction is a known risk factor for lung cancer development, it was not associated with the clinical aggressiveness of lung cancer; however, smoking-induced lung destruction was. Thus, smoking-induced lung destruction and dysfunction may play different roles in the development and progression of lung cancer.

Chapter IV - Alpha-1-antitrypsin (AAT) is an important serine protease inhibitor in human plasma that is encoded by the protease inhibitor (Pi) locus on chromosome 14q and shows a co-dominant pattern of inheritance. It is a highly polymorphic gene with approximately 125 single nucleotide polymorphisms (SNPs) reported in public databases. AAT variants may be classified by their effect on AAT level and function as normal, deficient, null (nil detectable) or dysfunctional. The PiM allele is the wild type, and is the most prevalent. The PiZ and PiS allele are more common deficiency variants. Deficient alleles are responsible to lung diseases (emphysema, chronic bronchitis, and bronchiectasis), liver disease (neonatal jaundice and liver cirrhosis), vasculitis and panniculitis whilst the rare null alleles are responsible only to lung disease. Dysfunctional alleles code for an abnormal form of AAT, which, whilst present at a detectable level, does not function normally.

Elastases form a subfamily of serine proteases that hydrolyze many proteins in addition to elastin. Humans have six elastase genes that encode the structurally similar proteins. Neutrophil elastase is present in azurophil granules in the neutrophils and released at inflammatory sites when they are stimulated by a variety of compounds, including cytokines and chemoattractants. This important protease is enzyme that when expressed aberrantly can cause emphysema or emphysematous changes. This involves breakdown of the lung structure and increased airspaces.

Physiologically these protease and antiprotease are closely connected and present inseparable duet in patophysiology of lung injury. The major physiological role of AAT is to inhibit NE in the lower respiratory tract and protect lung tissue from destruction, with a smaller role in defending against damage by other serine proteases, such as cathepsin G and proteinase 3.

It is well known that imbalance in activity between NE and AAT in favor of NE play a role in the development of emphysema in smokers or in patients with inherited alpha-1-antitrypsin deficiency (AATD). A number of studies indicated etiological role of NE and AAT separately in lung cancer development. However, the rare investigations have been focused on their association as it relates to lung cancer. Some of them have been shown that AATD subjects with high plasma level of NE have a significant risk for lung cancer. It was postulated that the imbalance between NE and AATD was generally considered as a cause of tissue damage, which could be a favorable tissue environment for the action of carcinogens and tumor progression.

On the other hand, both of these proteins are tumor promoters. Namely, it was shown that lung-cancer cell lines produce elastase and the high levels of this enzyme in lung tumor tissue have been correlated with higher stage tumors and poor survival in lung cancer patients. It has been proposed that increase elastase and similar proteinases could destroy the barrier between tumor and the local circulatory system and results in facilitating cancer cell invasion. It has been obtained that higher stage of lung cancer was associated with high plasma level of AAT because increased transcription of AAT is response for the elevated elastase level or their activity.

Chapter V - Introduction: A new country-by-country report on tobacco use and control, co-published by the American Cancer Society, the World Health Organization and the International Union against Cancer, lends further support to the evidence that the tobacco industry is increasingly targeting women in developing countries, the largest remaining untapped market for cigarettes. Thus, tobacco's cancer burden is increasingly being shifted to developing countries. Serbia, a South East European country in transition, ranks among the top first several countries in Europe by tobacco use of its inhabitants: some 48% of the Serbian adult population smokes (men predominate), and in some urban areas this proportion is even higher, especially among women.

The aim of the chapter is to analyze the incidence rate and trend of lung cancer in Serbia in the period 1993-2005 with special regard to women and patients' tobacco smoking status.

Methods: In this descriptive study, annual collective data on newly- diagnosed cases of lung cancer, categorized by sex and tobacco smoking status (smokers, ex-smokers and non-smokers), have been analyzed for the 13-year period. The data represent a summary of all new cases of lung cancer in Serbia reported to the Research and Epidemiology Department of the Institute of Lung Diseases and Tuberculosis in Belgrade through the pulmonary facilities network. Population estimates were based on 1991 and 2002 census data with extrapolation.

Results: Total lung cancer incidence rate shows a slight increasing tendency ($y=27.554+0.1473x$) with a peak value of 33.8/100,000 population in the year 2003, and 26.7/100000 in the last year of analysis and significant differences among districts. Smokers, ex-smokers, and non-smokers account for 70.3%, 17% and 12.7%, respectively ($p<0.001$). Total number of lung cancer cases in women is doubled: a dramatic increase in tendency in smokers, but increase in former smokers, and even more in non smokers is found ($y=4.0535+0.5182x$). The male/female ratio in total was 4.25 but 6.9 in smokers, the latter showing a decreasing tendency in the observed period ($y=9.1615-0.3758x$).

Conclusion: Reducing smoking in the community will have a considerable positive effect on morbidity and mortality of lung cancer. As an example of a developing country in transition, Serbia needs urgent and continual increase of people's awareness towards tobacco smoking and other environmental harmful effects on human health, and health care workers' education on tobacco smoking as an addictive disease, its primary prevention and cessation. The relationship between tobacco smoking and lung cancer remains a challenge for further investigations that could lead to more effective therapy, and possibly a primary prevention of tobacco use.

Chapter VI - In industrialized countries, lung cancer is among the most common cancers in both genders. In the US (2007), this cancer was diagnosed in 213,380 men and women, and 160,390 men and women are expected die of it. The highest rates are still observed in North America and Europe, but lung cancer is already the most common fatal cancer worldwide, with 1.04 million new cases and 921,000 deaths yearly. Lung cancer accounts for more deaths than breast and colon cancer combined. Unlike breast and colon cancers, there is currently no recommendation in favor of lung cancer screening.

The rationale of lung cancer screening is debated mostly because basic principles are misinterpreted. Thus, we first discuss the rationale for lung cancer screening by reviewing the fundamental conditions needed in order to propose a screening intervention. The authors review fundamental concepts that are essential to appropriately design and interpret lung cancer screening studies, and will illustrate common systematic errors including lead time bias, length bias, and over-diagnosis.

They then review the available tools for lung cancer screening; we will show that, although each tool may detect lung cancer at an earlier stage compared with no intervention, all except low dose CT (LDCT) failed to reduce mortality. Screening studies from 1960 to now will be presented critically, including studies using LDCT, both and observational and experimental, in the US and Europe. Lastly, we will discuss lung cancer screening from ethical and social perspectives.

Since smoking is the major risk factor for lung cancer, some argue that the major intervention to decrease lung cancer is to prevent people from smoking or to make them quit, and have further argued that even if lung cancer screening trials report clear mortality reduction, resources should be allocated to smoking prevention rather than screening. The authors will argue that preventing tobacco use is the key element of lung cancer prevention, and must be therefore encouraged to reduce the incidence (primary prevention). However, this does not preclude the efforts to improve the treatment of lung cancer, and screening (secondary prevention) might be part of these efforts if effective.

Chapter VII - Second-hand smoke (SHS) is also referred as passive smoke, involuntary smoke, environmental tobacco smoke, and environmental cigarette smoke. The sources of SHS include exposure from relatives at home, work place, and in public. Experimental and epidemiologic studies have observed the intake and metabolism of SHS (National Research Council (U.S.).

Part of the importance of SHS stems from the fact that the levels of some carcinogens, e.g., polycyclic aromatic hydrocarbon (PAH), benzo(a)pyrene (BP) and 4-aminobiphenyl (4-ABP, an arylamine), are actually higher in undiluted SHS than in mainstream smoke (i.e., active smoke) (National Research Council 1986). In addition, the size of the particles in SHS is smaller than those in mainstream smoke and, therefore, these particles are more likely to be deposited in the lung (Dockery and Trichopoulos 1997; Hecht 1999). The association between SHS and lung cancer or childhood asthma has been studied extensively. While it is well-recognized that 80-90% of all lung cancer is attributable to cigarette smoking, only 15% of all smokers develop this disease and about 10% of all diagnosed lung cancers are never smokers (Hammond and Seidman 1980).

In summary, for different health effects, significant associations have been observed in genetic markers, including risk modification by germline polymorphisms, gene expression changes, and somatic alterations.

Some gaps in our knowledge of SHS health effects remain. The associations between sequence variants of genes involved in phase I and II metabolism and cell cycle pathways and the risk of lung cancer have been widely explored for SHS exposure and conclusive findings are not yet available.

Chapter VIII - Many studies have associated passive smoking with an increased risk of developing certain diseases. Smoking during pregnancy increases the risk of the newborn having a low birth weight (at term or pre-term), and of suffering impaired respiratory function and ischaemic heart disease etc. In children and adolescents, environmental exposure to tobacco smoke has been associated with abnormal lipid profiles and an increased risk of atherosclerosis. Passive smoking can also be the cause of reduced female fertility in the general population. The food habits of both active and passive smokers may also be negatively affected.

The diets of smokers tend to be less adequate than those of non-smokers. Exposure to tobacco smoke modifies the sense of taste and smell, leading to changes in food preferences and food intake, and eventually to a more imbalanced diet. Matters are made worse in that smokers may have greater needs of certain nutrients such as antioxidants. Thus, even with a normal intake of these nutrients, the nutritional status of smokers can be inadequate.

As with active smokers, passive smokers may show slightly unhealthy food habits and more imbalanced diets than non-smokers – either as a consequence of living with smokers (and therefore sharing their food habits) or via the direct modification of their food choices. Passive smokers consume fewer fruits and vegetables and have lower intakes of a number of nutrients, which might be reflected at the serum level. For example, exposure to tobacco smoke is associated with reduced folate levels, via which some of the effects of active and passive smoking on health may be made manifest. Like active smokers, passive smokers may have a greater need of certain nutrients. For example, they show lower plasma concentrations of antioxidants than do non-smokers not exposed to smoke, independent of the differences in dietary antioxidant intake.

The diet of passive smokers may be an important factor in the relationship between tobacco smoke exposure and health problems. Although the cessation of smoking and the avoidance of passive smoking is the ideal goal, it cannot always be attained. Dietary intervention may therefore be a useful and indeed necessary strategy to prevent or delay smoking-related pathologies.

Chapter IX - Lung cancer has reached nearly epidemic proportions in women; the incidence has quadrupled over the past 40 years. Multiple studies have been conducted to identify reasons for the dramatic increase in lung cancer over the past decades. Smoking behaviors, pathways of carcinogenesis and the impact of the hormonal milieu have all been examined as possible explanations. Although many studies have attempted to address these questions, they have been retrospective or case-control studies and results have been inconsistent. With the recognition that lung cancer may behave differently in men versus women, current studies are prospectively examining this question.

Chapter X - The proportion between smoking and radon related lung cancer incidences is discussed with focus on the real situation in a region with high radon concentrations in dwellings. Special emphasis has been put on the exposition of children where there is a lack of data. The risks from domestic radon seem to be highly coupled with the risks from smoking. Smoking is by far the most leading risk factor for primary lung cancer, and the risks from radon seem to be overemphasised. The most effective method to reduce the number of primary lung cancer incidences seems to be to stop smoking, both what concerns smoking related as well as radon related lung cancers. Campaigns for testing all homes for radon should also include campaigns against smoking.

In: Smoking and Lung Cancer
Editors: E. N. Powers and J. B. Cabbot

ISBN 978-1-60692-367-2

Expert Commentary

Screening for Lung Cancer: Benefit or Harm

Rodrigo Córdoba-García [*]
University of Zaragoza, Spain
redIAPP (Primary Care Research Network)

Abstract

Lung cancer exhibits symptoms only after the disease has made cure unlikely. Because early-stage disease can be successfully treated, a screening technique that can detect lung cancer before it has spread might be useful in decreasing lung cancer mortality. In this chapter, we review the evidence on the benefit and harm on the early detection of lung cancer, with a focus on three technologies: chest x-ray (CXR), sputum cytology, and low-dose CT (LDCT) scanning and offer recommendations regarding its usefulness for asymptomatic patients with no history of cancer. Studies of lung cancer screening with chest radiograph and sputum cytology have failed to demonstrate that screening lowers lung cancer mortality rates. Published studies of newer screening technologies such as low-dose CT and "biomarker" screening report primarily on lung cancer detection rates and do not present sufficient data to determine whether the newer technologies will benefit or harm. Although researchers are conducting randomized trials of low-dose CT, results will not be available for several years. In the meantime, cost-effectiveness analyses and studies of nodule growth are considering practical questions but producing inconsistent findings. Studies of symptomatic patients suggest that surgery causes morbidity and mortality. Overall, mortality rates range from 1.3% to 11.6% and morbidity rates from 8.8% to 44% and these figures might be higher among asymptomatic patients. Another potential harm of screening is false-negative findings with possible false reassurance. In current practice, the best estimate of the rate of false-negative results from chest x-rays comes from the CT studies, where false-negative rates as high as 75% were shown. In conclusion, for high-risk populations, no screening modality has been shown to alter mortality outcomes. Individuals undergo screening only

[*] rcordobag@papps.org.

when it is administered as a component of a well-designed clinical trial with appropriate protection for human subjects. Current smokers should be clearly informed that the most immediate preventive health priority is the elimination of tobacco use altogether, because smoking cessation offers the surest route at this time for reducing the risk of premature death from lung cancer.

Keywords: Lung cancer, screening, smoking

Screening for Lung Cancer: Benefit or Harm?

Over the last 50 years, a set of very consistent evidence has been compiled on the association between tobacco consumption and an excess risk of mortality for numerous causes, among them several types of cancer, cardiovascular disease and an elevated prevalence of chronic respiratory processes. Because of this, tobacco has been acknowledged by the scientific community as the most important single cause of premature and preventable morbidity and mortality.

All healthcare professionals should strongly advise smokers to give up tobacco. There is fullconsensus on this particular point [1]. Tobacco consumption is associated with the cause of 25 acute and chronic processes leading to avoidable suffering, serious illness and premature death [2]. Lung cancer (LC) is particularly significant among them. Between 1980 and 2020, 600,000 persons will have died of LC as a result of their addiction to tobacco. There may be hundreds more deaths related to factors such as radon or other environmental pollutants, but LC not related to either active or passive tobacco use is currently considered a rarity with the exception of inhabited areas with a high granite concentration.

LC is more common in males, in terms of both morbidity and mortality. The situation is different for females; however, the trends observed in other countries are causing concern. LC became the leading cause of cancer death in women in the US 20 years ago and led to 50% more deaths than breast cancer in 2002 [3]. A similar trend can be expected in other countries where women have taken up habits of tobacco later over the next few years.

In the United States, the incidence of lung cancer has decreased significantly, by 0.7% per year from 1991 to 2004 for men and women combined. It has also decreased significantly, by 1.8% per year from 1991 to 2004 among men, and remained level from 1998 to 2004 among women [4]. The only lung cancer prevention procedure currently accepted is not taking up smoking. Despite this, there are in the region of 10 million smokers in Spain (European Union). Although the prevalence of smoking in this country has been falling rapidly in recent years and a reduction in the incidence of LC in males has been observed, the numbers of women suffering from this form of cancer in Spain is expected to increase because different stage in tobacco epidemic model [5, 6]. In addition, it known that the increased risk is maintained for former smokers for a long period of time after having given up the habit, and for persons who persist, despite attempts to give up on different occasions, 40% are not successful and remain at risk for the rest of their lives. In fact, one out of every two smokers dies prematurely as a consequence of tobacco if they do not stop smoking, and of all of the causes of premature death, LC is one of the most dramatic given that average survival rate at 5 years is 7%. Faced with this panorama, clinicians and diagnostic imaging experts have spent years trying to identify a valid screening method in the hope of producing early detection. In this way, we would be in a position to treat greater number of cases during stage 1 where the survival rate at 5 years is 70%, compared to the meagre 5-10% of cases diagnosed as a result of early detection. The question being considered is: with the information available at present, is population screening feasible for early lung cancer detection?

In the 1960s and 70s, seven clinical trials were begun in which chest x-rays (CXRs), taken individually or in combination with sputum cytology, at different intervals were assessed. After several years, evaluation did not show differences in mortality rates between the experimental group and the control group [7, 8, 9, 10, 11,12]. Subsequently, results were published of the results from five studies carried out in Japan between 1992 and 2001 with a case-control design. Their results supported CXR screening (OR between 0.42 and 0.72)[13, 14, 15, 16, 17]. However, design weaknesses designs do not permit the influence of selection bias, such as the healthy volunteer, to be assessed, which may make the populations of both groups difficult to compare from the start.

Given the lack of results using these strategies, an attempt was made with CAT scanning. We have the data from several cohort studies that lack control groups. There is agreement in the suitability of reviewing the capacity of CT scanning to detect a greater number of cases and in earlier stages, but this does not allow conclusions to be drawn on the impact on mortality. It has been estimated that the percentage of cancers detected with stage I screening CT scans is somewhere between 55 and 85%, compared to 16% when diagnosis is made when following the usual clinical course of the disease [18]. Given the difference in expectations of cure depending on the stage of a tumour, it seems reasonable to assess intervention favourable. Data from the I-ELCAP study [19] have just been published along these lines. This is a broad, collaborative study that monitored a cohort of 31,567 asymptomatic subjects with risk of LC who underwent annual low-dose CT scanning as a screening test. Aspects relative to test performance and survival at 10 years were evaluated. LC detection on first screening was 1.3% and 0.3% on annual screening. Alterations requiring some type of follow up were detected in 13% of those initially screened (10% positive predictive value for first screening) and in 5.3% of subjects on annual screening (PPV 5.6%). 85% of the detected tumours were in stage I. This set of data raise hopes with regard to a potential method for early detection of lung cancer and the consequent improvement in the mortality of its natural process. However, studies available with CT, including I-ECAP, leave a number of important issues unresolved. The rate of false positives for the total of these studies is between 5 and 50% on first screening, not inconsiderable, and from 3 to 12% in subsequent screenings. Between 4.8 and 14.5% of patients are referred for biopsy, with 63 and 90% resulting in a cancer diagnosis. A false positive can produce potential side effects, in addition to anxiety and preoccupation - the results of the risk and evaluation tests that can lead to a biopsy and even organ resection. Mortality rates for surgery in symptomatic patients ranges between 1.3 and 11.6% and morbidity rates between 8.8% and 44% [20]. It is also a controversial issue owing the influence of possible bias on the results, in the absence of a control group and randomization. The role of potential over-diagnosis cannot be ruled out in the case of detection via screening of pre-clinical stage cancers that never would have become clinically manifest. Likewise, threats to the validity of these studies are lead time bias, resulting in a longer period of awareness of the disease that does not prolong survival, and length bias, providing greater opportunities for detecting slow-growth cancers in an early detection programme and therefore better prognosis. Both biases are particularly problematic when the final estimated variable is the survival rate, as is the case of I-ECAP.

Some of these concerns have not been completely mitigated in the wake of the publication of a recent study [21]. A contrast was made of the results observed after an annual CT scan screening on a cohort of 3,246 patients at risk (smokers and former smokers), compared to cases expected using a predictive model, where the same population had not been subject to screening. In the 3.9 years that the study lasted, 3.2 times more cases were diagnosed in the screened group than expected (144 observed v. 44.5 expected). The risk of undergoing a lung resection in the screened group was multiplied by 10 (109 v. 10.9). No decrease was observed in the number of advanced LC diagnoses (42 v. 33.4) or in the number of deaths from LC (38 v. 38.8). These data are not reassuring. While being inconclusive, they emphasise the concern over possible over-diagnosis and the consequent risks of the diagnosis and therapeutic cascade. It will be necessary to await the results of a number of studies in progress in order to resolve pending doubts. In 2009, the Lung Cancer Screening Trial by the US National Cancer Institute, where CT scanning and CXR are compared (unfortunately, there is no unscreened control group), and in 2010, a European study, comparing CT scanning and routine practice [22], may shed more light on this matter.

Positron emission tomography (PET) use in precision diagnosis of lung nodules has created certain expectations regarding its potential for LC screening. It is true that it improves the validity of CT scanning for the study of lung nodules [23]. However, PET lacks a randomized clinical trial that demonstrates lowering of lung cancer mortality.

Therefore, we can conclude that the CT scan screening studies available to date should be interpreted with due caution as their demonstrated capacity for detecting the disease in earlier stages has a still uncertain effect on mortality and more so as doubts raised on the demonstration of its cost-effectiveness are yet to be resolved. No benefits have been established for any group, and the risk/benefit ratio is still unfavourable for persons at low risk. The final recommendations for Low Dose CT are exposed in Table 1

Table 1. Low Dose CT for LC Screening

Summary of Recommendations.
1. We do not recommend that low-dose CT be used to screen for lung cancer except in the context of a well-designed clinical trial. Grade of recommendation, 2C
2. We recommend against the use of serial chest X-rays to screen for the presence of lung cancer. Grade of recommendation, 1A
3. We recommend against the use of single or serial sputum cytologic evaluation to screen for the presence of lung cancer. Grade of recommendation, 1A

Source: Bach PB, Jett JR, Pastorino U, et al. Computed Tomograph. Screening and Lung Cancer Outcomes. *JAMA* 2007;297:953-61.

The Best Prevention: Quit Smoking

In its 2004 update, the US Preventive Services Task Force concludes that available information does not allow it to declare itself in favour of or against LC screening and that the aggressive nature of some diagnostic tests must be taken into account together with a potentially high rate of false positives in certain populations.

Table 2. Guidelines on Screening for Lung Cancer

Recommending Body	Topic	Recommendation
National Cancer Institute (http://www.cancer.gov/cancertopics/pdq/screening/lung/healthprofessional)	CXR and sputum cytology	On the basis of fair evidence, screening does not reduce mortality from lung cancer. On the basis of solid evidence, screening would lead to false-positive results and unnecessary invasive diagnostic procedures and treatments
National Cancer Institute (http://www.cancer.gov/cancertopics/pdq/screening/lung/healthprofessional)	LDCT	The evidence is inadequate to determine whether screening reduces mortality from lung cancer. On the basis of solid evidence, screening would lead to false positive results and unnecessary invasive diagnostic procedures and treatments
American Cancer Society	CXR and sputum cytology	Lung cancer screening is not a routine practice for the general public or even for people who are at increased risk, such as smokers
US Preventive Services Task Force (http://www.ahrq.gov/clinic/uspstf/uspslung.htm)	CXR, sputum cytology, and LDCT	The evidence is insufficient to recommend for or against screening asymptomatic individuals for lung cancer with LDCT, CXR, sputum cytology, or a combination of these tests.
Canadian Coordination Office for Health Technology Assessment (http://www.cadth.ca/media/pdf/213_ct_cetap_e.pdf)	LDCT	Currently, the evidence does not exist to suggest that detecting early-stage lung cancer reduces mortality. At present, screening for lung cancer with multislice/helical CT would be premature.
Society of Thoracic Radiology	LDCT	Mass screening for lung cancer is not currently advocated. Suitable subjects who wish to participate should be encouraged to do so in controlled trials so that the value of CT screening can be ascertained

Source: Bach PB, Jett JR, Pastorino U, et al. Computed Tomography Screening and Lung Cancer Outcomes. *JAMA* 2007; 297:953-61.

The American Cancer Association has maintained for some time that smokers or persons exposed to carcinogens in the workplace must be given special attention by their doctors, who may choose selective LC screening based on potential benefit to the individual.

Other institutions such as the National Cancer Institute, el Canadian Coordination Office for Health Technology Assessment and the Society of Thoracic Radiology [24] do not advocate population screening for LC with any of the techniques put forward to date – sputum cytology, CXR, conventional CT, helical CT or a combination of these techniques (Table 2).

Discussion must come on whether these diagnostic techniques should be subject to 'aggressive promotion' for their indiscriminate use on the entire at-risk population. The ACS recommends caution and highlights the importance of informed decision-making for persons choosing a method of screening. Smokers should continue to receive a forceful and clear message: the preventive priority for protection of health is to completely eliminate tobacco use, because smoking cessation is the surest behaviour to reduce the risk of premature death from lung cancer[25] and 25 other chronic and fatal diseases. Would the fact that lung cancer screening might prove to reduce mortality and is cost-effective for the public health system change this message? No. The possibility to prevent lung cancer does not guarantee the prevention of 9 other types of tobacco-related diseases or the other 15 cardiovascular and respiratory diseases, some of which are caused by very low doses or exposure to smoking or even by passive smoking. LC is an almost totally preventable form of cancer. This is an uncommon and favourable option that must not be hidden behind the hope placed in complex and intricate statistics from clinical mega-trials. What is more logical and efficient – to rescue victims that fall into turbulent waters one by one with great difficulty or to stop the monster that is throwing them in by the hundreds upstream?

References

[1] Fiore M. Tobacco Use and Dependence Clinical Practice Guideline Panel, Staff and Consortium representatives. A clinical Practice Guideline for treating tobacco use and dependence. A US Public Health Report. *JAMA* 2000;283:3244-3254

[2] U.S. Departament of Health and Human Services. The Health Consequences of Smoking. A Report of the Surgeon General. Atlanta, GA: US Department of Health and Human Services, Centers for Disease Control Prevention and Health Promotion, Office on Smoking and Health, 2004.

[3] The GLOBOCAN 2002 database. Consulted 25th Fabruary 2007. http://www-dep.iarc.fr/

[4] http://www.cdc.gov/cancer/lung/statistics/trends.htm

[5] Lopez AD, Collishaw NE, Piha T.A descriptive model of the cigarette epidemic in developed countries. Tobacco Control, 1994; 3: 242-247

[6] Banegas JR, Diez L, Rodríguez-Artalejo F, González J, Graciani A y Villar F. Mortalidad atribuible al tabaquismo pasivo en España en 1998. *Med. Clin.* (Barc) 2001; 117:692-694.

[7] Brett GZ. The value of lung cancer detection by six-monthly chest radiographs. *Thorax* 1968;23(4):414-20.

[8] Dales LG; Friedman GD, Collen MF. Evaluating periodic multiphasic health checkups: a controlled trial. *J. Chron. Dis.* 1979;32(5):385-404.

[9] Melamed MR, Flehinger BJ, Zaman MB, et al. Screening for early lung cancer. Results of the Memorial Sloan-Kettering study in New York. *Chest* 1984;86(1):44-53.

[10] Levin ML, Tockman MS, Front JK, et al. Lung cancer mortality in males screened by chest X-ray and cytologic sputum examination: a preliminary report. Recent Results. *Cancer Res.* 1982;82:138-146.

[11] Marcus PM, Bergstralh EJ, Fagerstrom RM, et al. Lung cancer mortality in the Mayo Lung Project: impact of extended follow-up. *J. Natl. Cancer Inst.* 2000;92(16):1308-16.

[12] Kubik AK, Parkin DM, Zatloukal P. Czech Study on Lung Cancer Screening: post-trial follow-up of lung cancer deaths up to year 15 since enrolment. *Cancer* 2000; 89(11):2363-68.

[13] Okamoto N, Suzuki T, Hasegawa H, et al. Evaluation of a clinic-based screening program for lung cancer with a case-control design in Kanagawa, Japan. *Lung Cancer* 1999; 25(2):77-85.

[14] Sobue T. A case-control study for evaluating lung cancer screening in Japan. *Cancer* 2000: 89(11 Suppl): 2392-96.

[15] Sagawa M. Tsubono Y, Saito Y, et al. A case-control study for evaluating the efficacy of mass screening program for lung cancer in Miyagi Prefecture. Japan. *Cancer* 2001;92(3):588-94.

[16] Tsukada H, Kurita Y, Yokoyama A, et al. An evaluation of screening for lung cancer in Niigata Prefecture, Japan: a population-base case-control study. *Br. J. Cancer* 2001;85(9):1326-31.

[17] Nishii K, Ueoka H, Kiura K, et al. A case-control study of lung cancer screening in Okayama Prefecture, Japan. *Lung Cancer* 2001;34(3):325-332.

[18] Mulshine JL, Sullivan DC. Lung Cancer Screening. *N Eng J Med* 2005;352:2714-20.

[19] Henschke CI, Yankelevitz DF, Libby DM, et al. Survival of Patients with Stage I Lung Cancer Detected on CE Screening. The International Early Lung Cancer Action Program. *N Eng. J. Med.* 2006;355:1763-71

[20] Humphrey LL, Teutsch S, Johnson MS. Lung Cancer Screening: An Update of the U.S. Preventive Services Task Force. *Ann. Intern. Med.* 2004;140:740-53

[21] Bach PB, Jett JR, Pastorino U, et al. Computed Tomography Screening and Lung Cancer Outcomes. *JAMA* 2007;297:953-61

[22] Hirsh FR, Bunn PA, et al. IV International Conference on Prevention and Early Detection of Lung Cancer, Reykjavik, Iceland. *Lung Cancer* 2002;37:24-44.

[23] Pastorino U, Bellomi M, Landoni C, et al. Early lung-cancer detection with spiral CT and positron emission tomography in heavy smokers: 2-years results. *Lancet* 2003; 362:593-97.

[24] Aberle D, Gamsu G, Henschke C, et al. A consensus statement of the Society of Thoracic Society: screening for lung cancer with helical computed tomography. *J. Thorax Imaging* 2001; 16:65-68.

[25] Smith RA, Cokkinides V, Eyre HJ. American Cancer Society Guidelines for the Early Detection of Cancer, 2004. *CA Cancer J. Clin.* 2004;54:41-52.

Research and Review Studies

In: Smoking and Lung Cancer
Editors: E. N. Powers and J. B. Cabbot
ISBN 978-1-60692-367-2

Chapter I

Smoking and Lung Cancer

Hisamitsu Omori**, Mayumi Tsuji and Takahiko Katoh
Department of Public Health, Graduate School of Medical Sciences,
Kumamoto University, Kumamoto 860-8556, Japan

Abstract

Tobacco smoke is the single most important etiologic factor in the development of lung cancer, accounting for approximately 90% of all lung cancer deaths in men and approximately 60% in women, although a great deal of variation was present between countries. This review provides a current understanding of the epidemiologic evidence on lung cancer. The major objectives of this article were 3-fold: 1) to review the updated risk estimates associated with smoking for lung cancer by histologic type, 2) to summarize the relationship between passive smoking and lung cancer risk, 3) to describe the effect of smoking reduction and cessation on lung cancer risk. Lung cancer in never smokers is seventh leading cause of cancer deaths in the world. Epidemiological studies of lung cancer in never smokers have identified significant gender and geopraphic variations. This review also summarizes the epidemiological features of lung cancer in never smokers. Cigarette smoking plays a part in the development of Chronic Obstructive Pulmonary Disease (COPD) in only a proportion of smokers. The association of susceptibility to COPD and the prognostic outcome of smokers with early-stage lung cancer were also reviewed. In the present article, we also provide a summary of current understanding about the computed tomography screening for lung cancer and lung cancer outcomes.

* Correspondence to Hisamitsu Omori, TEL: +81 96 373 5112 FAX: +81 96 373 5113. E-mail: omorih@gpo.kumamoto-u.ac.jp.

Introduction

Every year, approximately 1.35 million people die of lung cancer worldwide. In women, lung cancer is the leading cause of cancer deaths with a mortality rate that is approximately 60% higher than that for breast cancer [1]. The annual female age-standardized lung cancer mortality increased by 4.2% between 1982 and 1990 and by 1.7% between 1990 and 1995. In men, the annual mortality rate increased by a very modest 0.4% between 1982 and 1991 and decreased by 1.9% between 1991 and 2001 [1].

Over the past 50 years, studies have shown an indisputable causal role of tobacco smoke in the worldwide epidemic of lung cancer. Lung cancer has been the most common cancer in the world since 1985. The annual number of new cases was estimated to be 12.4% of all new cancer cases [2, 3].

Tobacco smoke is the single most important etiologic factor in the development of lung cancer, accounting for approximately 90% of all lung cancer deaths in men and approximately 60% in women, although a great deal of variation was present between countries [2, 4, 5]. The risk of lung cancer rises with increasing pack-years. Although the pack-year is a convenient indicator for smoking intensity, this assumes that the duration of smoking and number of cigarette per day equally affect the risk of lung cancer, which is not the case [6].

This overview mainly provides as follows: ethnic and racial differences, women and lung cancer, the updated risk estimates associated with smoking for lung cancer by histologic type, the relationship between passive smoking and lung cancer risk, the effect of smoking reduction and cessation on lung cancer risk, the epidemiological features of lung cancer in never smokers, the association of susceptibility to COPD and the prognostic outcome of smokers with early-stage lung cancer, and the computed tomography screening for lung cancer and lung cancer outcomes.

Ethnic and Racial Differences

Haiman and colleagues reported the existence of ethnic and racial differences in the smoking-associated risk of lung cancer [7]. And they reported that among cigarette smokers, African Americans and Native Hawaiians are more susceptible to lung cancer than whites, Japanese Americans, and Latinos. They investigated differences in the risk of lung cancer associated with cigarette smoking among 183,813 African-American, Japanese-American, Latino, Native Hawaiian, and white men and women in the multiethnic Cohort Study. Their analysis contained 1979 cases of incident lung cancer identified prospectively over an eight-year period, between baseline (1993 through 1996) and 2001. They found significant differences in the association between cigarette smoking and risk of lung cancer among five self-reported ethnic and racial populations. Among participants who smoked no more than 30 cigarettes per day, African and Native Hawaiians had significantly greater risks of lung cancer than did the other groups. However, at levels exceeding 30 cigarettes per day, these differences were not significant. The findings could not be explained by differences between populations in known or suspected risk factors, including diet, occupation, and socioeconomic status as assessed according to the level of education. Differences in risk associated with smoking were observed among both men and women and for all histologic types of lung cancer.

Particularly in women with primary lung cancer, adenocarcinoma has been the most common histologic subtype [8, 9].

Women and Lung Cancer

Some case-control studies suggest that, given equal smoking exposure, women may have a higher relative risk of developing lung cancer than men [10-12]. The possibility that women are more susceptible than men to developing lung cancer after exposure to similar amounts of cigarette smoke has generated substantial controversy [10-12].

On the contrary, according to the Nurses' Health Study, women do not appear to have a greater susceptibility to lung cancer than men, given equal smoking exposure [13].

Regarding sex-related differences in the risk for lung cancer, there are major phenotypic and histologic differences in lung cancer between men and women [13]. Peripheral lung adenocarcinomas are common in women than in men; this is in contrast to squamous cell carcinomas, which are more common in men.

One of the important first steps in lung carcinogenesis is the formation of DNA adducts. DNA adducts alter DNA structure, which in turn modifies its ability to replicate, translate, and repair. Female smokers have higher adduct levels compared with male smokers, and this difference becomes even larger when the adduct levels are adjusted for cigarette smoking and expressed as adducts/pack-year or adducts/cigarettes consumed per day [14].

Estrogen and related compounds may up-regulate the expression of cytochrome P450 (CYP) enzymes in lungs and liver, which are involved in the metabolism of various constituents of cigarette smoke [15]. Epidemiologic studies have shown an association between exogenous estrogens and development of lung adenocarcinoma in women [15]. In a case control study by Taioli and colleagues showed that women who used estrogen therapy had a higher risk of lung cancer [16]. Women have been reported to have increased susceptibility to tobacco carcinogens but have a lower rate of fatal outcome of lung cancer compared with men [17].

Updated Risk Estimates Associated with Smoking for Lung Cancer by Histologic Type

Each of the three major histologic subtypes of lung cancer, including squamous cell carcinoma, adenocarcinoma, and small cell carcinoma, is associated with tobacco-smoking exposure [18, 19]. The influence of tobacco smoke on the risk of adenocarcinoma is not considered as great as that of the other two histologic types [20].

According to an analysis from a prospective cohort study of 41,836 Iowa women aged 55-69 years with 13 years of follow-up from 1986 through 1998, of the three major lung cancer subtypes, the excess risk for heavy smokers compared with never smokers was higher for adenocarcinoma than for squamous cell and small cell carcinomas [21]. This study suggested that adenocarcinoma of the lung is more strongly associated with tobacco smoke exposure than previously recognized [21].

Sobue and colleagues reported the update risk estimates associated with cigarette smoking for lung cancer by histologic type from Japan, based on a population-based prospective cohort study using incidence as an endpoint during 1990-1999 [6]. The relative risk for all incident cases associated with current smokers versus non-smokers was 4.5 (95% confidence interval (CI): 3.0-6.8) and 4.2 (95% CI: 2.4-7.2), for men and women, respectively. When divided by histologic type, relative risk for squamous cell carcinoma (SCC) and small cell lung cancer (SCLC) was 12.7 (95% CI: 4.7-34.7) and 17.5 (95% CI: 4.9-62.1), while for adenocarcinoma it was 2.8 (95% CI: 1.6-4.9) and 2.0 (95% CI: 0.8-5.0) for men and women, respectively [6].

Although the histological spectrum of lung cancer demonstrates geographic variations, there has been a major global trend with a decrease in SCC and a sharp rise in adenocarcinoma [22]. This changing histological pattern has occurred over a period of a few decades. This trend has been hypothesized to be due to the widespread usage in many countries of cigarettes with lowered tar and nicotine content [23]. Over the last 40 years, the type of cigarettes most frequently used has been changing, namely the increased use of low tar and nicotine cigarettes. This has been accompanied by an increased risk of lung cancer due to a smokers' need to maintain blood nicotine levels, which in turn causes the need for smoking more cigarettes per day and deeper inhalation [23]. This phenomena has led to the increasing rates of lung adenocarcinoma [23]. Cigarette smoke contains four thousand chemicals including over 60 identified as carcinogens according to assessments by the International Agency for Research in Cancer (IARC) [24]. The most potent carcinogens are the polycyclic aromatic hydrocarbons (PAHs), such as benzo[a]pyrene (BAP) and the tobacco-specific nitrosamine known as nicotine – derived nitrosoaminoketone (NNK). NNK is a potent tobacco-specific carcinogen, and readily induces KRAS mutation-associated adeocarcinoma in rodents [25].

The Relationship between Passive Smoking and Lung Cancer Risk

Passive smoking contains smoke from two sources: sidestream and exhaled mainstream smoke. Environmental tobacco smoke (ETS) has been classified as a known (Group A) human lung carcinogen by the United States Environmental Protection Agency (EPA) since 1993 [26].

At least 17 carcinogenic chemicals contained in tobacco smoke are emitted at higher levels in sidestream smoke than mainstream smoke [27]. One of the metabolites of tobacco smoke [benzo (a) pyrene diol epoxide], which shows a direct aetiological association with lung cancer, is found in both mainstream and sidestream smoke [28].

Numerous epidemiological studies since 1981 have examined the association between passive smoking and lung cancer. Taylor and colleagues reported meta-analysis of passive smoking and lung cancer, which included 55 studies (7 cohort studies, 25 population-based case-control and 23 non-population-based case-control studies [29]. They reviewed twenty previously published meta-analyses. Fixed and random effect models and meta-regression are used to obtain pooled estimates of RR and P-value functions are used to demonstrate consistency of results. The pooled RR for never-smoking women exposed to passive smoking from spouses is 1.27 (95% CI 1.17-1.37). The RR for North America is 1.15 (95% CI 1.03-1.28), Asia, 1.31 (95% CI 1.16-1.48) and Europe, 1.31 (1.24-1.52). Sequential cumulative meta-analysis shows no trend. There is no strong evidence of publication bias [29].

A population-based prospective study conducted in Japan demonstrated that passive smoking from husbands is a risk factor for lung cancer, especially for adenocarcinoma among Japanese women [30]. Compared with women married to never smokers, hazard ratio (HR) [95% confidence interval (CI)] for all lung cancer incidence in women who lived with a smoking husband was 1.34 (95% CI 0.81-2.21) [30]. According to their study, association was clearly identified for adenocarcinoma (HR 2.03, 95% CI 1.07-3.86), for which dose-response relationships were seen for both the intensity (p for trend = 0.02) and amount (p for trend = 0.03) of the husband's smoking. Passive smoking at the workplace also increased the risk of lung cancer (HR 1.32, 95% CI 0.85-2.04). Moreover, a higher risk of adenocarcinoma was seen for combined husband and workplace exposure (HR 1.93, 95% CI 0.88-4.23) [30].

The Effect of Smoking Reduction and Cessation on Lung Cancer Risk

For smokers, smoking cessation is the most effective measure to decrease the risk of lung cancer. The Copenhagen Centre for Prospective Population Studies [31] contained pooled data from 3 longitudinal population-based studies carried out in Copenhagen, Denmark and its vicinity during 1964 through 1993. In these studies, the association between smoking reduction and incidence of the major histologic subtypes of primary lung cancer was analyzed [31].

Participants were 11,151 men and 8,563 women aged 20 to 93 years, who attended 2 consecutive examinations with a 5- to 10-year interval between 1964 and 1988. Incident primary lung cancer cases were assessed by record linkage with the National Cancer Registry until 2003. There were 864 incident lung cancers during follow-up. The adjusted hazard ratio (HR) for lung cancer in reducers was 0.73 (95% CI: 0.54-0.98) compared with persistent heavy smokers. The HR for light smokers was 0.44 (95% CI: 0.35-0.56); for quitters, HR 0.50(95% CI: 0.36-0.69), for stable ex-smokers, HR 0.17 (95% CI: 0.13-0.23), and for never smokers, HR 0.09 (95% CI: 0.06-0.13) [31]. These studies concluded that among individuals who smoke 15 or more cigarette per day, smoking reduction by 50% significantly reduces the risk of lung cancer [31].

Doll R and colleagues [32] reported that there was a steady trend in lung cancer mortality ratio between lifelong non-smokers, ex-smokers who had stopped at 25-34, 35-44, 45-54, or 55-64, and continuing smokers. This trend was consistent with the findings from case-control studies [33] that there is substantial protection even for those who stop at 55-64, and progressively greater protection for those who stop earlier. None the less, those who had smoked until about 40 years of age before they stopped had some excess risk of lung cancer at older ages [32].

The Lung Health Study (LHS) is one of the largest randomized clinical trial of smoking cessation and inhaled bronchodilator (ipratropium) therapy in smokers 35 to 60 years of age who did not consider themselves ill but had evidence of mild to moderate airway obstruction [34].Although initial study was designed as a 5-year trial, the follow-up was subsequently extended to 14.5 years. After up to 14.5 years of follow-up, 731 patients of 5887 participants died: 33% of lung cancer, 22% of cardiovascular disease, 7.8% of respiratory disease other than cancer, and 2.3% of unknown causes [34]. All-cause mortality was significantly lower in the special intervention group than in the usual care group (8.83 per 1000 person-years vs. 10.38 per 1000 person-years; P=0.03). The hazard ratio for mortality in the usual care group compared with the special intervention group was 1.18 (95% CI, 1.02 to 1.37). In this study, the benefits of smoking cessation in retarding disease progression and attenuating morbidity and mortality were confirmed.

In the ACCP evidence-based clinical practice guidelines (2nd edition), the reduction in smoking prevalence in men that occurred in the late 1960s through the 1980s will continue to drive lung cancer mortality rates downward in men during the first portion of this century, but rates in women have not yet begun to decrease [35].

Lung Cancer in Never Smokers

Lung cancer is often viewed as solely a smoker's disease, and efforts to study the disease in never smokers have been limited [36]. An estimated 15% of lung cancer in men and 53% of lung cancer in women (25% of all cases) world wide are not attributable tobacco smoking. Lung cancer in never smokers is the seventh leading cause of cancer deaths in the world, killing more people every year than pancreatic or prostate cancers [36]. Epidemiological studies of lung cancer in never smokers have identified significant gender and geographic variations [36]. A consistent global observation is that lung cancer in never smokers occurs more frequently in women than men. In addition, it has been observed that the proportion of female lung cancer cases in never smokers varies considerably from region to region [36]. The proportion of females with lung cancer who are never smokers is as high as 83% in South Asia, whereas approximately 15% of females with lung cancer in the United States are never smokers. Among men, the proportion of never smokers is lower with less regional variation [36]. All major histological types of lung cancer are associated with smoking, although the association is stronger for small cell lung cancer (SCLC) and for squamous cell carcinoma (SCC) than for adenocarcinoma [19, 36]. By comparison, adenocarcinoma is the common form of lung cancer in never smokers [36].

According to this review, a number of different epidemiological, clinical and molecular differences between lung cancers which arise in never smokers and those which arise in smokers suggest that lung cancer in never smokers is a 'different' disease, with a different aetiology and a different natural history [36].

COPD and Lung Cancer

Chronic Obstructive Pulmonary Disease (COPD) is also an important risk factor for lung cancer. In both men and women, the risk of lung cancer increases with decreasing lung function [37]. There is good epidemiological data to indicate that COPD patients are at increased risk of cancer, especially lung cancer. Lange and colleagues showed that those with percentage-predicted forced expiratory volume in one second (FEV_1) <40 had a risk of lung cancer death 3.9 times higher than those with 80+; this study included smokers and non-smokers [38]. Eberly and colleagues demonstrated the strong predictive value of FEV_1 for lung cancer among cigarette smokers independent of smoking history [39].

Purdue and colleagues reported that mild COPD (GOLD stage 1) is associated with a 50% increase in the risk of lung cancer, moderate COPD (GOLD stage 2) is associated with a 2.1-fold increase and severe COPD is associated with a 2.7-fold increase in the risk, independent of the effects of smoking [40]. Other studies demonstrated that, after adjustment for age and smoking, reduced FEV_1 is associated with an increased risk of lung cancer [41-44].

Wasswa-Kintu and colleagues [45] reported a systemic review and meta-analysis of all published data of large population-based studies showing that reduced FEV_1 is strongly associated with lung cancer. They showed even a relatively modest reduction in FEV_1 is a significant predictor of lung cancer, especially among women [45]. The mechanisms linking COPD to lung cancer are unclear. Potential mechanism is by delayed clearance of inhaled carcinogens in COPD patients. With progressive airflow impairment, patients may not be able to fully clear the inhaled carcinogens in a timely manner, which increase the opportunity for carcinogenic materials to effect DNA mutagenesis [46]. Additionally, COPD has been associated with increased chronic and persistent oxidative stress and local inflammation, which have also been implicated in the pathogenesis of lung cancer [15].

Computed tomography (CT) has been shown to be a sensitive technique for evaluation of presence and severity of emphysema [47, 48]. In recent years, it has become apparent that COPD is a syndrome that encompasses a heterogeneous group of conditions that share the common characteristics of chronic airflow obstruction with varying conditions from emphysema, small-airway disease and chronic bronchitis [48, 49].

Patients with a predominance of small-airways disease are at greater risk of lung cancer compared with those with a predominance of emphysema for the same degree of FEV_1 Impairment and smoking history [50].

CT Screening for Lung Cancer

Screening for lung cancer with low-dose computed tomography (CT) is controversial [51]. It is well established that CT is far more sensitive than chest radiography in detecting lung cancer when it is small and asymptomatic [51]. In a large population-based lung cancer screening program of smokers (n=7,498 women and 9,427 men), women were almost twice as likely to be diagnosed with lung cancer on screening computed tomography compared with men (odds ratio, 1.9) [52]. Ueda and colleagues reported that computed tomography –

diagnosed emphysema, but not airway obstruction, is associated with poor prognosis in smokers with early-stage lung cancer [53].

In 1993, The Early Lung Cancer Action Project (ELCAP) initiated a study of the early diagnosis of lung cancer in cigarette smokers with the use of annual screening with spiral screening with spiral computed tomography (CT) [54]. In this large collaborative study, 31,567 asymptomatic persons at risk for lung cancer were screened from 1993 through 2005, and from 1994 through 2005. Repeated screenings of 27,456were performed 7 to 18 months after the previous screening. They reported as follows. Screening resulted in a diagnosis of lung cancer in 484 participants. Of these participants, 412 (85%) had Clinical stage 1 lung cancer, and the estimated 10-year survival rate was 88% in this subgroup (95% confidence interval [CI], 84 to 91). Among the 302 participants with clinical stage 1 cancer who underwent surgical resection within 1 month after diagnosis, the survival rate was 92% (95% CI: 88 to 95).They concluded that annual spiral CT screening can detect lung cancer that is curable. Thus, very high rates of survival were reported recently for screen-detected lung cancers in a large, multinational, single-arm observational study. However, a reduction in lung cancer mortality has not been demonstrated to date, and a recent longitudinal study with a simulated control group suggested little or no mortality reduction [51]. Ongoing RCTs should resolve this uncertainty in a few years [51].

Conclusion

This overview mainly provided as follows: ethnic and racial differences, women and lung cancer, the updated risk estimates associated with smoking for lung cancer by histologic type, the relationship between passive smoking and lung cancer risk, the effect of smoking reduction and cessation on lung cancer risk, the epidemiological features of lung cancer in never smokers, the association of susceptibility to COPD and the prognostic outcome of smokers with early-stage lung cancer, and the computed tomography screening for lung cancer and lung cancer outcomes.

Lung cancer is the leading cause of cancer death worldwide with over one million deaths each year. The disease is largely preventable because it is estimated that 90% of all lung cancers are attributed to smoking. Since the weight of all evidence indicates that smoking cessation decreases lung cancer risk, health care providers need to continue to provide smoking cessation intervention program for all smokers at all ages. A further effort is needed to identify the factors responsible for most lung cancers arising in never smokers worldwide.

References

[1] Jemal, A., Murray, T., Ward, E., Samuels, A., Tiwari, R.C., Ghafoor, A., Feuer, E.J., Thun, M.J. (2005). Cancer statistics, 2005. CA *Cancer J. Clin.* 55, 10-30.

[2] Pirozynski M. Historical Review 100 years of lung cancer. *Respiratory medicine* 2006; 100: 2073-2084.

[3] Parkin, D.M., Bray, F., Ferlay, J.and Pisani, P. (2005). Global cancer ststistics. CA *Cancer J. Clin.* 55, 74-108.

[4] Bray, F., Tyczynski, J.E., and Parkin, D.M. (2004). Going up or coming down? The changing phases of lung cancer epidemic from 1967 to 1999 in the 15 European Union countries. *Eur. J. Cancer* 40(1): 96-125.

[5] Pisani, P. (2000). Avoidable Cancer in Europe: Estimating Avoidable Fractions. Europe Against Cancer Programme (EU contrast SOC 96 200504), Lyon, December.

[6] Sobue, T., Yamamoto, S., Hara, M., et al. (2002). Cigarette smoking and subsequent risk of cancer by histologic type in middle-ages Japanese men and women: the JPHC study. 99, 245-251.

[7] Haiman,C.A., Stram,D.O., Wilkens,L.R., Pike,M.C., Kolonel,L.N., Henderson,B.E., and Marchand,L.L. (2006). Ethnic and racial differences in the smoking-related risk of lung cancer. *N. Engl. J. Med.,* 354(4), 333-342.

[8] Ernster, V.L. (1996). Female lung cancer. *Annu. Rev. Public Health* 17, 97-114.

[9] Franceschi, S., Bidoli, E. (1999). The epidemiology of lung cancer. NewYork, NY: Kluwer Academic Publishers, 1-6.

[10] Zang, E.A., Wynder, E.L. (1996). Differences in lung cancer risk between men and women: examination of evidence. *J. Natl. Cancer Inst.* 88: 183-192.

[11] Perneger, T.V. (2001). Sex, smoking, and cancer: a reappraisal. *J. Natl. Cancer Inst.* 93: 1600-1602.

[12] Thum, M.J., Henley, S.J., and Calle, E.E. (2002). Tobacco use and cancer: an epidemiologic perspective for geneticists. *Oncogene* 21: 7307-7325.

[13] Bain, C., Feskanich, D., Speizer, F.E., Thun, M., Hertzmark,E., Rosner, B.A., and Colditz, G.A. (2004). Lung cancer rates in men and women with comparable histories of smoking. *J. Natl. Cancer Inst.* 96: 826-834.

[14] Mollerup, S., Ryberg, D., Hewer, A., Phillips, D.H., Haugen, A. (1999). Sex differences in lung CYP1A1 expression and DNA adduct levels among lung cancer patients. *Cancer Res.* 59: 3317-3320.

[15] Cohen, S.B-Z., Pare, P.D., Sin, D.D. (2007). The growning burden of chronic obstructive pulmonary disease and lung cancer in women. Examining sex differences in cigarette smoke metabolism. *Am. J. Respir. Crit. Care Med.* 176: 113-120.

[16] Taioli, E., wynder, E.L. (1994).Re: endocrine factors and adenocarcinoma of the lung in women. *J. Natl. Cancer Inst.* 86, 869-870.

[17] International Early Lung Cancer Action Program Investigators. (2006). Women's susceptibility to tobacco carcinogens and survival after diagnosis of lung cancer. *JAMA* 296: 180-184.

[18] Blot, W.J., Fraumeni, J.F.Jr. (1996). Cancers of the lung and pleura. In: Schottenfeld, D., Fraumeni, J.F.Jr.,eds. Cancer epidemiology and prevention. New York, NY: Oxford University Press, Inc, 637-665.

[19] Khuder, S.A. (2001). Effect of cigarette smoking on major histological types of lung cancer: a meta-analysis. *Lung Cancer* 31, 139-148.

[20] Kabat, G.C. (1996). Aspects of the epidemiology of lung cancer in smokers and nonsmokers in the United States. *Lung Cancer* 15, 1-20.

[21] Yang, P., Cerhan, J.R., Vierkant, R.A., Olson, J.E., et al. (2002). Adenocarcinoma of the lung is strongly associated with cigarette smoking: further evidence from a prospective study of women. 156, 1114-1122.

[22] Gabrielson, E. (2006). Worldwide trends in lung cancer pathology. *Respirology* 11, 533-538.

[23] Shield, P.G. (2002). Molecular epidemiology of smoking and lung cancer. *Oncogene* 21, 6870-6876.

[24] Hoffmann, D., Hoffmann, I., and E.I. Bayoumy, K. (2001). The less harmful cigarette: a controversial issue. A tribute to Ernst L Wynder. *Chem. Res. Toxicol.* 14, 767-790.

[25] Hecht, S.S. (2002). Cigarette smoking and lung cancer: chemical mechanisms and approaches to prevention. *Lancet Oncol.* 3, 461-469.

[26] US Department of Health and Human Services EpA. (1993). Respiratory Health Effects of Passive Smoking: lung cancer and Other Disorders. Smoking and Tobacco Control Monograph 4. NIH Pub. 93-3605. Washington DC: DHHS.

[27] United States Environmental Protection Agency. (1992). Respiratory Health Effects of Passive Smoking: Lung Cancer and other Disorders. Washington DC: Office of Research and Development.

[28] Denissenko, M.F., Pao, A., Tang, M., and Pfeifer, G.P. (1996). Preferential formation of benzo[a]pyrene adducts at lung cancer mutational hotspots in P53. *Science* 274: 430-432.

[29] Taylor, R., Najafi, F., and Dobson, A. (2007). Meta-analysis of studies of passive smoking and lung cancer: effects of study type and continent. *Int. J. Epidemol.* 36: 1048-1059.

[30] Kurahashi, N., Inoue, M., Liu, Y., et al. (2008). Passive smoking and lung cancer in Japanese non-smoking women: A prospective study. *Int. J. Cancer* 122: 653-657.

[31] Godtfredsen, N.S., Prescott, E., Osler, M. (2005). Effect of smoking reduction on lung cancer risk. *JAMA* 294: 1505-1510.

[32] Doll, R., Peto, R., Boreham, J., and Sutherland, I. (2004). Mortality in relation to smoking: 50 years' observations on male British doctors. Jun 26; 328 (7455): 1519.

[33] Peto, R., Darby, S., Deo, H., et al. (2000). Smoking, smoking cessation, and lung cancer in the UK since 1950: combination of national statistics with two case-control studies. *BMJ* 321, 323-329.

[34] Anthonisen, N.R., Skeans, M.A., Wise, R.A., et al. (2005). The effects of a smoking cessation intervention on 14.5-year mortality: a randomized clinical trial. *Ann. Intern. Med.* 142, 233-239.

[35] Alberg, A.J., Ford, J.G., and Samet, J.M. (2007). Epidemiology of lung cancer. ACCP evidence-based clinical practice guidelines (2nd edition). 132, 29S-55S.

[36] Sun, S., Schiller, J.H., and Gazdar, A.F. (2007). Lung cancer in never smokers – a different disease. *Nature Reviews Cancer* 7, 778-790.

[37] Sin, D.D., and Man, S.F.P. (2008). Impact of cancers and cardiovascular diseases in chronic obstructive pulmonary disease. *Curr. Opin. Pulm Med.* 14, 115-121.

[38] Lange, P., Nyboe, J., Appleyard, M., et al. (1990). Ventilatory function and chronic mucus hypersecretion as predictors of death from lung cancer. *Am. Rev. Respir. Dis.* 141, 613-617.

[39] Eberly, L.E., Ockene, J., Sherwin, R., et al. (2003). Pulmonary function as a predictor of lung cancer mortality in continuing cigarette smokers and in quitters. *Int. J. Epid.* 32, 592-599.

[40] Purde, M.P., Gold, L., Jarvholm, B., et al (2007). Impaired lung function and lumg cancer incidence in a cohort of Swedish construction workers. *Thorax* 62: 51-56.

[41] Skillrud, D.M., Offord, K.P., and Miller, R.D. (1986). High risk of lung cancer in chronic obstructive pulmonary disease. A prospective, matched, controlled study. *Ann. Int. Med.* 105, 503-507.

[42] Mannino, D.M., Aguayo, S.M., Petty, T.L., and Redd, S.C. (2003). Low lung function and incident lung cancer in the United States: data from the first National Health and Nutrition Examination Survey follow-up. *Arch Int. Med.*163, 1475-1480.

[43] Wassawa-Kintu, S., Gan, W.Q., Man, S.F., et al. (2005). Relationship between reduced forced expiratory volume in one second and risk of lung cancer: a systematic review and meta-analysis. *Thorax* 60, 570-575.

[44] Young, R.P., Hopkins, R., and Eaton, T.E. (2007). Forced expiratory volume in one second: not just a lung function test but a marker of premature death from all causes. *Eur. Respire J.* 30, 616-622.

[45] Wasswa-Kintu, S., Gan, W.Q., Man, S.F., Pare, P.D., Sin, D.D. (2008). Relationship between reduced forced expiratory volume in one second and risk of lung cancer: a systematic review and meta-analysis. *Thorax* 60, 570-575.

[46] Yanai, M., Hatazawa, J., Ojima, F., et al. (1998). Deposition and clearance of inhaled 18FDG powder in patients with chronic obstructive pulmonary disease. *Eur. Respir. J.* 11: 1342-1348.

[47] Omori, H., Nakashima, R., Otsuka,N. (2006). Emphysema detected by lung cancer screening with low-dose spiral CT: prevalence, and correlation with smoking habits and pulmonary function in Japanese male subjects. *Respirology* 11, 205-210.

[48] Omori, H., Fujimoto, K., and Katoh, T. (2008) Computed-tomography findings of emphysema: correlation with spirometric values. Curr Opin Pulm Med. 14, 110-114.

[49] Celli, B.R. (2006). Chronic obstructive pulmonary disease phenotypes and their clinical relevance. *Proc. Am. Thorac. Soc.* 3, 461-466.

[50] Kishi,K., Gurney, J.W., Schroeder, D.R., et al. (2002). The correlation of emphysema or airway obstruction with the risk of lung cancer: a matched case-controlled study. *Eur. Respir. J.* 19: 1093-1098.

[51] Black, W.C. (2007). Computed tomography screening for lung cancer. Review of screening principles and update on current status. *Cancer* 110, 2370-2384.

[52] Henschke, C.I., Yip, R., Miettinen, O.S. (2006). Women's susceptibility to tobacco carcinogens and survival after diagnosis of lung cancer. *JAMA* 296, 180-184.

[53] Ueda, K., Jinbo, M., Li, T-S., et al. (2006). Computed tomography-diagnosed emphysema, not airway obstruction, is associated with the prognostic outcome of early-stage lung cancer. *Clin. Cancer Res.* 12(22), 6730-6736.

[54] The International Early Lung Cancer Action Program Investigators. (2006). Survival of patients with stage 1 lung cancer detected on CT screening. *N Eng. J. Med.* 355: 1763-1771.

In: Smoking and Lung Cancer
Editors: E. N. Powers and J. B. Cabbot

ISBN 978-1-60692-367-2

Chapter II

Smoking and Prognosis of Surgically Resected Non-Small Cell Lung Cancer

Haruyuki Kawai[1]*, Katsuyuki Hotta[2], Kazuhiko Watanabe[1], Mituru Muguruma[1], Masafumi Kataoka[3], Toshinori Ohara[3], Atsuhiko Tada[4] and Shin Kawahara[5]

[1]Department of Internal Medicine, Okayama Saiseikai General Hospital, Okayama 700-8511, Japan
[2]Department of Hematology, Oncology and Respiratory, Graduate School of Medicine, Dentistry and Pharmaceutical Sciences, Okayama University, Okayama 700-8558, Japan
[3]Department of Surgery, Okayama Saiseikai General Hospital
[4]Department of Internal Medicine, National Minami-Okayama Medical Center, Okayama 701-0304, Japan
[5]Kawahara Medical Clinics, Okayama 701-0304, Japan

Abstract

An estimated 85% of the lung cancer cases worldwide in men, and 47% in women, are attributable to tobacco smoking. In other words, smoking is an important risk factor for developing lung cancer. On the other hand, the impact of smoking status on survival after the diagnosis of lung cancer, especially in the surgical setting, has long been controversial, although numerous relevant studies have been conducted. Recently, we reported that the preoperative smoking history is an important clinical postoperative prognostic factor in patients with primary resected non-small cell lung cancer (NSCLC), and since then, several studies have reported identical findings. Furthermore, smoking cessation even after the diagnosis is associated with improved survival in early-stage

* Corresponding to Haruyuki Kawai M.D., Ph.D., Department of Internal Medicine, Okayama Saiseikai General Hospital, 1-7-18, Ifuku-cho, Okayama-shi, 700-8511, Japan. Phone: +81-86-252-2211, Fax: +81-86-255-2224. E-mail: ha-kawai@po.harenet.ne.jp

NSCLC patients. In addition, the longer the time has been since the cessation of smoking, the better the survival outcome. Interestingly, a possible association between exposure to passive smoking prior to diagnosis of early-stage NSCLC and survival after treatment has also been reported. Here, we review several studies investigating the relationship between smoking and prognosis of non-small cell lung cancer in surgical settings.

Keywords: smoking, prognosis, prognostic factor, non-small cell lung cancer, surgery, resected, review.

Introduction

Lung cancer is the leading cause of worldwide cancer mortality: an estimated 1.2 million people are diagnosed annually with lung cancer, and 1.1 million of them die from their disease [1]. The association between cigarette smoking and the risk of developing non-small cell lung cancer (NSCLC) is well established. An estimated 85% of the lung cancer cases worldwide in men, and 47% in women, are attributable to tobacco smoking [2].

Surgery is the best way to achieve a cure among the various treatment options in early-stage NSCLC. As compared with other cancers, however, long-term survival is relatively poor, with a 5-year survival rate of 49%, even though surgical approach was performed [3]. Thus, identification of prognostic factors is critical for optimizing additional or more aggressive treatment among the resected NSCLC patients to further improve outcomes. Such information would be useful for not only patients and their families, but also for the attending physicians in terms of assigning therapy in clinical practices and designing clinical trials.

To date, the prognosis of lung cancer patients with surgically resected NSCLC can be predicted from various pretreatment clinical characteristics including age, gender, stage at diagnosis, histologic type, performance status, and body weight loss [4]. In contrast, the clinical significance of smoking status on patient prognosis has long been a matter of debate. In 1997, experts reached agreement on general criteria regarding the importance of different prognostic variables in NSCLC [5].

In this report, clinical stage, performance status, and body weight loss were definite prognostic factors, and gender, age, histology, lactate dehydrogenase, albumin, hemoglobin, white blood cell count, platelet count, and biologic factors were possible prognostic factors. However, this proposal did not clearly mention whether smoking status was indeed prognostic in lung cancer patients. More recently, we reported that the preoperative smoking history is an important clinical postoperative prognostic factor in patients with primary resected NSCLC using a large data set [6]. Since then, several studies have reported identical findings, and numerous bodies of evidence have been accumulated regarding the harmful effect of smoking on patient survival in the surgical setting.

Objectives

The purpose of this work was to review the modern literature investigating the role of smoking status on prognosis in patients with surgically resected non-small cell lung cancer (NSCLC).

Search Strategy for Identification of Studies

Articles were identified by an electronic search on Medline (PubMed System) using the keywords "smoking", "smoker", "non-small cell lung cancer", "surgery", "surgically", "resected", "operated", "operation", "prognosis", "prognostic factor", and "survival". The search ended in December 2007. In addition, relevant articles that were quoted in the original search results were also reviewed.

Results

We identified a total of 29 studies evaluating the prognostic significance of smoking status in resected NSCLC patients. We here introduce these studies with regard to how they address the following questions: (1) Would smoking status affect long-term survival after surgical resection? (2) Would smoking cessation even after the diagnosis be beneficial in terms of survival prolongation? (3) Would the duration of smoking abstinence relate to prognosis? (4) Would even secondhand smoke exposure influence patient prognosis?

Smoking Status and Prognosis of Resected Non-Small Cell Lung Cancer

Several studies have reported that cigarette smoking is a negative prognostic factor in resected NSCLC cases [6-24], whereas other reports have found no association between lung cancer and smoking cigarettes [25-29]. Early studies found no association between smoking status and lung cancer survival in the surgical setting [25-27]. Clee et al. described that in a retrospective survey of 337 patients who had resection for lung cancer, there was no significant difference ($P = 0.9$) in survival between ever smokers, ex-smokers, and never smokers [27]. However, a large majority of the patients (92.4%) were ever smokers, whilst only 4% of patients were never smokers, and those with small cell lung cancer were included in the study. Gail et al. reported that there was no significant association between smoking status and survival in stage I NSCLC patients who were treated with thoracotomy [26]. Harpole et al. reported a prognostic model of recurrence and death in stage I NSCLC, in which smoking history did not affect patient survival [28].

Since the appearance of these preliminary studies, an increasing number of reports have been published concerning this issue. In the modern literature, there were many reports of a positive correlation between smoking status and prognosis in resected NSCLC patients. In a study of 587 patients undergoing surgical resection for adenocarcinoma, current smokers, defined in many studies as those currently smoking or who had quit less than one year before diagnosis, were 2.38 times more likely to die following surgical resection compared to nonsmokers [7] Isobe et al. conducted a multivariate analysis using the Cox proportional hazards model and revealed that a history of smoking was an independent unfavorable prognostic factor in lung adenocarcinoma patients who underwent potentially curative resection [8]. Fujisawa et al. also investigated a correlation between long-term survival and cigarette smoking in patients with primary, resected lung carcinoma [11]. They employed a multivariate analysis and showed that smoking history is a prognostic factor for long-term overall survival in patients with stage I primary resected NSCLC. It is noteworthy that six patients who died within 1 month after surgery were excluded from survival analyses in that study. Sioris et al. reported that in resected NSCLC patients with squamous cell carcinoma, stage and heavy smoking (> 38 pack-years) had prognostic significance for overall survival [13].

In a randomized, controlled chemoprevention trial comparing isotretinoin and placebo in patients with stage I non-small cell lung cancer, recurrence and mortality rates were significantly increased among those who were current smokers at entry compared with never smokers in the isotretinoin arm, in multivariate analysis [15]. Wu et al. reported that in their surgically treated patients, smoking status as well as the number of totally removed lymph nodes during thoracotomy, and tumor size in the multivariable analysis significantly affected both overall and cancer-related survival rates [18]. Myrdal et al. demonstrated that current smoking as well as positive lymph node at operation, higher age, earlier period for operation, impaired lung function, and major operative complication were all related to poorer prognosis [17]. In 2004, Haque et al reported a poor survival in those with smoking history of > 40 pack-years as compared with that in those with lower pack-years. They discussed that this may be due to the inactivation of the protective p53 pathway [19].

Recently, we showed a significant correlation between cigarette smoking and long-term cancer-specific survival in resected patients with stage IA NSCLC in 3,082 cases (6) (Figure).

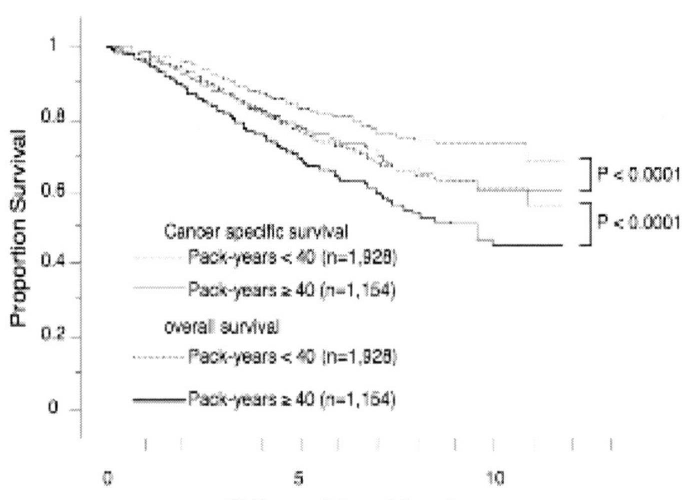

Figure. Overall and cancer-specific survival curves in patients with surgically resected stage IA NSCLC evaluated by pack-years. (Data from Kawai H et al. Smoking history before surgery and prognosis in patients with stage IA non-small-cell lung cancer--a multicenter study. Lung Cancer. 2005 Jul;49(1):63-70).

The Table shows the overall and disease-specific 5- and 10-year survival rates according to several variables. Significant differences in overall survival were demonstrated with age ($P<0.0001$), sex ($P<0.0001$), histologic type ($P=0.0041$), performance status ($P<0.0001$), and pack-years ($P<0.0001$). In a subgroup analysis in male patients, disease-specific survival demonstrated a significant association with age ($P = 0.0120$), PS ($P = 0.0022$), and pack-years ($P = 0.0463$). The reports by Yoshino et al. and Sawabata et al. support our results in stage I NSCLC patients [23, 24].

Table. Overall and cancer-specific survival, According to Clinical Prognostic Factors

		Overall Survival (%)			Cancer-Specific Survival (%)		
Clinical Feature	No. of patients	5 Years	10 Years	$P^{a)}$	5 Years	10 Years	$P^{a)}$
Age, years							
<70	2,115	77.3	60.6	< 0.0001	83.1	70.9	0.0003
ε70	961	64.4	36.3		76.1	60.7	
Sex							
Male	1,861	70.7	47.3	< 0.0001	79.2	63.0	< 0.0001
Female	1,221	78.1	66.7		84.5	76.7	
Histology [b)]							
Squamous cell carcinoma	840	69.8	49.8	0.0041	79.8	61.5	0.0831
Nonsquamous cell carcinoma	2,242	75.1	56.6		81.8	71.2	
Performance status[c)]							
0	2,467	76.8	58.1	< 0.0001	82.3	69.9	< 0.0001
ε1	595	61.0	41.8		76.5	62.0	
Pack-years [d)]							
<40	1,928	76.5	60.5	< 0.0001	83.4	73.6	< 0.0001
ε40	1,154	69.0	45.7		77.8	60.3	

[a)] p-value for the log-rank test.

[b)] Nonsquamous cell carcinoma is comprised of adenocarcinoma and large cell carcinoma.

[c)] Performance status was classified according to the criteria of Eastern Cooperative Oncology group.

[d)] number of cigarette packs per day, and years of smoking (Data from Kawai H et al. Smoking history before surgery and prognosis in patients with stage IA non-small-cell lung cancer--a multicenter study. Lung Cancer. 2005 Jul;49(1):63-70.)

Timing and Duration of Smoking Abstinence and Prognosis

As described in the previous section, we have demonstrated the potential significance of smoking status before the diagnosis on the prognosis after the surgical resection. How important would smoking cessation before the surgery be for those with smoking habits at the time of diagnosis? Sardari Nia et al. reported that in surgically resected stage I-III NSCLC patients, those who quit smoking after the diagnosis and before the surgery have a lower risk of dying when compared with current smokers who continued smoking at the time of surgery, suggesting that smoking cessation is beneficial for lung cancer patients at any time point prior to surgery [21]. They classified the patients into four categories based on the cigarette smoking status at the time of surgery: (1) non-smokers, (2) former smokers, i.e., patients who had stopped smoking prior to developing lung cancer, (3) recent quitters, i.e., patients who had stopped smoking soon after the diagnosis, and (4) current smokers. They showed that recent quitters, former smokers, and non-smokers have a better prognosis in the multivariable analyses for disease-free and overall survival than do current smokers, though this study included both early and locally advanced stage NSCLC patients.

The importance of duration of smoking cessation has also been investigated in terms of its survival advantage in early-stage, resected NSCLC patients [30]. Interestingly, the risk of death due to smoking history can gradually decrease as the period of smoking cessation is prolonged, with the adjusted hazard ratios for ex-smokers who quit 1-8, 9-17, $\geq$ 18 years and never smokers of 0.82 (95% confidence interval, 0.59-1.13), 0.69 (0.4-0.97), 0.66 (0.45-0.95), and 0.54 (0.29-0.996), respectively, when compared with current smokers ($P = 0.004$). However, a brief period of abstinence does not always reduce the risk of postoperative pulmonary complications [31, 32]. A recent systematic review of the literature has suggested that there was no increased risk in postoperative complications by short-term smoking cessation (4-8 weeks) in 12 prospective cohort studies [33]. Thus, the minimum duration of smoking abstinence that can improve outcome seems to remain undetermined.

Passive Smoking and Prognosis of Resected NSCLC Patients

The association between exposure to passive smoking (secondhand smoke, or SHS) prior to the diagnosis and treatment outcome in the surgical setting has hardly been investigated. Zhou et al. investigated its relationship in 393 patients with early-stage NSCLC (stages Ia-IIb) [34]. The information about SHS was obtained by interviewing each patient at the time of diagnosis, mainly focusing on the duration and location of exposure. Even after adjusting for covariates including pack-years of smoking, SHS exposure is still associated with worse survival in early-stage NSCLC patients, especially for SHS exposure in the workplace.

Discussion

We and other investigators have demonstrated an inverse correlation between cigarette smoking and survival in surgically resected NSCLC patients. Several possible reasons may be considered. First, current cigarette smokers have an increased risk for postoperative pulmonary complications. However, Fujisawa et al and we excluded patients who died within one month after surgery from survival analysis [6, 11]. Therefore, postoperative pulmonary complications might not be a major cause of poor prognosis in those with smoking habits.

A second possible reason is that smoking may lead to death through comorbidity, which may be one of the most important prognostic factors in cancer patients, as smoking is strongly associated with numerous serious diseases such as chronic obstructive pulmonary disease, coronary heart disease, and stroke [35]. To offset the influence of comorbidities on survival, disease-specific survival might be superior to overall survival. We indeed showed a significant correlation between cigarette smoking and long-term disease-specific survival in the large cohort of over 3,000 resected NSCLC cases. Tammemagi et al. also showed the negative effect of smoking on survival [36]; even adjusted for 18 deleterious comorbidities as well as other baseline covariates, the hazard ratio for smoking was significant (1.38 with 95% confidential interval from 1.18 to 1.60 [$p < 0.001$]). Finally, the authors mentioned that the poor outcome in smokers was not explained directly by comorbidity. Additionally, in a Singaporean study [37], no difference in the frequency or patterns of comorbidity was noted between never smokers and ever smokers. All these findings would indicate that smoking potentially but not definitively leads to death through comorbidity.

A third and, we believe most likely reason for the inverse correlation between cigarette smoking and survival is that never smokers may be different biologically from ever (current and former) smokers. Increased exposure to tobacco carcinogens may lead to an accumulation of genetic abnormalities that result not only in the evolution into cancer but also in the progression towards biologically aggressive cancers. Striking differences in the epidemiological, clinical, and molecular characteristics of lung cancers arising between never smokers and smokers have been identified [37-40], suggesting that they would be separate entities [41, 42]. Three points of molecular differences were reported in the reviews, which examined molecular alterations, DNA methylation profiles, and gene expression profiles, as discussed below.

Regarding molecular alterations, researchers from Boston described mutations in the epidermal growth factor receptor (EGFR) that were present in those who responded to the EGFR-tyrosine kinase (TK) inhibitor gefitinib, and subsequent research groups, including those at Memorial Sloan-Kettering, have described the same phenomenon with responders to erlotinib, another type of EGFR-TKI [43-45]. The somatic mutations in EGFR are found more frequently in patients without any smoking habits than in smokers [46, 47]. Furthermore, striking differences in the molecular alterations of two major genes involved in the pathogenesis of lung cancers, KRAS and TP53, have been found in lung cancers in never and ever smokers, providing evidence that these cancers arise through different molecular mechanisms [46, 48].

Regarding DNA methylation, the profile of lung cancer in never smokers and smokers is very different [49]. In human NSCLC, it has also been demonstrated that the hypermethylation of the p16/CDKN2A8, 9 and the RASSF1A genes was significantly associated with tobacco smoking, suggesting that the carcinogens in tobacco smoke induce hypermethylation in the promoter lesions of the tumor-suppressor genes. Kim et al. reported that hypermethylation of the RASSF1A genes was significantly associated with tobacco smoking (16). Furthermore, hypermethylation of the RASSF1A promoter was found to be associated with a poor prognosis in NSCLC patients at stage I and II. Although the clinical significance of the hypermethylation of tumor suppressor genes (TSGs) in lung cancer has been examined in a number of studies, most of these studies have focused on single genes in a small cohort of patients. The results have been inconsistent, with each study showing a significant association between a single TSG methylation and survival. In addition, most of these reported associations with NSCLC have not been reproduced in a second independent study. Gu et al. reported that a combination of hypermethylation of multiple genes exhibited a significant differential effect on NSCLC patient survival [22].

Regarding using gene expression arrays, several studies have identified distinct differences between smokers and never smokers [50]. Sanchez-Cespedes et al. demonstrated that widespread chromosomal abnormalities are frequent in lung adenocarcinoma from smokers, whereas these abnormalities are infrequent in such tumors arising in nonsmokers [50]. Powell et al. showed that there were many differences in gene expression in smokers and non-smokers, suggesting different pathways of cell transformation and tumor formation [51].

All these findings regarding molecular alterations, DNA methylation profiles, and gene expression profiles show that never smokers may be different biologically from ever (current and former) smokers in molecular settings. Unfortunately, there is no consensus yet regarding biological parameters that can be established as independent prognostic factors in patients with NSCLC.

Smoking cessation is a very effective way to not only decrease the risk of developing lung cancer but also improve the survival of lung cancer patients. Currently, effective aids for the treatment of tobacco dependence are available, including nicotine gum, nicotine patch, nicotine nasal spray, nicotine inhalar, bupropion, nortriptyline, and varenicline [52-54]. Tobacco dependence treatment remains the most cost-effective way to prevent morbidity and mortality from lung cancer. As introduced in the results section, smoking cessation even at the time of diagnosis of lung cancer is beneficial for those who have a smoking habit and will receive thoracotomy soon, and the diagnosis of lung cancer seems to provide a teachable moment to motivate patients to attempt tobacco abstinence. Therefore, clinicians should advise their patients to quit smoking.

Conclusion

We reviewed several studies that investigated smoking and prognosis in cases of non-small cell lung cancer in surgical settings. Smoking not only causes lung cancer, but it is also considered to be an important prognostic factor. Smokers need to be more aggressively treated and more frequently followed up after undergoing resection. This means that future efforts should focus on conducting studies to refine treatment strategies for ever smokers and never smokers. We want to stress that smoking cessation is essential to prolong survival of lung cancer patients as well as to prevent any carcinogenesis, so every effort must be made to promote smoking cessation vigorously as one of the global tobacco control policies [55].

References

[1] Parkin DM, Bray F, Ferlay J, Pisani P. Global cancer statistics, 2002. CA *Cancer J. Clin.* 2005 Mar-Apr;55(2):74-108.

[2] Pisani P, Parkin DM, Bray F, Ferlay J. Estimates of the worldwide mortality from 25 cancers in 1990. *Int. J. Cancer*. 1999 Sep 24;83(1):18-29.

[3] Jemal A, Siegel R, Ward E, Murray T, Xu J, Thun MJ. Cancer statistics, 2007. CA *Cancer J. Clin.* 2007 Jan-Feb;57(1):43-66.

[4] Jones DR, Detterback FC. Surgery for Stage I Non-Small Cell Lung Cancer: An Evidence-Based Guide for the Practicing Clinician. In: Detterback FC, Rivera MP, Socinski MA, Rosenman JG, editors. *Diagnosis and Treatment of LUNG CANCER*. Philadelphia: W. B. SAUNDERS COMPANY; 2001. p. 177-90.

[5] Feld R, Abratt R, Graziano S, Jassem J, Lacquet L, Ninane V, et al. Pretreatment minimal staging and prognostic factors for non-small cell lung cancer. *Lung Cancer*. 1997 Jun;17 Suppl 1:S3-10.

[6] Kawai H, Tada A, Kawahara M, Nakai K, Maeda H, Saitou R, et al. Smoking history before surgery and prognosis in patients with stage IA non-small-cell lung cancer--a multicenter study. *Lung Cancer*. 2005 Jul;49(1):63-70.

[7] Sobue T, Suzuki T, Fujimoto I, Doi O, Tateishi R, Sato T. Prognostic factors for surgically treated lung adenocarcinoma patients, with special reference to smoking habit. *Jpn. J. Cancer Res*. 1991 Jan;82(1):33-9.

[8] Isobe T, Hiyama K, Yoshida Y, Fujiwara Y, Yamakido M. Prognostic significance of p53 and ras gene abnormalities in lung adenocarcinoma patients with stage I disease after curative resection. *Jpn. J. Cancer Res*. 1994 Dec;85(12):1240-6.

[9] Hendriks J, Van Schil P, Van Meerbeeck J, Gdeedo A, Van Marck E, Vanmaele R, et al. Short-term survival after major pulmonary resections for bronchogenic carcinoma. *Acta Chir. Belg*. 1996 Nov-Dec;96(6):273-9.

[10] Suzuki K, Nagai K, Yoshida J, Nishimura M, Takahashi K, Yokose T, et al. Conventional clinicopathologic prognostic factors in surgically resected nonsmall cell lung carcinoma. A comparison of prognostic factors for each pathologic TNM stage based on multivariate analyses. *Cancer*. 1999 Nov 15;86(10):1976-84.

[11] Fujisawa T, Iizasa T, Saitoh Y, Sekine Y, Motohashi S, Yasukawa T, et al. Smoking before surgery predicts poor long-term survival in patients with stage I non-small-cell lung carcinomas. *J. Clin. Oncol*. 1999 Jul;17(7):2086-91.

[12] de Perrot M, Licker M, Bouchardy C, Usel M, Robert J, Spiliopoulos A. Sex differences in presentation, management, and prognosis of patients with non-small cell lung carcinoma. *J. Thorac. Cardiovasc. Surg*. 2000 Jan;119(1):21-6.

[13] Sioris T, Husgafvel-Pursiainen K, Karjalainen A, Anttila S, Kannio A, Salo JA, et al. Survival in operable non-small-cell lung cancer: role of p53 mutations, tobacco smoking and asbestos exposure. *Int. J. Cancer*. 2000 May 15;86(4):590-4.

[14] Shiba M, Kohno H, Kakizawa K, Iizasa T, Otsuji M, Saitoh Y, et al. Ki-67 immunostaining and other prognostic factors including tobacco smoking in patients with resected nonsmall cell lung carcinoma. *Cancer*. 2000 Oct 1;89(7):1457-65.

[15] Lippman SM, Lee JJ, Karp DD, Vokes EE, Benner SE, Goodman GE, et al. Randomized phase III intergroup trial of isotretinoin to prevent second primary tumors in stage I non-small-cell lung cancer. *J. Natl. Cancer Inst.* 2001 Apr 18;93(8):605-18.

[16] Kim DH, Kim JS, Ji YI, Shim YM, Kim H, Han J, et al. Hypermethylation of RASSF1A promoter is associated with the age at starting smoking and a poor prognosis in primary non-small cell lung cancer. *Cancer Res.* 2003 Jul 1;63(13):3743-6.

[17] Myrdal G, Lambe M, Gustafsson G, Nilsson K, Stahle E. Survival in primary lung cancer potentially cured by operation: influence of tumor stage and clinical characteristics. *Ann. Thorac. Surg.* 2003 Feb;75(2):356-63.

[18] Wu YC, Lin CF, Hsu WH, Huang BS, Huang MH, Wang LS. Long-term results of pathological stage I non-small cell lung cancer: validation of using the number of totally removed lymph nodes as a staging control. *Eur. J. Cardiothorac. Surg.* 2003 Dec;24(6):994-1001.

[19] Haque AK, Au W, Cajas-Salazar N, Khan S, Ginzel AW, Jones DV, et al. CYP2E1 polymorphism, cigarette smoking, p53 expression, and survival in non-small cell lung cancer: a long term follow-up study. Appl Immunohistochem. *Mol. Morphol.* 2004 Dec;12(4):315-22.

[20] Okada M, Nishio W, Sakamoto T, Uchino K, Yuki T, Nakagawa A, et al. Effect of histologic type and smoking status on interpretation of serum carcinoembryonic antigen value in non-small cell lung carcinoma. *Ann. Thorac. Surg.* 2004 Sep;78(3):1004-9; discussion 9-10.

[21] Sardari Nia P, Weyler J, Colpaert C, Vermeulen P, Van Marck E, Van Schil P. Prognostic value of smoking status in operated non-small cell lung cancer. *Lung Cancer.* 2005 Mar;47(3):351-9.

[22] Gu J, Berman D, Lu C, Wistuba, II, Roth JA, Frazier M, et al. Aberrant promoter methylation profile and association with survival in patients with non-small cell lung cancer. *Clin. Cancer Res.* 2006 Dec 15;12(24):7329-38.

[23] Yoshino I, Kawano D, Oba T, Yamazaki K, Kometani T, Maehara Y. Smoking status as a prognostic factor in patients with stage I pulmonary adenocarcinoma. *Ann. Thorac. Surg.* 2006 Apr;81(4):1189-93.

[24] Sawabata N, Miyoshi S, Matsumura A, Ohta M, Maeda H, Sueki H, et al. Prognosis of smokers following resection of pathological stage I non-small-cell lung carcinoma. *Gen. Thorac. Cardiovasc. Su*rg. 2007 Oct;55(10):420-4.

[25] Anthony HM, Madsen KE, Mason MK, Templeman GH. Lung cancer, immune status, histopathology and smoking. Is oat cell carcinoma lymphodependent? *Br. J. Dis. Chest.* 1981 Jan;75(1):40-54.

[26] Gail MH, Eagan RT, Feld R, Ginsberg R, Goodell B, Hill L, et al. Prognostic factors in patients with resected stage I non-small cell lung cancer. A report from the Lung Cancer Study Group. *Cancer.* 1984 Nov 1;54(9):1802-13.

[27] Clee MD, Hockings NF, Johnston RN. Bronchial carcinoma: factors influencing postoperative survival. *Br. J. Dis. Chest.* 1984 Jul;78(3):225-35.

[28] Harpole DH, Jr., Herndon JE, 2nd, Wolfe WG, Iglehart JD, Marks JR. A prognostic model of recurrence and death in stage I non-small cell lung cancer utilizing

presentation, histopathology, and oncoprotein expression. *Cancer Res.* 1995 Jan 1;55(1):51-6.

[29] Tsuchiya T, Akamine S, Muraoka M, Kamohara R, Tsuji K, Urabe S, et al. Stage IA non-small cell lung cancer: vessel invasion is a poor prognostic factor and a new target of adjuvant chemotherapy. *Lung Cancer.* 2007 Jun;56(3):341-8.

[30] Zhou W, Heist RS, Liu G, Park S, Neuberg DS, Asomaning K, et al. Smoking cessation before diagnosis and survival in early stage non-small cell lung cancer patients. *Lung Cancer.* 2006 Sep;53(3):375-80.

[31] Nakagawa M, Tanaka H, Tsukuma H, Kishi Y. Relationship between the duration of the preoperative smoke-free period and the incidence of postoperative pulmonary complications after pulmonary surgery. *Chest.* 2001 Sep;120(3):705-10.

[32] Warner MA, Offord KP, Warner ME, Lennon RL, Conover MA, Jansson-Schumacher U. Role of preoperative cessation of smoking and other factors in postoperative pulmonary complications: a blinded prospective study of coronary artery bypass patients. *Mayo Clin. Proc.* 1989 Jun;64(6):609-16.

[33] Theadom A, Cropley M. Effects of preoperative smoking cessation on the incidence and risk of intraoperative and postoperative complications in adult smokers: a systematic review. *Tob. Control.* 2006 Oct;15(5):352-8.

[34] Zhou W, Heist RS, Liu G, Asomaning K, Miller DP, Neuberg DS, et al. Second hand smoke exposure and survival in early-stage non-small-cell lung cancer patients. Clin *Cancer Res.* 2006 Dec 1;12(23):7187-93.

[35] Ogle KS, Swanson GM, Woods N, Azzouz F. Cancer and comorbidity: redefining chronic diseases. Cancer. 2000 Feb 1;88(3):653-63.

[36] Tammemagi CM, Neslund-Dudas C, Simoff M, Kvale P. Smoking and lung cancer survival: the role of comorbidity and treatment. *Chest.* 2004 Jan;125(1):27-37.

[37] Toh CK, Gao F, Lim WT, Leong SS, Fong KW, Yap SP, et al. Never-smokers with lung cancer: epidemiologic evidence of a distinct disease entity. *J. Clin. Oncol.* 2006 May 20;24(15):2245-51.

[38] Bryant A, Cerfolio RJ. Differences in epidemiology, histology, and survival between cigarette smokers and never-smokers who develop non-small cell lung cancer. *Chest.* 2007 Jul;132(1):185-92.

[39] Nordquist LT, Simon GR, Cantor A, Alberts WM, Bepler G. Improved survival in never-smokers vs current smokers with primary adenocarcinoma of the lung. *Chest.* 2004 Aug;126(2):347-51.

[40] Subramanian J, Velcheti V, Gao F, Govindan R. Presentation and stage-specific outcomes of lifelong never-smokers with non-small cell lung cancer (NSCLC). *J. Thorac. Oncol.* 2007 Sep;2(9):827-30.

[41] Subramanian J, Govindan R. Lung cancer in never smokers: a review. *J. Clin. Oncol.* 2007 Feb 10;25(5):561-70.

[42] Sun S, Schiller JH, Gazdar AF. Lung cancer in never smokers--a different disease. *Nat. Rev. Cancer.* 2007 Oct;7(10):778-90.

[43] Lynch TJ, Bell DW, Sordella R, Gurubhagavatula S, Okimoto RA, Brannigan BW, et al. Activating mutations in the epidermal growth factor receptor underlying

responsiveness of non-small-cell lung cancer to gefitinib. *N. Engl. J. Med.* 2004 May 20;350(21):2129-39.

[44] Paez JG, Janne PA, Lee JC, Tracy S, Greulich H, Gabriel S, et al. EGFR mutations in lung cancer: correlation with clinical response to gefitinib therapy. *Science.* 2004 Jun 4;304(5676):1497-500.

[45] Pao W, Miller V, Zakowski M, Doherty J, Politi K, Sarkaria I, et al. EGF receptor gene mutations are common in lung cancers from "never smokers" and are associated with sensitivity of tumors to gefitinib and erlotinib. *Proc. Natl. Acad. Sci. USA.* 2004 Sep 7;101(36):13306-11.

[46] Janne PA, Engelman JA, Johnson BE. Epidermal growth factor receptor mutations in non-small-cell lung cancer: implications for treatment and tumor biology. *J. Clin. Oncol.* 2005 May 10;23(14):3227-34.

[47] Hotta K, Kiura K, Toyooka S, Takigawa N, Soh J, Fujiwara Y, et al. Clinical significance of epidermal growth factor receptor gene mutations on treatment outcome after first-line cytotoxic chemotherapy in Japanese patients with non-small cell lung cancer. *J. Thorac. Oncol.* 2007 Jul;2(7):632-7.

[48] Shigematsu H, Gazdar AF. Somatic mutations of epidermal growth factor receptor signaling pathway in lung cancers. *Int. J. Cancer.* 2006 Jan 15;118(2):257-62.

[49] Toyooka S, Tokumo M, Shigematsu H, Matsuo K, Asano H, Tomii K, et al. Mutational and epigenetic evidence for independent pathways for lung adenocarcinomas arising in smokers and never smokers. *Cancer Res.* 2006 Feb 1;66(3):1371-5.

[50] Sanchez-Cespedes M, Ahrendt SA, Piantadosi S, Rosell R, Monzo M, Wu L, et al. Chromosomal alterations in lung adenocarcinoma from smokers and nonsmokers. *Cancer Res.* 2001 Feb 15;61(4):1309-13.

[51] Powell CA, Spira A, Derti A, DeLisi C, Liu G, Borczuk A, et al. Gene expression in lung adenocarcinomas of smokers and nonsmokers. *Am. J. Respir Cell Mol. Biol.* 2003 Aug;29(2):157-62.

[52] Kawai H, Shibayama T, Tada A, Kawahara S, Soda R, Takahashi K. [Factors affecting the success or failure of smoking cessation using nicotine patches]. *Nihon Kokyuki Gakkai Zasshi.* 2005 Mar;43(3):144-9.

[53] Hotta K, Kinumi K, Naito K, Kuroki K, Sakane H, Imai A, et al. An intensive group therapy programme for smoking cessation using nicotine patch and internet mailing supports in a university setting. *Int. J. Clin. Pract.* 2007 Dec;61(12):1997-2001.

[54] Ebbert JO, Sood A, Hays JT, Dale LC, Hurt RD. Treating tobacco dependence: review of the best and latest treatment options. *J. Thorac. Oncol.* 2007 Mar;2(3):249-56.

[55] American Society of Clinical Oncology policy statement update: tobacco control--reducing cancer incidence and saving lives. 2003. *J. Clin. Oncol.* 2003 Jul 15;21(14):2777-86.

In: Smoking and Lung Cancer
Editors: E. N. Powers and J. B. Cabbot

ISBN 978-1-60692-367-2

Chapter III

Smoking-Induced Lung Destruction, Not Dysfunction, is Associated with Recurrence and Death from Early-Stage Lung Cancer

Kazuhiro Ueda,[1,1] Toshiki Tanaka,[1] Nobuyuki Tanaka,[2] and Kimikazu Hamano[1]

[1] Department of Surgery and Clinical Science, Division of Chest Surgery, Yamaguchi University Graduate School of Medicine, Japan

[2] Department of Radiopathology and Science, Division of Radiology, Yamaguchi University Graduate School of Medicine, Japan

Abstract

Background: Cigarette smoking-induced lung damage is one of the most important factors predisposing to lung cancer with aggressive clinical features. However, the relationship between lung damage and the clinical features of lung cancer is still unclear.

Methods: The subjects of this study were a consecutive series of 72 smokers who underwent complete resection of pathological stage I non-small-cell lung cancer. Pulmonary emphysema and airflow limitation was diagnosed based on the findings of quantitative computed tomography and spirometry, respectively. We compared the clinicopathological features of smokers with, and smokers without lung damage.

Results: Pulmonary emphysema and airflow limitation were diagnosed in 39 and 30 patients, respectively. Pulmonary emphysema was associated with higher risks of death and recurrence, whereas airflow limitation was not. Male gender and poorly differentiated type were more common in patients with emphysema than in those without emphysema. However, according to a multivariate analysis, emphysema, tumor size, and microvessel invasion were the independent predictors of survival and recurrence.

[1] Reprint requests to: K. Ueda, Department of Surgery and Clinical Science, Division of Chest Surgery, Yamaguchi University Graduate School of Medicine, 1-1-1 Minami-Kogushi, Ube, Yamaguchi, 755-8505, Japan. Tel: +81-836-22-2259, Fax: +81-836-22-2423, E-mail: kaueda@c-able.ne.jp.

Conclusion: Although smoking-induced lung dysfunction is a known risk factor for lung cancer development, it was not associated with the clinical aggressiveness of lung cancer; however, smoking-induced lung destruction was. Thus, smoking-induced lung destruction and dysfunction may play different roles in the development and progression of lung cancer.

Keywords: smoking, pulmonary emphysema, lung cancer, prognosis

Introduction

Cigarette smoking induces pathological changes in the lung, resulting in various combinations of alveolar destruction and bronchiolar remodeling, leading to airway obstruction. Although cigarette smoking-induced lung damage is one of the most important factors predisposing to lung cancer with aggressive clinical features, the relationship between lung pathological or functional abnormalities and the clinical features of smoker's lung cancer remains controversial. Alveolar destruction can be evaluated by computer-assisted quantification of the low-attenuation area on chest computed tomography [1,2], and airway obstruction can be measured by spirometry [3,4]. We conducted this retrospective study to clarify the relationship between the presence or absence of alveolar destruction or airway obstruction and the clinicopathological features of smoker's lung cancer.

Materials and Methods

Patients

Between January, 2000 and December, 2003, 163 patients underwent surgery for primary lung cancer at our institution. The subjects of this study were a consecutive series of 72 of these patients who underwent lung lobectomy with hilar and mediastinal lymph node dissection for pathological stage I non-small cell lung cancer, and that who had a smoking history before surgery. Operability was determined according to the existing guidelines for pulmonary resection [5]. The criteria for resection included a partial pressure of arterial carbon dioxide ($PaCO2 < 50$ mmHg, a mean pulmonary arterial pressure < 30 mmHg, and a calculated predicted postoperative forced expiratory volume in 1 second > 500 ml. The preoperative patient data included age, sex, performance status, presence or absence of breathlessness, smoking habit, spirometric variables, arterial blood gas values, tumor size, and the extent of emphysema. Smoking data were based on the pack-years smoked, with the smoking index calculated by the average number of packs of cigarettes smoked per day multiplied by the number of years the person had smoked. The extent of emphysema was determined by CT densitometry. Spirometric variables were obtained within the preoperative month and included vital capacity (VC) and forced expiratory volume in 1 second (FEV_1). VC and FEV_1 were expressed as percentages of predicted values for age, sex, and height.

Pathological data obtained after surgery included histological subtype, histological grade, microvessel invasion, lymphatic vessel invasion, and pathological TNM status. The tumors were classified histologically as squamous cell carcinoma or non-squamous cell carcinoma, and graded as well, moderately, or poorly differentiated carcinoma according to the World Health Organization classification [6]. Likewise, microvessel invasion and lymphatic vessel invasion were diagnosed histologically using Hematoxylin-Eosin and Elastica Van Gieson stains. The patients' clinicopathological characteristics are summarized in Table 1. The mean smoking index was 51 ± 29 pack-years (median, 50 pack-years), and the mean number of resected segments was 4.0 ± 1.1. Preoperatively, 20 patients complained of slight breathlessness, defined as inability to keep up with healthy persons of equivalent age on hills or stairs [7]), and 17 patients had restricted physically strenuous activity, defined as Eastern Co-operative Oncology Group-performance status grade 1 [8]).

Table 1. Patient characteristics (n = 72)

Variables		Number, Percentage, or Mean ± SD
Age	(years)	70.1 ± 8.3
Gender	(male / female)	62 / 10
PS	(0 / 1 / 2)	54 / 13 / 4
Breathlessness	(yes / no)	20 / 52
Pack-year smoked		51 ± 29
PaO_2	(mmHg)	80.5 ± 8.9
VC	(%)	98.9 ± 18.9
FEV_1	(%)	70.8 ± 14.0
Tumor size	(mm)	24.3 ± 12.1
Stage	(IA / IB)	48 / 24
Extent of emphysema	(%)	8.1 ± 7.5
Resection	(lobectomy / bilobectomy)	69 / 3
Histologic subtype	(Sq / non-Sq)	20 / 52
Histologic grade	(well / moderate / poor)	27 / 28 / 17
Vessel invasion	(present / absent)	13 / 59

PS, European Cancer Organization Group-performance status; Breathlessness, inability to keep up on hills or stairs; PaO2, Partial pressure of arterial oxygen; VC, vital capacity; FEV1, forced expiratory volume in 1 second; Sq, squamous cell carcinoma; Vessel invasion was diagnosed microscopically and includes lymphatic vessel invasion. VC and FEV1 are expressed as a percentage of the predicted value.

Table 2. Patient characteristics according to the presence or absence of emphysema

Variables		Emphysema (n = 39) Number or Mean ± SD	Non-emphysema (n = 33) Number or Mean ± SD	P
Age	(years)	70.3 ± 8.2	70.0 ± 8.6	.875[a]
Gender	(male / female)	36 / 3	26 / 7	.0984[b]
PS	(0 / 1 / 2)	30 / 6 / 3	25 / 7 / 1	.5949[b]
Breathlessness	(yes / no)	28 / 11	24 / 9	.9299[b]
Pack-year smoked		54 ± 30	47 ± 27	.2605[a]
PaO_2	(mmHg)	80.5 ± 9.6	80.5 ± 8.1	.9927[a]
VC	(%)	100.7 ± 19.2	96.9 ± 18.5	.3910[a]
FEV_1	(%)	66.9 ± 13.0	75.5 ± 14.0	.0083[a]
Tumor size	(mm)	25.3 ± 12.3	23.2 ± 11.9	.4526[a]
Clinical stage	(IA / IB)	25 / 14	23 / 10	.6158[b]
Resection	(lobectomy / bilobectomy)	37 / 2	32 / 1	.6571[b]
Histologic subtype	(Sq / non Sq)	13 / 26	7 / 26	.2526[b]
Histologic grade	(well / moderate / poor)	12 / 14 / 13	15 / 14 / 4	.0988[b]
Vessel invasion	(present / absent)	8 / 31	5 / 28	.5557[b]

[a] compared by the unpaired Student's t test, [b] compared by the X^2 test.

PS, European Cancer Organization Group-performance status; Breathlessness, inability to keep up on hills or stairs; PaO_2, Partial pressure of arterial oxygen; VC, vital capacity; FEV_1, forced expiratory volume in 1 second; Sq, squamous cell carcinoma; p-T status, pathological T status; p-N status, pathological N status.

Vessel invasion was diagnosed microscopically and includes lymphatic vessel invasion. VC and FEV_1 are expressed as a percentage of the predicted value.

Diagnosis of Emphysema

CT was performed with a Siemens Volume Zoom Scanner (Siemens-Asahi Medical Technologies, Ltd., Tokyo, Japan) in the helical mode, without intravenous contrast material. With the patient in the supine position, scans were done during full inspiration with the following measurements: 120 - 140 kVp, 280 - 320 mA, 10-mm collimation, and a pitch of 1.5. Scan volumes extended from the thoracic inlet to the lung base and were acquired in one-breath-hold periods. Lung images were reconstructed in a 512 (512 matrix with a lung algorithm. We constructed volume-rendering three-dimensional (3D) models of the lungs using imaging software (M900 QUADRA, ZioSoft K.K., Osaka, Japan). Threshold limits of -600 to -1024 Hounsfield units (HU) were applied to segment the lung parenchyma and to exclude the soft tissue surrounding the lung and the large vessels within the lung. The trachea, mainstem bronchi, and gastrointestinal structures were manually and selectively removed from the model, using volume-adding and multifusion imaging techniques. The total number of voxels with any selected specific attenuation number (in HU) in the lung model was counted automatically by the computer. The percentage of voxels with attenuation values lower than -910 HU among the total number of voxels in the entire lung was considered to be the extent of emphysema because the low-attenuation thresholds that have been used most often to identify emphysema on conventional 10-mm-thick CT sections are -900 or -910 HU [9-12]. Emphysema was confirmed if it occupied more than 5% of the lung, because 95% of non-smokers in our preliminary series had lungs with less than 5% emphysematous involvement.

Postoperative Follow up

All 72 patients were followed up in our outpatient clinic at 3- or 4-month intervals during the first 2 years after their operation, then at 6-month intervals, by chest CT and if necessary, head and abdominal CT.

Statistical Analysis

We compared continuous variables by the unpaired Student's t test, and categorical variables by the X^2 test. Dependence between two continuous variables was tested by linear regression analysis. Survival analysis was done using a univariate Cox regression model. Variables with $p < 0.1$ at univariate analysis were then used as independent variables in a stepwise Cox regression analysis, with a $p = 0.05$ criterion for retention of variables in the final model. All tests were two-tailed, with significance defined as 0.05, and were performed using the statistical software, Statview 5.0 (SAS Inc., Cary, NC).

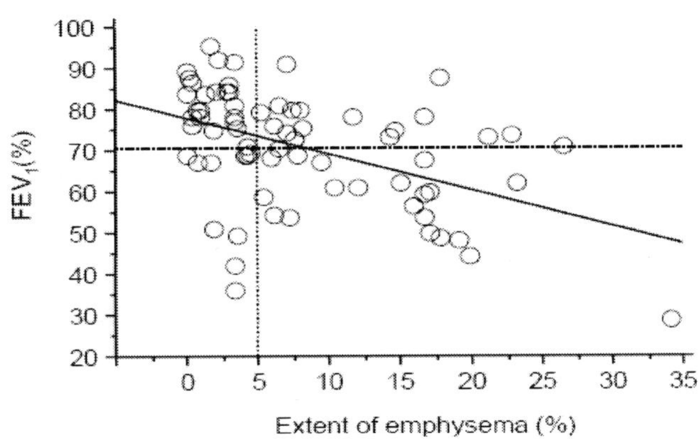

Figure 1. Dependence between the extent of emphysema and the percentage of predicted forced expiratory volume in 1 second (FEV_1%). The dotted line expresses X = 5, representing the boundary between the presence and absence of emphysema. Regression equation, Y = 77.9 - 0.88 X, $R^2 = 0.223$, $P < 0.0001$.

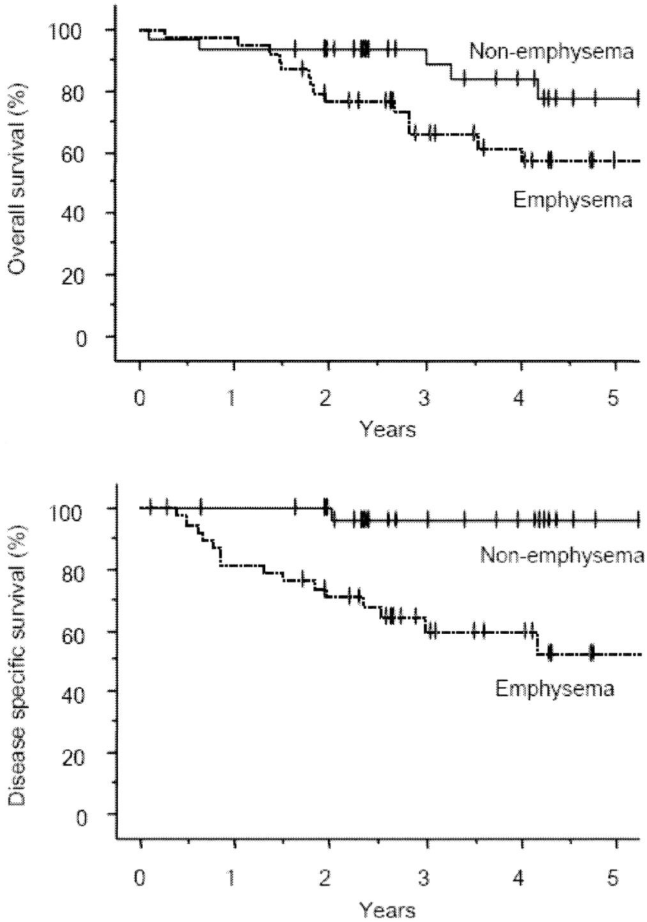

Figure 2. The overall survival (upper) and disease-specific survival (lower) curves according to the presence or absence of emphysema diagnosed by computed tomography. Significantly different survival rates were seen between the patients with and those without emphysema in both overall survival (logrank test, p = 0.0398) and disease-specific survival (logrank test, p = 0.0004).

Results

We diagnosed emphysema in 39 (54%) of the 72 patients. There were no significant differences between the patients with and those without emphysema in age, pack-year smoked, performance status, incidence of breathlessness, gas exchange capacity, vital capacity, tumor size, pathological stage, surgical procedure, histological subtype, histological grade, and microvessel invasion; however, we noted male predominance (P = 0.0984), a poorer histological grade (P = 0.0988), and a poorer FEV_1 (P = 0.0083) in the patients with emphysema (Table 2). The dependence between the extent of emphysema and the FEV_1 is shown in Figure 1. The presence or absence of emphysema affected both overall survival (5-year overall survival rate of 56.9% for patients with emphysema and 77.6% for patients without emphysema, p = 0.0398, Figure 2) and disease-free survival (5-year disease-free survival rate of 52.5% for patients with emphysema and 96.3% for patients without emphysema, p = 0.0004, Figure 2); whereas FEV_1 did not affect overall survival (5-year overall survival rate of 61.6% for patients with $FEV_1 \geq 70\%$ and 72.5% for patients with $FEV_1 < 70\%$, p = 0.5540 , Figure 3) and disease-free survival (5-year disease-free survival rate of 75.6% for patients with $FEV_1 \geq 70\%$ and 68.0% for patients with $FEV_1 < 70\%$, p = 0.8377, Figure 3).

Using the univariate Cox regression model, tumor size, the presence or absence of emphysema, and microvessel invasion were significantly associated with overall survival; whereas the presence or absence of breathlessness, tumor size, the presence or absence of emphysema, and microvessel invasion were significantly associated with disease-free survival (Table 3). Using the stepwise Cox regression analysis, the presence of emphysema, together with tumor size, and microvessel invasion, was considered to be an independent poor prognosticator for both overall and disease free survival (Table 4).

Table 3. Univariate Cox regression analysis of clinicopathological variables for overall and disease-specific survival

Variables		Overall survival		Disease-specific survival	
		HR	p	HR	p
Age	(years)	1.027	.3943	1.001	.9648
Gender	(female)	2.498	.0793	0.986	.9846
PS	(0)	1.186	.7454	1.457	.5578
Breathlessness	(no)	0.526	.1590	0.338	.0302
Pack-year smoked		0.998	.8108	0.999	.9132
PaO2	(mmHg)	0.985	.5460	0.998	.9508
VC	(%)	0.988	.3662	0.996	.7811
FEV1	(%)	0.999	.9256	0.982	.2319
Tumor size	(mm)	1.050	.0049	1.046	.0149
Stage	(IA)	0.566	.2067	0.566	.2592
Emphysema	(no)	0.361	.0488	0.066	.0084
Resection	(bilobectomy)	3.316	.1095	1.502	.6938
Histologic subtype	(non-Sq)	0.643	.3480	0.521	.2071
Histologic grade	(well)	0.354	.0647	0.329	.0830
Vessel invasion	(absent)	0.381	.0403	0.304	.0219

HR, hazard ratio; PS, European Cancer Organization Group-performance status; Breathlessness, inability to keep up on hills or stairs; PaO_2, Partial pressure of arterial oxygen; VC, vital capacity; FEV_1, forced expiratory volume in 1 second; Sq, squamous cell carcinoma; p-T status, pathological T status; p-N status, pathological nodal status. Vessel invasion was diagnosed microscopically and includes lymphatic vessel invasion. VC and FEV_1 are expressed as a percentage of the predicted value.

Table 4. Stepwise Cox regression analysis of clinicopathological variables for overall and disease-specific survival

Variables		Overall survival		Disease-specific survival	
		HR	p	HR	p
Tumor size	(mm)	1.058	.0025	1.056	.0060
Emphysema	(no)	0.300	.0239	0.051	.0046
Vessel invasion	(absent)	0.281	.0100	0.181	.0028

HR, hazard ratio; Vessel invasion was diagnosed microscopically and includes lymphatic vessel invasion.

Comment

The findings of this retrospective study suggest that cancer arising in the smoker's damaged lung has aggressive clinical features. This notion has long been overlooked because of the lack of a universal method to diagnose alveolar destruction on preoperative chest imaging. In contrast, pulmonary function is measured routinely to assess risk after major lung resection surgery. Pulmonary dysfunction is attributed to both alveolar destruction and bronchiolar remodeling; however, only 67% of our patients with pulmonary dysfunction had alveolar destruction, whereas as many as 45% of those without pulmonary dysfunction had alveolar destruction (Figure 1). Because there is a discrepancy between the grade of pulmonary dysfunction and that of alveolar destruction [13], we must be aware of the various phenotypes in smoking-induced lung damage.

It remains unclear why lung cancer arising in the smoker's damaged lung has such aggressive clinical features, although it is possible that the damaged lung promotes tumor progression. Indeed, a previous study found that the tumor microenvironment plays an important role in tumor cell invasion and metastasis [14]. Ishikawa et al. reported that matrix metalloproteinase-2 (MMP-2) expression in stromal fibroblasts, but not in tumor cells, is associated with poor prognosis in lung cancer [15]. It is known that MMP-2 in stromal fibroblast is activated in response to membrane-type-1-matrix metalloproteinase (MT-1-MMP) in tumor cells [16], but it has not been proven that MT-1-MMP expression in lung cancer cells is a prognostic marker [17]. This suggests that MMP-2 expression in stromal cell is not always a consequence of tumor-to-stroma interaction (paracrine loop), but is regulated by host lung pathology. This speculation is supported by the fact that MMP-2 and MT-1-MMP are more over-expressed in emphysematous lungs than in non-emphysematous lung [18].

Gender was not identified as a prognostic factor with respect to disease-specific survival in our series, which is inconsistent with the literature [19]. Despite little supportive evidence [20], we believe that the poor prognosis of men with lung cancer is attributable to the aggressive biological characteristics of lung cancer in men, and to the higher susceptibility of men to smoking-induced emphysema: in our series, 58% of male smokers vs. only 30% of female smokers had emphysema ($P = 0.0984$). There is also wide geographical variation in the incidence of emphysema [21, 22].

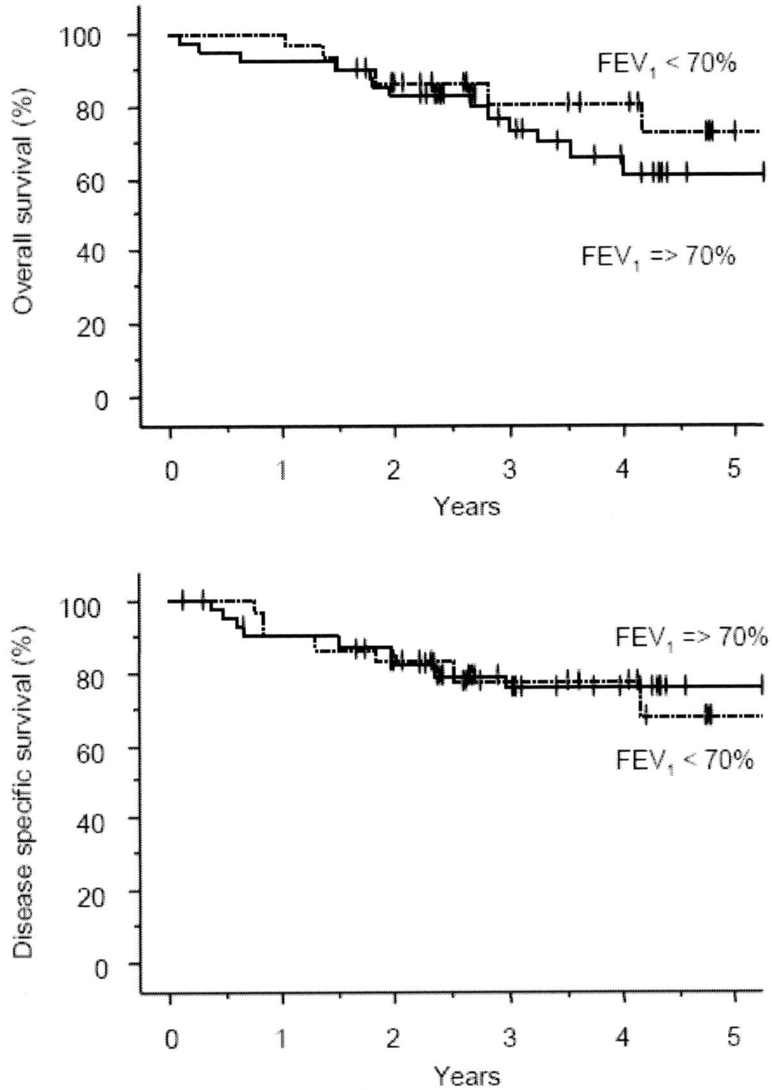

Figure 3. The overall survival (upper) and disease-specific survival (lower) curves according to the presence or absence of airflow limitation, based on the percentage of predicted forced expiratory volume in 1 second (FEV1 ≥ or < 70%). Similar survival rates were seen between the patients with and those without airflow limitation in both overall survival (logrank test, $p = 0.5539$) and disease-specific survival (logrank test, $p = 0.8377$).

Japan has a much lower incidence of emphysema than US or UK. Thus, in addition to TNM classification, the presence or absence of emphysema should be an important stratification factor, not only to evaluate the outcome of clinical trials, but to compare the survival of lung cancer patients among different countries. Such assessment may help us understand how geographic differences affect the therapeutic efficacy of various cytotoxic or cytostatic drugs, including epidermal growth factor receptor antagonists.

Between January, 2000 and December, 2003, we performed lung lobectomy for pathological stage I cancer in 33 never-smokers. The 5-year disease-specific survival rate of these never-smokers (96.7%) was consistent with that of smokers without lung destruction

(96.3%). This suggests that smoking may be associated with the aggressive clinical characteristics of lung cancer only in those patients with susceptibility to smoking-induced lung destruction.

Many molecular markers, such as vascular endothelial growth factor (VEGF), fragile histidine triad (FHIT), retinoblastoma (Rb), p16, p53, c-myc, and K-ras, have been reported to influence the clinical characteristics of smoking-induced lung cancer [23]. However, the definitive role of these markers as prognosticators remains unclear because of the lack of large-scale, prospective studies or meta-analyses. This is partly attributable to the inconsistent reproducibility or reliable determination of these markers. Conversely, quantitative CT is an objective technique, which uses computer software to distinguish voxels with abnormally low attenuation, representing emphysema, from those representing normal lung tissue. The user-friendly computer software allows us to establish, within a few minutes, the proportion of voxels with attenuation values representative of emphysema, without the need for extensive technical training, by creating a 3D-CT lung model and imputing a defined threshold. The results are reproducible for viewers of varying expertise and experience and across institutions, enabling accurate comparisons of results among different centers. Thus, we must further clarify the biological characteristics of lung cancer arising in the damaged lung by examining the expression of various molecular markers.

FEV1 is a well-known prognostic marker in patients with COPD and is thus used to grade COPD [24]. Limited FEV1 was not associated with a poor prognosis in our patients, who were followed up for 5 years, but longer follow up is needed to confirm its effect on their extended survival. In contrast to lung function, lung destruction may be associated with early recurrence and death from lung cancer because both overall and disease-specific survival differed in the patients with, and those without emphysema in this study. Furthermore, four patients without emphysema and only one with emphysema died without cancer recurrence. According to one case-controlled study, limited FEV1 was associated with an increased risk of death from lung cancer [25,26], whereas pulmonary emphysema was not a risk factor for lung cancer [27]. Although both lung destruction and dysfunction can be used to grade COPD, these conditions may be linked to lung cancer differently.

Major prospective studies have shown a rising trend in lung cancer death with increasing smoking exposure [28-30]. In our series, the amount of smoking exposure was not associated with the prognosis of patients with lung cancer, or with the level of FEV1, or the grade of lung destruction. These findings suggest that increased smoking exposure is associated with the development of lung cancer, but it is not associated with the clinical characteristics of smoking-induced lung cancer. However, we must clarify what effect the degree of smoking exposure has on the therapeutic outcome of smoker's lung cancer by comparing the data of survivors and non-survivors after longer follow up.

In conclusion, although it has been overlooked for too long, lung cancer arising in a smoker's damaged lung is associated with devastating entities. Thus, we must clarify the biological characteristics in this population. Prophylaxis or treatment of pulmonary emphysema may substantially decrease the incidence of this devastating disease, resulting in improved lung cancer survival.

References

[1] Goldin JG. Quantitative CT of emphysema and the airways. *J. Thorac Imaging* 2004; 19: 235-40.

[2] Bakker ME, Stolk J, Putter H, et al. Variability in densitometric assessment of pulmonary emphysema with computed tomography. *Invest Radiol.* 2005; 40: 777-83.

[3] Thurlbeck MW, Henderson JA, Fraser RG, Bates DV. Chronic obstructive lung disease - a comparison between clinical, roentgenologic, functional and morphological criteria in chronic bronchitis, emphysema, asthma and bronchiectasis. *Medicine* (Baltimore). 1970; 49: 81-145.

[4] Berend N, Woolcock AJ, Martin GE. Correlation between the function and structure of the lung in smokers. *Am. Rev. Respir. Dis.* 1979; 119: 695-705.

[5] Celli BR. What is the value of preoperative pulmonary function testing? *Med. Clin. North Am.* 1993; 77: 309-25.

[6] Travis WD, Brambilla E, Muller-Hermelink K and Harris CC: World Health Organization Classification of Tumours. Pathology and Genetics of Tumours of the Lung, Pleura, Thymus and Heart. Lyon (France): IARC Press, 2004.

[7] Stoller JK, Ferranti R, Feinstein AR. Further specification and evaluation of a new clinical index for dyspnea. *Am. Rev. Respir. Dis.* 1986; 134: 1129-34.

[8] Oken MM, Creech RH, Tormey DC, et al. Toxicity and response criteria of the Eastern Cooperative Oncology Group. *Am. J. Clin. Oncol.* 1982; 5: 649-55.

[9] Park KJ, Bergin CJ, Clausen JL. Quantitation of emphysema with three-dimensional CT densitometry: comparison with two-dimensional analysis, visual emphysema scores, and pulmonary function test results. *Radiology* 1999; 211: 541-7.

[10] Kinsella M, Muller NL, Abboud RT, Morrison NJ, DyBuncio A. Quantitation of emphysema by computed tomography using a "density mask" program and correlation with pulmonary function tests. *Chest* 1990; 97: 315-21.

[11] Lamers RJ, Thelissen GR, Kessels AG, Wouters EF, van Engelshoven JM. Chronic obstructive pulmonary disease: evaluation with spirometrically controlled CT lung densitometry. *Radiology* 1994; 193: 109-13.

[12] Knudson RJ, Standen JR, Kaltenborn WT, et al. Expiratory computed tomography for assessment of suspected pulmonary emphysema. *Chest* 1991; 99: 1357-66.

[13] Gelb AF, Hogg JC, Muller NL, et al. Contribution of emphysema and small airways in COPD. *Chest* 1996; 109: 353-9.

[14] Taniwaki K, Fukamachi H, Komori K, Ohtake Y, Nonaka T, Sakamoto T, Shiomi T, Okada Y, Itoh T, Itohara S, Seiki M, Yana I. Stroma-derived matrix metalloproteinase (MMP)-2 promotes membrane type 1-MMP-dependent tumor growth in mice. *Cancer Res.* 2007; 67: 4311-9.

[15] Ishikawa S, Takenaka K, Yanagihara K, et al. Matrix metalloproteinase-2 status in stromal fibroblasts, not in tumor cells, is a significant prognostic factor in non-small-cell lung cancer. *Clin. Cancer Res.* 2004; 10: 6579-85.

[16] Itoh Y, Takamura A, Ito N, Maru Y, Sato H, Suenaga N, Aoki T, Seiki M. Homophilic complex formation of MT1-MMP facilitates proMMP-2 activation on the cell surface and promotes tumor cell invasion. *EMBO J.* 2001; 20: 4782-93.

[17] Yamamura T, Nakanishi K, Hiroi S, Kumaki F, Sato H, Aida S, Kawai T. Expression of membrane-type-1-matrix metalloproteinase and metalloproteinase-2 in nonsmall cell lung carcinomas. *Lung Cancer* 2002; 35: 249-55.

[18] Ning W, Dong Y, Sun J, Li C, Matthay MA, Feghali-Bostwick CA, Choi AM. Cigarette smoke stimulates matrix metalloproteinase-2 activity via EGR-1 in human lung fibroblasts. *Am. J. Respir. Cell Mol. Biol.* 2007; 6: 480-90.

[19] de Perrot M, Licker M, Bouchardy C, Usel M, Robert J, Spiliopoulos A. Sex differences in presentation, management, and prognosis of patients with non-small cell lung carcinoma. *J. Thorac. Cardiovasc. Surg.* 2000; 119: 21-6.

[20] Chapman KR.Chronic obstructive pulmonary disease: are women more susceptible than men? *Clin. Chest Med.* 2004; 25: 331-41.

[21] Yamanaka A. Pulmonary emphysema in Japan. *Pathol. Microbiol.* (Basel) 1970; 35: 161-6.

[22] Hasleton PS. Incidence of emphysema at necropsy as assessed by point-counting. *Thorax* 1972; 27: 552-6.

[23] Duarte RL, Paschoal ME. Molecular markers in lung cancer: prognostic role and relationship to smoking. *J. Bras. Pneumol.* 2006; 32: 56-65.

[24] Hole DJ, Watt GC, Davey-Smith G, Hart CL, Gillis CR, Hawthorne VM. Impaired lung function and mortality risk in men and women: findings from the Renfrew and Paisley prospective population study. *BMJ* 1996; 313: 711-5.

[25] Skillrud DM, Offord KP, Miller RD. Higher risk of lung cancer in chronic obstructive pulmonary disease. A prospective, matched, controlled study. *Ann. Int. Med.* 1986; l06: 503-507.

[26] Tockman MS, Anthonisen NR, Wright EC, Donithan MG. The intermittent positive pressure breathing trial group, The Johns Hopkins lung project for the early detection of lung cancer. Airway obstruction and the risk for lung cancer. *Ann. Int. Med.* 1987; 106: 512-518.

[27] Kishi K, Gurney JW, Schroeder DR, Scanlon PD, Swensen SJ, Jett JR. The correlation of emphysema or airway obstruction with the risk of lung cancer: a matched case-controlled study. *Eur. Respir. J.* 2002; 19: 1093-8.

[28] Hammond EC. Smoking in relation to the death rates of one million men and women. *Natl. Cancer Inst. Monogr.* 1966; 19: 127-204.

[29] Doll R, Peto R. Mortality in relation to smoking: 20 years' observations on male British doctors. *Br. Med. J.* 1976; 2: 1525-36.

[30] Rogot E, Murray JL. Smoking and causes of death among U.S. veterans: 16 years of observation. *Public Health Rep.* 1980; 95: 213-22.

In: Smoking and Lung Cancer
Editors: E. N. Powers and J. B. Cabbot
ISBN 978-1-60692-367-2

Chapter IV

Inseparable Duet of Alpha-1-Antitrypsin and Neutrophil Elastase in Lung Cancer Development

Aleksandra Topic
Institute of Medical Biochemistry, Faculty of Pharmacy, Belgrade, Serbia

Abstract

Alpha-1-antitrypsin (AAT) is an important serine protease inhibitor in human plasma that is encoded by the protease inhibitor (Pi) locus on chromosome 14q and show a co-dominant pattern of inheritance. It is a highly polymorphic gene with approximately 125 single nucleotide polymorphisms (SNPs) reported in public databases. AAT variants may be classified by their effect on AAT level and function as normal, deficient, null (nil detectable) or dysfunctional. The PiM allele is the wild type, and is the most prevalent. The PiZ and PiS allele are more common deficiency variants. Deficient alleles are responsible to lung diseases (emphysema, chronic bronchitis, and bronchiectasis), liver disease (neonatal jaundice and liver cirrhosis), vasculitis and panniculitis whilst the rare null alleles are responsible only to lung disease. Dysfunctional alleles code for an abnormal form of AAT, which, whilst present at a detectable level, does not function normally.

Elastases form a subfamily of serine proteases that hydrolyze many proteins in addition to elastin. Humans have six elastase genes that encode the structurally similar proteins. Neutrophil elastase is present in azurophil granules in the neutrophils and released at inflammatory sites when they are stimulated by a variety of compounds, including cytokines and chemoattractants. This important protease is enzyme that when expressed aberrantly can cause emphysema or emphysematous changes. This involves breakdown of the lung structure and increased airspaces.

Physiologically these protease and antiprotease are closely connected and present inseparable duet in patophysiology of lung injury. The major physiological role of AAT is to inhibit NE in the lower respiratory tract and protect lung tissue from destruction, with a smaller role in defending against damage by other serine proteases, such as cathepsin G and proteinase 3.

It is well known that imbalance in activity between NE and AAT in favor of NE play a role in the development of emphysema in smokers or in patients with inherited alpha-1-antitrypsin deficiency (AATD). A number of studies indicated etiological role of NE and AAT separately in lung cancer development. However, the rare investigations have been focused on their association as it relates to lung cancer. Some of them have been shown that AATD subjects with high plasma level of NE have a significant risk for lung cancer. It was postulated that the imbalance between NE and AATD was generally considered as a cause of tissue damage, which could be a favorable tissue environment for the action of carcinogens and tumor progression.

On the other hand, both of these proteins are tumor promoters. Namely, it was shown that lung-cancer cell lines produce elastase and the high levels of this enzyme in lung tumor tissue have been correlated with higher stage tumors and poor survival in lung cancer patients. It has been proposed that increase elastase and similar proteinases could destroy the barrier between tumor and the local circulatory system and results in facilitating cancer cell invasion. It has been obtained that higher stage of lung cancer was associated with high plasma level of AAT because increased transcription of AAT is response for the elevated elastase level or their activity.

Introduction

Worldwide, lung cancer is the most common cancer in terms of both incidence and mortality with 1.35 million new cases per year and 1.18 million deaths, with the highest rates in Europe and North America [1]. This malignancy remains the most common cause of cancer-related death in men and the second most common in women [2]. It is well accepted that 85 to 90 % of all lung cancer are attributable do cigarette smoking [3]. Three main approaches in struggle against this serious disease are prevention (discovering risk factors), early diagnosis of the risk populations and efficacy therapies (targeted therapies).

Although it is known that many proteases are involved in tumor growth at both the primary and metastasis sites, the roles of proteases and their inhibitors are still not well-investigated [4]. For the past 30 years, investigators have been studying the expression and activity of proteases in the final steps of tumor progression, invasion and metastasis. However, recent studies indicate that increased expression, increased activity and altered localization of many proteases are associates with early tumor progression. It was thought that only proteases outside the tumor cell were important in tumor invasion, but recent studies have shown that proteases inside the tumor cell also participate in local proteolysis by digesting phagocytosed extracellular matrix. To date, most investigators have focused on the role of proteases in the final step of tumor progression like as invasion and metastasis [4].

This chapter is focused on protease-antiprotease imbalance, which is involved in early stage of lung cancer development. Clinical studies indicated that imbalance between neutrophil elastase (NE) and their main circulating inhibitor alpha-1-antitrypsin (AAT) developed both panacinar emphysema and chronic obstructive pulmonary disease (COPD), particularly in smokers [5-7]. Besides of the well-documented facts that COPD is host factor related to the risk of lung cancer (LC), these lung diseases shares common etiologic factors, particularly cigarette smoking. Recent familial lung-cancer linkage studies tried to identify genes for lung function, COPD and susceptibly for LC.

Alpha-1-Antitrypsin

Structure and Physiological Role of AAT

Alpha-1-antitrypsin is a highly polymorphic, acute-phase glycoprotein (53 kD), synthesised in hepatocytes [8] and subsequently secreted into the plasma. It is also produced in smaller quantities by alveolar macrophages, circulating monocytes [9] and in lung-derived epithelial cells [10].

The mature AAT protein is 394 amino acids, with the active site residue belong to methionine at position 358, with isoelectric point in the range of 4.4 to 4.6. Crystalographic analysis of the mature protein reveals that it is a globular structure with tree carbohydrates on the external surface of the one end of the molecule [11].

The side chains are composed of N-acetylglukosamine, mannose, galactose and sialic acid and they are N-linked to amino acids Asn^{46}, Asn^{83} and Asn^{247}. The difference in carbohydrate side chains at position of Asn^{83} is responsible for the two major bands of AAT when serum focused at pH 4-4.9 on thin-layer polyacrilamide gel. The internal structure of AAT is highly ordered with 30 percent α-helices and 40 percent β-pleated sheets. There are nine α-helices (A→I) and three β-sheets (A→I).

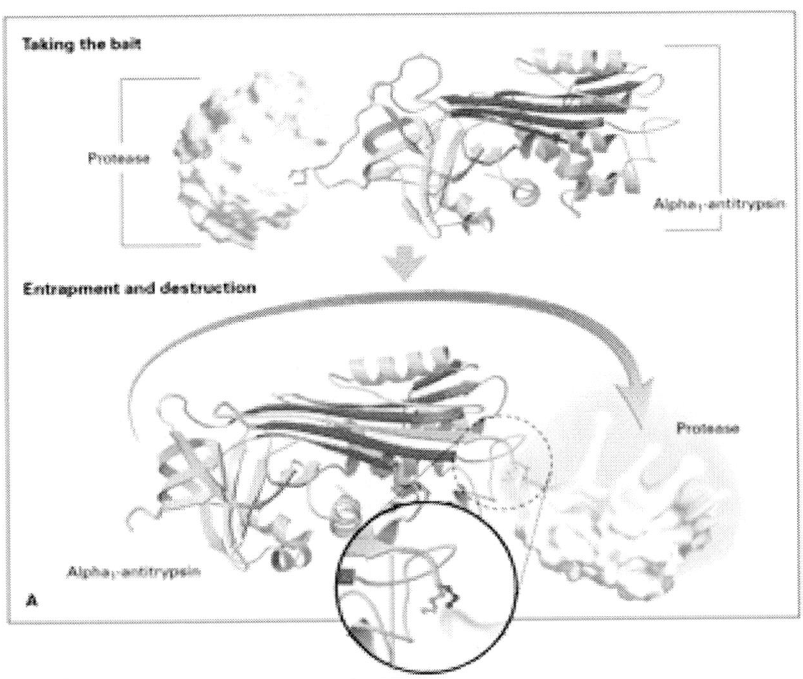

Figure 1. Mechanism of Inhibition of Proteases by Serpins. The protease attacks the reactive center loop (yellow) of AAT, with the active serine of the protease (small red side chain) forming a link to the amino acid at the base of the reactive center (small green side chain) of AAT. The resulting cleavage of the reactive loop allows it to snap back into the main β-sheet (red ribbons with arrows) of AAT. This spring-like movement flings the tethered protease to the opposite end of the AAT molecule, distorting its active site (inset) and altering its structure so that it can be destroyed. [From reference 17 with permission].

AAT is the archetype of the serpin family of proteins. SERPINs (SER*ine* P*roteinase* IN*hibitors*) are the superfamily of structurally related proteins that control many physiological reactions such as blood coagulation, fibrinolysis, programmed cell death, development and inflammation [12]. The target proteases of AAT are from the azurophilic granules of polymorphonuclear neutrophils, which contain three serine proteinases: elastase, cathepsin G, and proteinase 3. These proteases participate in lysosomal bacterial digestion and neutrophil migration through the extracellular matrix at sites of inflammation. The main physiological role of AAT is to inhibit NE in the lower respiratory tract to protect the connective tissue from NE released from triggered neutrophiles [13] with a smaller role in defending against damage by other serine proteases, such as cathepsin G [14] and proteinase 3 [15].

AAT inhibits proteases at its active site centered at residue Met^{358}-Ser^{359}, a part of a highly stressed external loop protruding from the molecule. The docking of the serpin and the protease is the beginning of the inhibitory process. The mechanism of inhibition of the AAT is like that of mousetrap with spring-like shift from a metastable to a hyperstable state (Figure 1.) [16, 17].

The Genetics, Heredity and Geographical Distribution of AAT Phenotypes

AAT is encoded by the protease inhibitor (Pi) locus on chromosome 14q32.1 [18, 19]. In humans, the protein is synthesized primarily in the liver and to a lesser extent in the alveolar macrophages and circulating monocytes. The Pi locus is 12.2 kb in length and consists of 4 coding exons (II, III, IV, and V), 3 non-coding exons (IA, IB, IC) and 6 introns; the region coding for the reactive loop is within exon V. The AAT mRNA is translated on ribosome bound to the rough endoplasmatic reticulum. Within the cisterna, the three carbohydrate chains are added and the protein begins to take on the globular configuration. Complete protein maturation is accomplished within the Golgi apparatus and protein is secreted.

Hepatic AAT gene expression as acute phase protein is under control by different cytokines, such as interleukin-1, tumor necrosis factor and most effectively by the interleukin-6 family of cytokines (interleukin-6, leukemia inhibitory factor, oncostatin M) [20].

However, in the alveolar macrophages neutrophil elastase may regulate AAT synthesis. In addition, it have been identified several regulatory regions in the promoter region of the AAT gene. AAT gene has been fully sequenced and cloned [21] and shows a co-dominant pattern of inheritance. The Pi locus is a highly polimorphic and approximately 125 single nucleotide polymorphisms (SNPs) reported in public SNP databases [22].

The variants of AAT are classified by the Pi (P*rotese* i*nhibitor*) system and each variant is identified by its speed of migration on agarose gel electrophoresis, and these differences in migration relate to variations in protein charge resulting from amino acid alterations [23, 24]. The most common forms of AAT are F (fast), M (medium), S (slow) and Z (very slow) [25]. The PiM allele is the wild type, and is the most prevalent. Using isoelectric focusing in narrow range of pH (4.2-4.9) it was able to identification, more AAT variants then in agarose gel electrophoresis. All the AAT variants categorized according the AAT serum level and function as normal, deficient, null and dysfunctional variants. Details about variants could be seeing in OMIM TM database [26]. Normal variants of AAT have a normal serum level and functional activity to inhibit neutrophil elastase. These variants represent the largest group of AAT alleles. More than 95 percent of normal variants are the "common" M1 (Ala213) which is the oldest, "classic" AAT variant, M1 (Val213), M2 and M3. The "rare" normal variants with frequencies of less than one pecent are M4, $B_{alhambra}$, F, $P_{StAlbans}$ and $X_{chirstchurch}$. Usually, rare variants are named by place names locating the birthplace of the oldest individual tested in pedegree. Deficient variants, associated with lower serum level of AAT than in normal variants.

Association between marked reduction of alpha -1-globulin peak on serum electrophoresis and the development of emphysema was first described in 1963.by Carl-Bertil Laurell and Sten Eriksson [6]. AAT deficiency (AATD) occurs because of alterations in gene expression or translation, or abnormal intracellular processing. Several mutations associated with AATD have been identified and the most common being the Z and S. Rare AATD variants are: M_{Malton}, $M_{MineralSprimgs}$, $M_{Procida}$,P_{Lowell}. The gene-mapping studies have shown that the PiZ allele probably arose in Northern Europe [27], until PiS originated in Iberia peninsula [28].

Individuals who are homozygous for AATD gene alleles can develop liver or lung disease; however, AATD heterozygotes, whith one normal allele, have sufficient amounts of AAT and they are protected from an increased risk of disease.

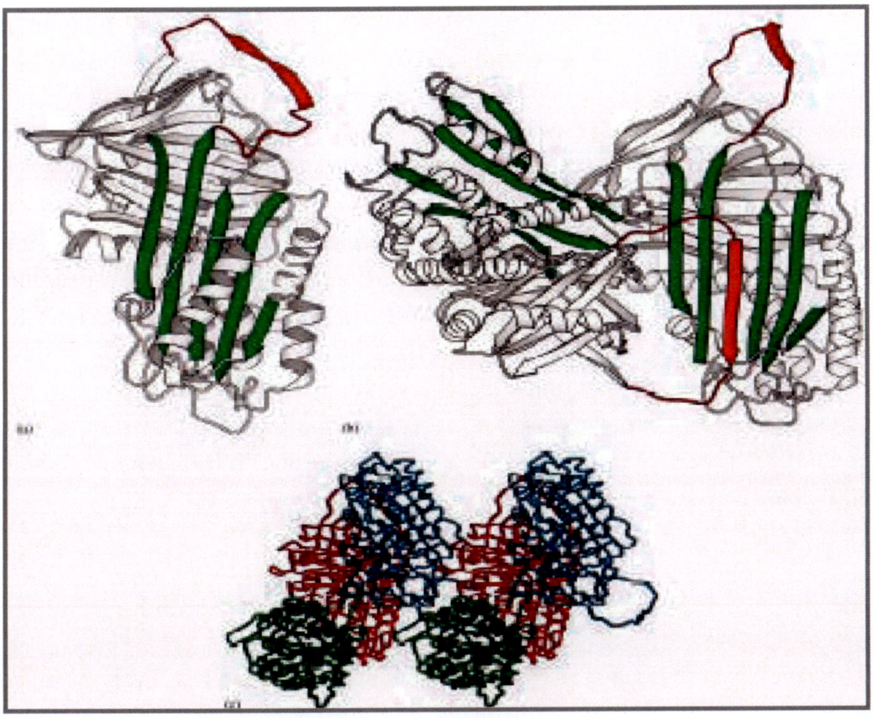

Figure 2. The molecular basis of loop-sheet polymerization. (a) The reactive loop of AAT (red) is held as a β-strand than can insert into β-sheet A of a second molecule (green). (b) A dimer of AAT showing the reactive centre loop of one molecule inserting into β-sheet A of a second. (c) Polymers of AAT (each molecule of AAT is shown in a different colour). [From reference 32 with permission].

Z Variant

The Z variant is"classic"AAT deficiency variant which occurs. It is derived from M1 (Ala^{213}) following a point mutation which is the same for the all Z individuals who are probably descendants of a single ancestral progenitor. The result of mutation is the substitution of a *G*AG that codes for Glu^{342} with an *A*AG that code for Lys^{342} [29].

This mutation causes a conformational change in the reactive loop that opens up β-sheet A and allows the reactive loop of a second molecule to insert at this point (Figure. 2.) [30-32].

This abnormality in posttranslational modification of protein causes accumulation of the protein polymers (Figure 2. c) in the cisterna of the rough endoplsmatic reticulum with a drastic reduction in secretion rates. The abnormal protein accumulates in the endoplsmatic reticulum of hepatocytes and form inclusion bodies (aggregates) which are PAS-positive and visible on microscopy. The process of accumulation of AAT aggregates causes hepatocyte death and ultimately liver disease in AATD as juvenile cirrhosis and hepatocellular carcinoma [33].

In addition, the expression of liver disease varies widely, from jaundice only at birth, through to cirrhosis, perhaps because of other genetic influences on this aspect of the clinical phenotype [34]. The large epidemiology study of Sveger [35] showed that up to 10 % of PiZZ newborns develop a clinically manifest cholestasis during the first 3-4 months of life. About half of these infants develop severe juvenile liver disease, but the other half become clinically, biochemically and hystologicaly healthy over a varying amount of time. During inflamation serum level of AAT rise and in AATD individuals formation of polymers overwhlem the degradative patway thereby exacerbating the formation of hepatic aggregates and the associated hepatocellular damage. Importance of understending mechanism of polymerisation is in discovering rational drug to block protein-protein linkage and so ameliorate the associated disease. Consequently, hepatocytes of ZZ homozygotes secreted only 10–15 % the normal quantity of AAT. Pi MZ heterozygotes have about 50 % of normal AAT concentration. Besides, to its low circulation level, the Z protein is also functionally less efficient in inhibiting elastase [36]. So that AATD in the ZZ individuals shows combination of quantitative and qualitative defects which leading in early-onset COPD including emphysema and chronic bronchitis.

Mechanism of loop-sheet polymerisation of AAT in this way also underlies the PiM_{malton} (52Phe deleted) [37], and S_{iiyama} (Ser53Phe) [38] forms of AATD, that are common in Sardinia and Japan, respectively.

S Variant

The S variant is more common and clinicaly less important than the Z variant. In contrast to Z allele, the S allele causes only mild plasma deficiency. The genetic sequenceof the S variant derives from M1 (Val^{213}) as a result of a mutation which cause substiotution of G*A*A that codes for Glu^{264} with an G*T*A that codes for Val^{264} [39, 40]. This single mutation of the S-type AAT gene results in reduced cellular secretion AAT because the newly synthesized protein is degraded intracellular prior to secretion [41, 42]. Carriers of S allele, Pi SS, Pi SZ and Pi MS have mean levels of 52 %, 32 % and 75 % of normal, respectively. If an individual has the genotype PiSZ, then they have clinical manifestation as a liver disease [43] and lung disease in smokers [44].

Null Variants

Null variants are characterized by the modification of an important part of the gene, which does not express AAT at all. Null-allelic variants are denoted as QO rather than Pi. It is highly rare variants; their frequencies among Caucasians are estimated to be less than 0.1 percent [45]. Although, all the AAT Null genes have identical phenotypic consequences (i.e. no detectable alpha 1AT in the serum), there are different genotypic mechanisms which cause the Null state. In homozygotes, AAT is not detectable in the serum and they are at very high risk of pulmonary emphysema. Logically, they are not at risk for developing liver disease [46]. It will be mentioned some examples of null variants. The Pi $Null_{Bellingham}$ differs from the normal M1 (Val^{213}) gene by the mutation in exon II where the codon for Lys^{217} (*A*AG) is altered to Stop codon (*T*AG). Pi $Null_{Bellingham}$ homozygotes with complete absence of AAT develop premature emphysema not having smoked or after only minimal exposure, and much earlier than the more common Pi Z individuals who have the usual form of AATD [47].

The $Null_{\text{isola di procida}}$ caused by complete deletion of the AAT coding exons. Cloning and mapping of the $Null_{\text{isola di procida}}$ gene demonstrated a deletion of a 17-kb fragment that included exons II-V of the AAT structural gene. Because of the deletion, the normal noncoding exons (IA-IC) were followed by exons II-V of the downstream AAT gene [48]. The $Null_{\text{granite falls}}$ allele derives from the M1 (Ala^{213}) by the deletion of a single base in exon II in the codon for Tyr^{160} (TA*C*) with deletion of the *C*. Consequently, there is 5' frame shift of the downstream nucleotides, moving the G form the next codon, Val^{161} G*T*C in place of the normal Tyr^{160} [49].

Sequencing of exons Ic-V and all exon-intron junctions of the $Null_{mattawa}$ gene demonstrated it was identical to the common normal M1(Val^{213}) AAT gene except for the insertion of a single nucleotide within the coding region of exon V, causing a 3' frameshift with generation of a premature stop signal [50].

Dysfunctional Variants

Dysfunctional variants are functional defective protein. These variants synthesized in normal quantities, but do not function normally. Amongst the dysfunctional AAT described, those associated with poor inhibition of NE may be associated with lung disease. An example of this is $M_{\text{mineral springs}}$ [51] caused by a single amino acid substitution ($Gly^{67} \rightarrow Glu^{67}$) with intracellular aggregation of AAT.

Table 1. Mean gene frequencies in 11 Geographic Region of the world [from reference 55 with permission]

Geographic Region	Cohorts	Mean gene Frequencies			Population at Risk				
					Carriers of Deficiency Alleles		Deficiency Allele Combinations		
	Size	PiM	PiS	PiZ	PiMS	PIMZ	PiSS	PiSZ	PiZZ
Central Europe	31,122	0.9708	0.0192	0.0074	10,499,896	3,933,048	118,791	85,661	17,514
Northern Europe	21,005	0.9577	0.0176	0.0153	1,064,350	1,027,452	10,775	21,150	11,578
Southern Europa	33,769	0.9272	0.0564	0.0125	20,148,269	3,946,672	915,593	262,780	27,515
Western Europa	6,941	0.9370	0.0451	0.0128	5,337,818	1,495,680	128,199	71,983	10,146
North America	33,147	0.9529	0.0328	0.0092	18,469,434	7,155,901	346,047	257,708	53,173
Africa	3,887	0.9444	0.0310	0.0048	17,334,307	1,404,344	607,616	75,096	6,412
Middle East and North Africa	3,859	0.9738	0.0133	0.0056	1,669,090	903,232	25,619	32,266	10,657
Central Asia	6,151	0.9872	0.0043	0.0040	6,499,962	4,506,979	23,283	40,815	20,504
Far East Asia	8,685	0.9937	0.0007	0.0004	1,911,276	607,460	2,244	3,553	1,771
Southeast Asia	4,547	0.9732	0.0159	0.0036	4,063,472	1,605,298	44,424	37,898	10,706
Australia and New Zealand	8,243	0.9410	0.0395	0.0151	1,816,658	639,174	41,624	28,231	5,476
Total	161,356	0.9727	0.0295	0.0107	88,814,533	27,225,242	2,260,801	929,014	175,268

The F allel is expressed in serum at normal levels but is dysfunctional in its ability to inhibit NE. Individuals who coinherit the F and a deficiency allele such as Z or Null, are likely to have a high risk for the development of emphysema [52]. In addition, Pi $E_{Franklin}$ form of A1AT is expressed at normal levels in serum but is functionally impaired as an inhibitor of NE [53].

PiPittsburgh is example of structure mutation in the PI gene that alters its function such that it becomes an antithrombin with anticoagulant effect by way of inhibition of factor IXa, kallikrein and factor XIIf and leads to a bleeding disorder [54].

Epidemiology of AATD

Genetic epidemiology studies on the general population predict a number of individuals with the genetic disease and are essential for planning public health coast. In the genetic epidemiologic surveys by deSerres [55] were including 11 Geographic Region of the world. The major findings of this study are: AATD affects all major racial subgroups worldwide and that there are at least 116 million carriers (PiMZ and PiMS) and 3.4 million-deficiency allele's combinations (PiSS, PiSZZ and PiZZ) worldwide (Table 1.). The database in that study also permits the conclusion that AATD may be one of the most common serious hereditary disorders in the world. The mean gene frequencies of Z and S allele vary in different geographic regions of the world and they were shown in the Table 1.

Estimated numbers and prevalence of AATD alleles in European countries in Blanco at al study [56] has been shown a large variation with calculating prevalence of Pi ZZ homozygotes ranged from 1: 354 in Latvia to 1:86,065 in Russia.

AAT and Lung Diseases

Since that Laurell and Eriksson [6] first recognized that absence of the α-globulin fraction on protein electrophoresis of serum taken from a patient at a local respiratory hospital had an increased prevalence of emphysema, many studies have confirmed that emphysema is strong associated with AATD homozygous state [57, 58].

Several case-control studies have a higher prevalence of MZ heterozygotes among COPD patients than in the healthy control [59-64]. Also, a few longitudinal lung function studies showed that PiMZ phenotype is a risk factor for the development of emphysema [65-67].

Chronic obstructive pulmonary disease (COPD) with high frequency of panacinar emphysema in AATD individuals or centriacinar emphysema in smokers with normal AAT variants is caused by well-accepted postulation of protease-antiprotease imbalance.

The protease-antiprotease hypothesis suggest that emphysema in AATD occurs because of an imbalance between antielastase defense by AAT and the relatively excessive activity of neutrophil elastase, which leading to degradation of elastin and other extracellular matrix components of the lower respiratory tract. This hypothesis has been corroborated by a range of studies and remains a prevailing concept in emphysema.

However, it was shown that many AATD individuals does not developed emphysema which mean that AAT deficiency, alone is not enough to induce emphysema [68]. The additional factors which may induce emphysema develops are inflammation, when elastin repair mechanisms are overwhelmed by a massive attack of elastase from triggered neutrophils and cigarette smoke. Emphysema, along with lung cancer and cardiovascular disease is major disease associated with cigarette smoking.

Damage to AAT in lung fluid could occur by several mechanisms involving species delivered to the lung by cigarette smoke and /or stimulated inflammatory cells [69]. Oxidative damage of AAT active site on Met^{358} is the main cause of functional inactivation of AAT. Namely, the methionyl residue in the reactive bond of the AAT (Met_{358}–Ser_{359}) can be converted by oxidation to methionine sulfoxide in biological systems containing peroxide, hydroxyl radicals, hypochloride, chloramines and peroxynitrite liberated by activated phagocytes [70]. Oxidation of the Met_{358} leading to decreasing the second order rate constant for association with NE [71, 72]. Furthermore, AAT polymers were detected in bronchoalveolar lavage liquid in PiZZ patients with emphysema [73]. Therefore, in AATD, oxidants contained in cigarette smoke could further impair a quantitatively and qualitatively functionally AAT. Cigarette smoke also plays a significant role in inflammatory cell recruiting. Patients with AATD have a more neutrophils in air spaces than in lungs [74].

Non-smoking individuals with severe AATD have a significant delayed onset of symptoms, thus the exact prevalence of AATD in most population remains unknown and many affected individuals remain undiagnosed [75]. Many of the AATD symptoms are non-specific like cough, wheeze and chest infections, which may contribute to the delay in diagnosis experienced by many patients, which is 5.6 years on average from onset of symptoms [76]. It is important to early diagnostic AATD because there are many preventive measures that could be apply, like not smoking, adequate immunization against influenza and pneumococcal infection, to minimize breathing polluted air, appropriate treatment of respiratory infection and atopic disease. Therefore, WHO recommended [77] that all patients with COPD (adults and adoscelents) and asthma be screened for AATD.

Recent studies suggest that the proinflammatory effects of polymeric AAT, in addition to loss of inhibitory activity, may contribute directly to the development of inflammation and COPD in individuals with AAT-Z deficiency [78-79]. Even, under specific conditions of pH, temperature, and concentration, wild-type M AAT is reported to form polymers *in vitro* and generate a proinflammatory form of the molecule which stimulated neutrophil adhesion and chemotaxis [80].

The proinflammatory effects of native and polymeric AAT may be critically dependent on the presence of other cell activators, bacterial or otherwise, while pure preparations of AAT appear to exert predominantly antiinflammatory activity [81].

Human Neutrophil Elastase

Human neutrophil elastase (HNE: EC 3.4.21.37) belongs chymotrypsin family of serine proteases besides proteinase 3 (PR3: EC 3.4.21.76) and cathepsin G (CG: EC 3.4.21.20), that are stored in the primary (azurophil) granules of polymorphonuclear neutrophils (PMNs)

[82]. NE was first recognized as degradative enzymes that act either intracellular to degrade ingested host pathogens or extracellularly in the breakdown of extracellular matrix components at inflammatory sites [83-85]. Neutrophils are one of the first lines of host defense against infection. These defence cells achieving their anti-bacterial function through a series of coordinated responses (intracellular sequestration of microorganisms into the phagosome, fusion of neutrophil granules with the phagolysosome, release of proteases and antimicrobial peptides into the phagolysosomes, release of large quantities of reactive oxygen species generated by the activation of the membrane bound NADPH oxidase system) that culminate in the destruction of pathogens [86].

Gene Structure, Regulation, Expression and Post-translational Modification of Neutrophil Elastase

All the three proteases, HNE, PR3 and CG have evolved from a common ancestor by gene duplication [reviewed in 87].

The gene for HNE, *ELA,* is located within a 50 kb segment in the terminal region of the short arm of chromosome 19p13.3 [88]. In humans, *ELA2* gene expression occurs within bone marrow, during promyelocytic differentiation. The enzyme genes are "switched on" early during differentiation at the promyelocyte stage and are "switched off" at the myelocyte stage [89]. Thereafter, there is no further production of these enzymes. The expression of *ELA2* gene is mainly regulated in transcription level [90]. The active enzyme is stored within cytoplasmatic azurophilic granules of the neutrophil until extruded into phagolysosomes.

HNE mRNA cannot be detected in mature PMNs isolated from the systemic circulation because mature circulating neutrophils cannot synthesize NE. *ELA2* promoter region also displays a binding sites for the transcription factors c-Myb, C/EBP, PU.1 and LEF-1 [91-92].

The HNE gene encodes a 267-residue preproprotein that is post-translational processed at both ends. The presence of an amino-terminal prodipeptide that maintains the enzyme in an inactive conformation is a typical feature of myeloid serine proteases. The HNE propeptide is removed in the post-Golgi organelles by the cysteine protease cathepsin C. Removal of this amino-terminal prodipeptide allows the free amino-terminus to be inserted into the interior of the molecule, where it interacts with the aspartic acid residue adjacent to the serine of the active site. The C-terminus consists of a 20-residue tail that is normally excised and is required neither for location in granules with no enzymatic activity [93]. The enzyme responsible for cleaving off the C-terminal propeptide is not known.

Mutations in *ELA2* have been associated with severe congenital neutropenia and cyclic neutropenia, a rare autosomal dominant disease characterized by oscillations in the production of PMNs (and other blood cells) [94]. There are about 20 different single nucleotide polymorphisms discovered. Elastase purified from granules and elastase from sputum showed that the enzyme several isoforms (E1, E2, E3) that differ in the extent of their glycosylation.

Biological Functions of NE

The NE stored in huge amounts as active enzymes in specialized granules, play a central role in the biological function of neutrophils, especially at inflammatory sites to which these cells are recruited and activated. NE exhibits antibacterial activity killing of Gram-negative, but not Gram-positive bacteria [95].

In addition to their degradative-bactericidal properties, NE is also important regulators of the local inflammatory response. NE can modulate biological functions such as the control of cellular signaling through the processing of chemokines, modulating the cytokine network and activating specific cell surface receptors [reviewed in 96]. In addition, NE is able to degrade most of the components of the pulmonary extracellular matrix (ECM), including elastin, collagens, proteoglycans [97, 98], and laminin [99], and to induce apoptosis of human lung epithelial cells via activation of surface receptors such as proteinase activated receptor 1 (PAR-1) [100]. The interaction between NE and cytokine includes: (a) the release of active cytokines from their inactive precursor molecules, (b) proteolytic cleavage, and thus inactivation of active cytokines, (c) proteolysis of cell surface-bound cytokine receptors, (d) proteolysis of the cytokine binding proteins, and finally, (e) the activation of specific cell surface receptors (such as PARs or Toll-like receptor 4) [reviewed in 101].

Neutrophil Elastase in Lung Diseases

The lung destructive actions of NE have been firmly established after Laurell and Eriksson reported the link between alpha-1-antitrypsin deficiency and airflow obstruction and emphysema [6]. This degradative potential was further demonstrated in the *in vivo* studies which have shown that two serine proteinases, elastase and proteinase-3, which are released by neutrophils [102-104], which can induce in animals pathologic changes that resemble human emphysema. It is believed that NE play a particularly important pathogenic role in several lung conditions including pulmonary emphysema [105], acute lung injury, acute respiratory distress syndrome [106,107], chronic inflammatory airway diseases [108]. Also, NE contribute to the matrix degradative potential that occurs in emphysema and in other lung diseases as well in the other tissue inflammatory diseases in which there is recruitment of blood PMNs to inflammatory sites [reviewed in 109]. The different rates at which individual proteases are controlled by their natural inhibitors, as well as the dysregulation of the extracellular protease–antiprotease balance that occurs during inflammation, lead to the activation of proinflammatory mediators. These favor the recruitment of more PMNs via increased IL-8 production, and thus explain the chronic inflammatory diseases [reviewed in 110]. The secretagogue activity of NE that normally allows the binding and removal of bacteria may also explain the excessive mucus production in COPD and the plugging of the airways with mucus in cystic fibrosis [111].

Neutrophil Elastase and Cancer

Tumour progression is a step-wise process and recent studies indicate that many proteases are involved in tumor growth both at the primary and metastasis sites [4]. During the invasion and metastasis, cancer cells must passes a variety of natural tissue barriers *in vivo*, such as basement membranes and surrounding tissue stromal matrices composed of elastins, collagens, and proteoglycans. It is thus necessary for cancer cells to enhance their invasiveness through an increased proteolytic activity. The production of tumor cell proteases has been implicated in the invasion of tumor cells into adjacent host tissues and metastasis [112,113]. Recent experimental and clinical studies on neutrophil elastase and cancer proved that those neoplasm metastases produce various degradative enzymes including NE [114, reviewed in 115].

Yamashita at al. [116] first reported that immunoreactive polymorphonuclear leukocyte elastase (*ir*-PMN-E) is produced by lines of non-small cell lung cancer *per se* with higher concentration in squamous cell carcinoma than in adenocarcinoma or large cell carcinoma. Consequently, author suggests that is plausible that the *ir*-PMN-E produced by lung cancer cell may facilitate the invasion of cancer cell either by directly dissolving the tumor matrix or by indirectly activating a protease cascade. In another study, the same author [117] showed that tumor NE may contribute to the direct extension of the tumor into aorta and may have direct pathological role in facilitating cancer cell invasion. In addition, in the case-control study Tanigushi at al [118] demonstrated that the polymorphism in the promoter region of the neutrophil elastase gene is associated with lung cancer development. In this study has been shown that individuals with a combination of the two single nucleotide polymorphism's (the -903 T and -741 G allele) in the NE promoter had a higher risk of developing lung cancer than the other allele types, which support an etiological role of NE in lung cancer development.

Biological Interrelationship between AAT and NE

There are several levels of interrelationship between AAT and NE. As already was mentioned, the main role of AAT is to protect normal tissue from the destructive capacity of NE. Besides the hepatocytes as the main source of AAT and the neutrophils itself are able to modulate the extracellular activity of NE by synthesizing and secreting AAT [119]. Thus, despite the fact that the neutrophils cannot synthesize NE, it can synthesize and secrete AAT and can modulating NE activity in the local environment without the help of antiproteases from other cells. NE may be permanently present at the surface of activated neutrophils and its activity tightly controlled by AAT in bronchoalveolar lavage fluids (BALF) [120-122]. But this control may be hampered once triggered neutrophils adhere and define a zone of restricted accessibility for inhibitors at the cell-subjacent substrate interface. In this case it is important a local modulating NE activity.

There is now a growing body of evidence that NE from azurophilic granules of nonadherent PMNs, remains in large part bound to the external surface of the plasma membrane (mNE), where it cleaves biologically relevant and synthetic substrates [123]. Recent study was shown that the mNE is fully controlled by AAT [124]. Further, it was shown that the AAT inhibits free NE and mNE stoichiometrically at the same rate. Therefore, any NE activity at the surface of neutrophils circulating in blood must be immediately inhibited by circulating AAT.

Inflammatory lung diseases are due, at least in part, to the impaired regulation of protease activities by endogenous inhibitors at inflammatory sites. The NE brought by infiltrating neutrophils and other inflammatory cells including bacteria and/or by the oxidative inactivation of critical Met residues by halogenated oxidants and by proteolysis may overwhelm the local binding capacity of these inhibitors.

AAT and NE in Lung Cancer Development

Despite the known associations of AATD with COPD and COPD with LC [125] and their interaction with environmental exposures, particularly cigarette smoking have not been adequately studied in LC etiology. Only a few studies examined the association of AATD alleles and LC. Recent three case-control studies proved that AATD is a risk factor for LC. In the study of Yang at al [126] was compared LC patients to the reported AATD carrier rate in Caucasians in the United States and they obtained higher AATD allele carriers in squamous cell or bronchoalveolar carcinoma LC patients than expected in USA whites. The same author [127] in larger case-control study using a haplotype analysis indicated an overall strong association between the two ELA2 markers and lung cancer risk. They showed significant and independent effects of the AAT-deficient allele (OR, 2.095% CI, 1.4 to 3.0) and the ELA2 T-G haplotype (OR, 4.1; 95% CI, 1.9 to 8.9) on lung cancer risk, and an increased risk (OR, 2.6; 95% CI, 2.4 to 2.8) for individuals carrying both an AAT-deficient allele and a G-G haplotype. Authors concluded that the AATD genotypes and/or an excess of neutrophil elastase are significantly associated with lung cancer risk. In the case-control study Topic at al [128] was obtained significant higher AATD phenotypes (PiMZ and PiMS) in squamous cell LC patients than in healthy control with the main conclusion that moderate AAT deficiency is a risk factor for squamous cell LC development (OR= 4.43. 95 % CI=1.46-13.43).

In the prevention of lung cancer, the early diagnose of risk group is the key of the adequate therapy. Because of that, nowadays efforts are steering to discovering a genetic determinant of susceptibility to lung cancer. Especially, investigators trying to explore the role of familial risk in lung cancer, linkage to familial risk for COPD and finally, the potential for shared genetic susceptibility for the lung.

In the Yang et al study [129] the segregation analysis provide indirect evidence for a common underlying genetic determinant of susceptibility to lung disease in families of nonsmoking lung cancer cases younger than 60 years modified by family history of lung cancer, smoking, and a personal history of COPD. Also, a number of linkage studies have been done with the aim to prove causality between gene regions and lung function [reviewed in 130].

It is well known that ZZs homozygotes are at high risk of COPD. The deficiency state results in unneutralized neutrophil elastase, and breakdown of lung tissue elastin, which leading to early-onset severe emphysema. Cigarette smoking contributes to faster tissue destruction through stimulation of neutrophils and increased secretion of elastase and further inactivation AAT. Moreover, it has been hypothesized that a proteinase-antiproteinase imbalance contributes to the development of COPD, as well as lung cancer [131].

Neutrophil elastase itself has been evaluated as a candidate in lung cancer etiology. As mentioned above, Taniguchi et al study [118] identified two polymorphisms in the promoter (T-903G [REP-a] and G-741A [REP-b]) and evaluated the contribution to lung cancer risk from these polymorphisms in a case-control setting. The TT genotype at REP-a was associated with 2.3-fold increased risk of lung cancer (95% CI, 1.2–4.7), whereas the GG genotype at REP-b was associated with a 1.4-fold increased risk (95% CI, 1.0–2.0). Higher promoter activity was associated with the risk genotypes. Similar finding for the TT genotype at REP-a was reported by Park et al [132]. They confirmed that the NE −903 polymorphism may increase lung cancer risk (OR = 3.2, 95% CI = 1.03–10.4) and that predicted high NE activity genotypes are associated with increased risk for lung cancer.

The role of neutrophil elastase in COPD development has not been evaluated.

It has been posulated several mechanisms of tumorigenesis in the AATD [131], as follows: excess neutrophil elastase, the counterpart of AAT, may facilitate cancer development by causing tissue damage and air trapping that fosters longer carcinogen exposure; may promote cancer progression by degrading the intercellular matrix barrier; and may lead to cancer development through the tumor necrosis factor signaling pathway.

The computer experts show a growing interest to device a computer strategy that can explore numbering gene interactions. One of them is the intriguing study of Edgerton et all study [133] which use Backward Chaining Role Induction (BCRI) method for hypothesizing causative mechanism between lung cancer gene expression and survival. BCRI is the role induction algorithms which have been used multiple studies to analyze gene array data to discover the conditions that predict a clinical outcome, long versus short survival periods for lung cancer patients. Authors implemented BCRI in C45W-BCRI rules using PubMed study [134], LocusLink study [135,136] and GeneCards [137] as a sources for peer-reviewed literature, chromosomal location and annotation, respectively. The first roles mean that elastase (ELA2 gene) is in low-risk tumors and for its association with AAT (SERPINA1 gene) is in high-risk tumors. Using C45W-BCRI method it could be predicted higher stage lung cancer results from lower levels of elastase transcript and higher level of AAT gene transcript. The association between AAT and NE discovered in their model is more interesting since both gene products have been implicated separately in lung cancer research. At first appear these results could be contradicted with the results by Yamashita et al study [116]. Authors explain contradiction: the decreasing of the elastase transcript may be secondary to negative feedback in the setting of a high concentration of elastase; the increase in transcribed AAT may be in response to the elevated elastase concentration or activity. The discovery of authors` role in the increased elastase activity or increased survival of the translated protein could be hypothesized as a mechanism for the higher level of both NE and AAT with poor survival. This conclusion is in correspondence with earlier experimental and clinical studies on NE and cancer. Neoplasm metastasizes because of a complex series of events. This process requires various degradative enzymes including proteases. Excessive NE results in digestion of not only elastin, but also other extracellular matrix proteins. It has been postulated that increased elastase [reviewed in reference 4] and similar proteases destroy the barrier between tumor and the local circulatory system and result in at least local or regional metastases. Further, author suppose that the increase in AAT level may have a role in promoting aggressive behavior in addition to that of elastase, or it may be simply in correlation with aggressive tumor behavior because of its up-regulation secondary to elastase activity. This explanation could be in correlation with results obtained in Higashiyama et al study [138]. In this study, high levels of AAT in adenocarcinomas were associated with higher stage disease. Advantage of C45W-BCRI algorithm is in construction of unifying model that explains several separate publications on both AAT and NE. The practical value of this kind of investigation is in advantage of molecularly target therapy. Namely, a major problem of LC therapy is resistance, because there is lack of knowledge about the numbering of gene interactions. This study identifies the coupling of gene networks relevant to cancer progression.

Conclusion

This chapter tried to present actual knowledge about association between NE and AAT as an inseparable duet in lung cancer development and progression. There was not easy because lack of definitive scientific conclusions about role of elastase production by lung tumor cells and the purpose of interplay between NE and AAT in LC, especially in late-stage.

The chronic obstructive pulmonary disease with high frequency of panacinar emphysema in heredity AATD or centriacinar emphysema in smokers with normal AAT variants are caused by protease-antiprotease imbalance a well-accepted postulation. In addition, there are firmly established important pathogenic role of NE in several lung conditions including pulmonary emphysema, acute lung injury, acute respiratory distress syndrome and chronic inflammatory airway diseases. It seems that the both protein could be involved in the LC development, but on the complex way. Now accepted, protease-antiprotease imbalance theory can explain lung cancer development by causing tissue damage and air trapping that fosters longer carcinogen exposure, but the main unresolved question is individuals` susceptibilities to lung disease.

Further research could be better explain the role of AAT-NE duet in lung carcinogenesis and their role as biological markers in order to provide opportunities for lung cancer risk reduction among smokers and individuals with existing COPD.

References

[1] Commonly diagnosed cancers worldwide. Cancer Research UK (Apr 2005). Retrieved on 2008-01-11.

[2] World Health Organization (2004). Deaths by cause, sex and mortality stratum. World Health Organization. Retrieved on 2007-06-01.

[3] Samet, JM; Wiggins, CL; Humble, CG; Pathak, DR. Cigarette smoking and lung cancer in New Mexico. *Am. Rev. Respir. Dis.*, 1988, 137, 1110–1113.

[4] Koblinski, JE; Ahram, M; Sloane, BF. Unravelling the role of proteases in Cancer. *Clin Chim. Acta*, 2000, 291, 113-135.

[5] Eriksson, S. Studies in alpha-1-antitrypsin deficiency. *Acta Med. Scand. Suppl.*, 1965, 432, 1-85.

[6] Laurell, CB; Eriksson, S. The electrophoretic alpha-1-globulin paterrn of serum in alpha-1-antitrypsin deficiency. *Scand. J. Clin. Lab. Invest.*, 1963, 15, 132-140.

[7] Lieberman, J; Benjamin, W; Sastre, A. Alpha1-antitrypsin Pi-Types in 965 COPD patients. *Chest*, 1989; 89, 3, 370-373.

[8] Koj, A; Regoeczi, E; Toews, CJ; Leveille, R; Gauldie, J. Synthesis of antithrombin III and 1-antitrypsin by the perfused rat liver. *Biochim. Biophys. Acta*, 1978, 539, 496-504.

[9] Mornex, JF; Chytil-Weir, A; Martinet, Y; Courtney, M; LeCocq, JP; Crystal, RG. Expression of the α-1-antitrypsin gene in mononuclear phagocytes of normal and α-1-antitrypsin-deficient individuals. *J. Clin. Invest.*, 1986, 77, 1952-1961.

[10] Cichy, J; Potempa, J; Travis, J. Biosynthesis of α1-proteinase inhibitor by human lung-derived epithelial cells. *J. Biol. Chem.*, 1997, 272, 8250-8255.

[11] Loebermann, H; Tokuoka, R; Deisenhofer, J; Huber, R. Human α1 -proteinase inhibitor: crystal modifications, molecular model and preliminary analysis of the implications for function. *J. Mol. Biol.*, 1984, 177, 531-556.

[12] Potempa, J; Korzus, E; Travis, J. The serpin superfamily of proteinase inhibitors: structure, function and regulation. *J. Biol. Chem.*, 1994, 269, 15957-15960.

[13] Travis, J; Salvesen, GS. Human plasma proteinase inhibitors. *Ann. Rev. Biochem.*, 1983, 52, 655-709.

[14] Duranton, J; Adam, C; Bieth JG. Kinetic mechanism of the inhibition of cathepsin G by alpha 1-antichymotrypsin and alpha 1-proteinase inhibitor. *Biochemistry*, 1998, 37, 11239-11245.

[15] Rao, NV; Wehner, NG; Marshall, BC; Gray, WR; Gray, BH; Hoidal, JR. Characterization of proteinase-3 (PR-3), a neutrophil serine proteinase. Structural and functional properties. *J. Biol. Chem.*, 1991, 266, 9540 - 9548.

[16] Hunington, JA; Read, RJ; Carrell, RW. Structure of a serpin-protease complex shows inhibition by deformation. *Nature*, 2000, 407, 923-926.

[17] Carrell, RW; Lomas, DA. Alpha1-Antitrypsin Deficiency — A Model for Conformational Diseases. *N. Engl. J. Med.*, 2002, 346, 45 – 53.

[18] Schroeder, WT; Miller, MF; Woo, SL; Saunders, GF. Chromosomal localization of the human α1-antitrypsin gene (PI) to 14q31-32. *Am. J. Hum. Genet.,* 1985, 37, 868-872.

[19] Billingsley, GD; Walter, MA; Hammond, GL; Cox, DW. Physical mapping of four serpin genes: α1 -antitrypsin, α1 -antishymotrypsin, corticosteroid-binding globulin, and proteinC inhibitor, within a 280-kb region on chromosome 14q32,1. *Am. J. Hum. Genet.*, 1993, 52, 343-353.

[20] Richards, CD; Gauldie, BB. Cytokine control of acute phase protein expression. Eur Cytokine Network., 1991, 2, 89-98.

[21] Lai, EC; Kao, FT; Law, ML; Woo, SL. Assignment of the 1-antitrypsin gene and a sequence-related gene to human chromosome 14 by molecular hybridization. *Am. J. Hum. Genet.*, 1983, 35, 385-392.

[22] Entrez SNP. http://www.ncbi.nlm.nih.gov/projects/SNP/ .

[23] Axelsson, U; Laurell, CB. Hereditary variants of serum alpha-1-antitrypsin. *Am. J. Hum. Genet.*, 1965, 17, 466-472.

[24] Laurell, CB. Electrophoretic microheterogenity of serum α1 antitrypsin. *Scand. J. Clin. Lab. Invest.*, 1965, 17, 271-274.

[25] Fagerhol, MK. The Pi system. Genetic variants of serum alpha-1-antitrypsin. *Ser. Haematol.*, 1968, 1, 153-161.

[26] OMIM™ - Online Mendelian Inheritance in Man™ database.

[27] Cox, DW; Woo, SL; Mansfield T. DNA restriction fragments associated with alpha 1-antitrypsin indicate a single origin for deficiency allele PI Z. *Nature*, 1985, 316, 79-81.

[28] Seixas, S; Garcia, O; Trovoada, MJ; Santos MT; Amorim, A; Rocha, J. Patterns of haplotype diversity within the serpin gene cluster at 14q32.1: insights into the natural history of the alpha1-antitrypsin polymorphism. *Hum. Genet.*, 2001, 108, 20-30.

[29] Nukiwa, T; Satoh, K; Brantly, ML; Ogushi, F; Fells, GA; Courtney, M; Crystal, RG . Identification of a second mutation in the protein-coding sequence of the Z type alpha 1-antitrypsin gene. *J. Biol. Chem.*, 1987, 262, 11999-12004.

[30] Lomas, DA; Evans, DL; Finch, JJ; Carell, RW. The mechanism of Z α1- antitrypsin accumulation in the liver. *Nature*, 1992, 357, 605-607

[31] Elliott PR, Lomas DA, Carrell RW, Abrahams JP: Inhibitory conformation of the reactive loop of 1-antitrypsin. *Nat. Struct. Biol.*, 1996, 3, 676-681.

[32] Lomas, DA. Loop-sheet polymerization: the mechanism of alpha1-antitrypsin deficiency. *Respir. Med.*, 2000, 94, Suppl C, S3-6.

[33] Eriksson, S; Carlson, J; Velez, R. Risk of cirrhosis and primary liver cancer in alpha1-antitrypsin deficiency. *N. Engl. J. Med.*, 1986, 314, 736-739.

[34] Wu, Y; Whitman, I; Molmenti, E; Moore, K; Hippenmeyer, P; Perlmutter, DH. A lag in intracellular degradation of mutant 1-antitrypsin correlates with the liver disease phenotype in homozygous PiZZ α1-antitrypsin deficiency. *Proc. Natl. Acad. Sci. USA*, 1994, 91, 9014-9018.

[35] Sveger, T. Liver disease in alpha1- antitrypsin deficiency detected by screening of 200,000 infants. *N. Engl. J. Med.*, 1976, 294, 1316-1321.

[36] Ogushi, F; Fells, GA; Hubbard, RC; Straus, SD; Crystal, RG. Z-type α1- antitrypsin is less competent then M1-type α1- antitrypsin as an inhibitor of neutropfil elastase. *J. Clin. Invest.,* 1987, 80, 1366-1374.

[37] Lomas, AD; Elliott, PR; Sidhar, SK; Foreman, RC; Finch, JT; Cox, DW; Whisstock, JC; Carrell, RW. α1-Antitrypsin Mmalton (Phe52-deleted) forms loop-sheet polymers in vivo: evidence for the C sheet mechanism of polymerization. *J. Biol. Chem.*, 1995, 270, 16864–16870.

[38] Seyama, K; Nukiwa, T; Takabe, K; Takahashi, H; Miyake, K; Kira, S. Siiyama (serine 53 (TCC) to phenylalanine 53 (TTC)): a new 1-antitrypsin-deficient variant

with mutation on a predicted conserved residue of the serpin backbone. *J. Biol. Chem.*, 1991, 266, 12627-12632.

[39] Owen, MC; Carrell, RW; Brennan, SO.The abnormality of the S variant of human alpha-1-antitrypsin. *Biochim. Biophys. Acta.*, 1976, 453, 257-261.

[40] Yoshida, A; Ewing, C; Wessels, M; Lieberman, J; Gaidulis. L. Molecular abnormality of PI S variant of human alpha1-antitrypsin. *Am. J. Hum. Genet.*, 1977, 29, 233-239.

[41] Curiel, DT; Chytil, A; Courtney, M; Crystal, RG. Serum alpha 1-antitrypsin deficiency associated with the common S-type (Glu264----Val) mutation results from intracellular degradation of alpha 1-antitrypsin prior to secretion. *J. Biol.Chem.*, 1989, 264, 10477-10486.

[42] Elliott, PR.; Stein, PE; Bilton, D; Carrell, RW; Lomas, DA. Structural explanation for the deficiency of S α1-antitrypsin. *Nat. Struct. Biol.,* 1996, 3, 910-911.

[43] Mahadeva, R; Chang, WS; Dafforn, TR; Oakley, DJ; Foreman, RC; Calvin, J; Wight, DG; Lomas, DA. Heteropolymerization of S, I, and Z α1-antitrypsin and liver cirrhosis. *J. Clin. Invest.*, 1999, 103, 999-1006.

[44] Turino, GM; Barker, AF; Brantly, ML; Cohen, AB; Connelly, RP; Crystal, RG; Eden, E; Schluchter, MD; Stoller, JK. Clinical features of individuals with PI*SZ phenotype of 1-antitrypsin deficiency. 1-Antitrypsin Deficiency Registry Study Group. *Am. J. Respir. Crit. Care. Med.*, 1996, 154, 1718-1725.

[45] Laurell, CB; Sveger; T Mass screening of newborn Swedish infants for alpha antitrypsin deficiency. *Am. J. Hum. Genet.*, 1975, 27, 213-217.

[46] Feldmann, G; Martin, JP; Sesboue, R; Ropartz, C; Perelman, R; Nathanson, M; Seringe, P; Benhamou, JP. The ultrastructure of hepatocytes in alpha-1-antitrypsin deficiency with the genotype Pi--. Gut, 1975, 16, 796-799.

[47] Cook, L; Janus, ED; Brenton, S; Tai, E; Burdon; J . Absence of alpha-1-antitrypsin (Pi Null Bellingham) and the early onset of emphysema. *Aust. N. Z. J. Med.*, 1994, 24, 263-269.

[48] Takahashi, H; Crystal, RG. Alpha 1-antitrypsin Null(isola di procida): an alpha 1-antitrypsin deficiency allele caused by deletion of all alpha 1-antitrypsin coding exons. *Am. J. Hum. Genet.*, 1990, 47, 403-413.

[49] Holmes, M; Curiel, D; Brantly, M; Crystal, RG. Characterization of the intracellular mechanism causing the alpha-1-antitrypsin Nullgranite falls deficiency state. *Am. Rev. Respir. Dis.*, 1989, 140, 1662-1667.

[50] Curiel, D; Brantly, M; Curiel, E; Stier, L; Crystal RG. Alpha 1-antitrypsin deficiency caused by the alpha 1-antitrypsin Nullmattawa gene. An insertion mutation rendering the alpha 1-antitrypsin gene incapable of producing alpha 1-antitrypsin. *J. Clin. Invest.*, 1989, 83, 1144-11452.

[51] Curiel, DT; Vogelmeier, C; Hubbard, RC; Stier, LE; Crystal RG. Molecular basis of α1-antitrypsin deficiency and emphysema associated with the α1-antitrypsin Mmineral springs allele. *Mol. Cell. Biol.*, 1990, 10,47-56.

[52] Cook L; Burdon, JG; Brenton, S; Knight, KR; Janus, ED. Kinetic characterisation of alpha-1-antitrypsin F as an inhibitor of human neutrophil elastase. *Pathology*, 1996, 28, 242-247.

[53] Cook L; Knight, KR; Burdon, JG; Brenton, S; Hunt, JM. Function of a rare variant of alpha-1-antitrypsin, phenotype Pi EFranklin S, a poor inhibitor of human neutrophil elastase. *Res. Exp. Med.*, 1996, 196, 355-362.

[54] Scott, CF; Carrell, RW; Glaser, CB; Kueppers, F; Lewis, JH; Colman, RW. α-1-antitrypsin-Pittsburgh: a potent inhibitor of human plasma factor XIa, kallikrein, and factor XIIf. *J. Clin .Invest.*, 1986, 77, 631-634.

[55] De Serres, FJ. Worldwide Racial and Ethnic Distribution of α1-Antitrypsin Deficiency: Summary of an Analysis of Published Genetic Epidemiologic Surveys. *Chest*, 2002, 122, 1818-1829.

[56] Blanco, I; de Serres, FJ; Fernandez-Bustillo, E; Lara, B; Miravitlles, M. Estimated numbers and prevalence of PI*S and PI*Z alleles of a1-antitrypsin deficiency in European countries. *Eur. Respir.J*, 2006, 27, 77-84.

[57] Tobin, MJ; Cook, PJ; Hutchinson, DC. Alpha 1-antitrypsin deficiency: the clinical and physiological features of pulmonary emphysema in subject homozygous for PiZ: a survey by the British Thoracic Association. *Br. J. Dis. Chest.*, 1983, 77, 14-27.

[58] Brantly, ML; Paul, LD; Miller, BH; Falk, RT; Wu, M; Crystal, RG. Clinical features and history of the destructive lung disease associated with alpha-1-antitrypsin deficiency of adults with pulmonary symptoms. *Am. Rev. Respir. Dis.*, 1988, 138, 327-336.

[59] Lieberman, J; Mittman, C; Schneider, AS. Screening for homozygous and heterozygous alpha1-antitrypsin deficiency. *J. Am. Med. Assoc.*, 1969, 210, 2055-2060.

[60] Buist, AS; Sexton, GJ; Azzam, AMH; Adams, BE. Pulmonary function in heterozygotes for alpha$_1$-antitrypsin deficiency: a case-control study. *Am. Rev. Respir. Dis.*, 1979, 120, 759-766.

[61] Mittman, C; Lieberman, J; Rumsfeld, J. Prevalence of abnormal protease inhibitor phenotypes in patients with chronic obstructive lung disease. *Am. Rev. Respir. Dis.*, 1974, 109, 295-296.

[62] Shigeoka, JW; Hall, WJ; Hyde, RW; Schwartz, RH; Mudholkar, GS; Speers, DM; Lin, CC.The prevalence of alpha1-antitrypsin heterozygotes (PiMZ) in patients with obstructive pulmonary disease. *Am. Rev. Respir. Dis.,* 1976, 114, 1077-1084.

[63] Janus, ED. Alpha1-antitrypsin Pi types in COPD patients. Chest, 1988, 94, 446-447.

[64] Bartman, K; Fooke-Achterrath, M; Koch, G; Nagy,I. Heterozygosity in the Pi system as a pathogenic cofactor in chronic obstructive pulmonary disease (COPD). *Eur. J. Resp. Dis.*, 1985, 66, 284-296.

[65] Dahl, M; Tybjærg-Hansen, A; Lange, P; Vestbo, J; Nordestgaard, BG. Change in Lung Function and Morbidity from Chronic Obstructive Pulmonary Disease in 1-Antitrypsin MZ Heterozygotes: A Longitudinal Study of the General Population. *Ann. Intern. Med.*, 2002, 136, 270 - 279.

[66] Madison, R; Zelman, R; Mittman, C. Inherited risk factors for chronic lung disease. *Chest,* 1980, 77, 255-257 :

[67] Tárjan, E; Magyar, P; Váczi, Z; Lantos, Å; Vaszár, L. Longitudinal lung function study in heterozygous PiMZ phenotype subjects. *Eur. Respir. J.*, 1994, 7, 2199-2204.

[68] Silverman, EK ; Pierce, JA; Province, MA; Rao, DC; Campbell, EJ. Variability of pulmonary function in α-1-antitrypsin deficiency: clinical correlates. *Ann. Intern. Med.*, 1989, 111, 982-991.

[69] Evans, MD;. Pryor, W. A.Cigarette smoking. emphysema. and damage to alpha 1-proteinase inhibitor *Am. J. Physiol. Lung. Cell. Mol. Physiol.*,1994, 266, L593-L611.

[70] Johnson, D; Travis, J. The oxidative inactivation of human alpha-1-proteinase inhibitor. Further evidence for methionine at the reactive center. *J. Biol. Chem.*, 1979, 254, 4022–4026.

[71] Padrines, M; Schneider-Pozzer, M; Bieth, JG . Inhibition of neutrophil elastase by alpha-1-proteinase inhibitor oxidized by activated neutrophils. *Am. Rev. Respir. Dis.*, 1989, 139, 783–790.

[72] Taggart, C; Cervantes-Laurean, D; Kim, G; McElvaney, NG; Wehr, N; Moss, J; Levine RL. Oxidation of either methionine 351 or methionine 358 in alpha 1-antitrypsin causes loss of anti-neutrophil elastase activity. *J. Biol. Chem.*, 2000, 275, 27258–27265.

[73] Elliott, PR; Bilton, D; Lomas, DA. Lung Polymers in Z α1 -Antitrypsin deficiency-related Emphysema. *Am. J. Respir. Cell. Mol. Biol.*, 1998, 18, 670-674.

[74] Morrison, HM; Kramps, JA; Burnett, D; Stockley, RA. Lung lavage fluid from patients with alpha 1-proteinase inhibitor deficiency or chronic obstructive bronchitis: anti-elastase function and cell profile. *Clin. Sci.* (Lond), 1987, 72, 373-381.

[75] American Thoracic Society/European Respiratory Society Statement: Standards for the Diagnosis and Management of Individuals with Alpha-1 Antitrypsin Deficiency. *Am. J. Respir. Crit. Care Med.*, 2003, 168, 818-900.

[76] Stoller, JK; Sandhaus, RA; Turino, G; Dickson, R; Rodgers, K; Strange, C. Delay in diagnosis of α1-antitrypsin deficiency: a continuing problem. *Chest*, 2005, 128, 1989-1994.

[77] A WHO Meeting on Alpha1-Antitrypsin Deficiency. Geneva. 1996, 18-20.

[78] Mahadeva, R; Atkinson, C; Li, Z; Stewart, S; Janciauskiene, S; Kelley, DG; Parmar, J; Pitman, R; Shapiro, SD; Lomas, DA. Polymers of Z α1-antitrypsin co-localize with neutrophils in emphysematous alveoli and are chemotactic in vivo. *Am. J. Pathol.*, 2005, 166, 377-386.

[79] Mulgrew, AT; Taggart, CC; Lawless, MW; Greene, CM; Brantly, ML; O'Neill, SJ; McElvaney, NG. Z α1-antitrypsin polymerizes in the lung and acts as a neutrophil chemoattractant. *Chest*, 2004, 125, 1952-1957.

[80] Parmar, JS; Mahadeva, R; Reed, BJ et al. Polymers of (1)-antitrypsin are chemotactic for human neutrophils: a new paradigm for the pathogenesis of emphysema. *Am. J. Respir. Cell. Mol. Biol.*, 2002, 26, 723-730.

[81] Persson, C; Subramaniyam, D; Stevens T; Janciauskiene S. Native and Polymeric α1-Antitrypsin Activate Human Neutrophils In Vitro? *Chest,* 2006, 129, 1683-1692.

[82] Korkmaz, B; Moreau, T; Gauthier, F. The Neutrophil elastase, proteinase 3 and cathepsin G: physicochemical properties, activity and physiopathological functions. *Biochimie*, 2008, 90, 227-242.

[83] Pham, CT. Neutrophil serine proteases: specific regulators of inflammation. *Nat. Rev. Immunol.*, 2006, 6, 541–550.

[84] Janoff, A; Scherer J. Mediators of inflammation in leukocyte lysosomes. IX. Elastinolytic activity in granules of human polymorphonuclear leukocytes. *J. Exp. Med.*, 1968, 128, 1137–1155.

[85] Baggiolini, M; Schnyder, J; Bretz, U; Dewald, B; Ruch, W. Cellular mechanisms of proteinase release from inflammatory cells and the degradation of extracellular proteins. *Ciba. Found. Symp.*, 1979, 105-121.

[86] Nathan C. Neutrophils and immunity: challenges and opportunities. *Nat. Rev. Immunol.*, 2006, 6, 173-182.

[87] Salvesen, G; Enghild, JJ. Zymogen activation specificity and genomic structures of human neutrophil elastase and cathepsin G reveal a new branch of the chymotrypsinogen superfamily of serine proteinases. *Biomed. Biochim. Acta*, 1991, 50, 665–671.

[88] Zimmer, M; Medcalf, RL; Fink, TM; Mattmann, C; Lichter, P; Jenne, DE. Three human elastase-like genes coordinately expressed in the myelomonocyte lineage are organized as a single genetic locus on 19pter. *Proc. Natl. Acad. Sci. USA.*, 1992, 89, 8215-8219.

[89] Farret,P; Dubois, RM; Bernaudin, J-F et al. Expression of the neutrophil elastase gene driving human bone marrow cell differentiation. *J. Exp. Med*, 1989, 169, 833-845.

[90] Yoshimura, K; Crystal, RG. Transcriptional and posttranscriptional modulation of human neutrophil elastase gene expression. *Blood*, 1992, 79, 2733-2740.

[91] Li, FQ; Person, RE; Takemaru, K; Williams, K; Meade-White, K; Ozsahin, AH; Gungor, T; Moon, RT; Horwitz, M. Lymphoid enhancer factor-1 links two hereditary leukemia syndromes through core-binding factor alpha regulation of ELA2. *J. Biol. Chem.*, 2004, 279, 2873-2884.

[92] Lausen, J; Liu, S; Fliegauf, M; Lubbert, M; Werner, MH. ELA2 is regulated by hematopoietic transcription factors, but not repressed by AML1-ETO. *Oncogene*, 2006, 25, 1349-1357.

[93] Gullberg, U; Lindmark, A; Lindgren, G; Persson, AM; Nilsson, E; Olsson, I. Carboxyl-terminal prodomain-deleted human leukocyte elastase and cathepsin G are efficiently targeted to granules and enzymatically activated in the rat basophilic/mast cell line RBL. *J. Biol. Chem.*, 1995, 270, 12912-12918.

[94] Horwitz, M; Benson, KF; Person, RE; Aprikyan, AG; Dale, DC. Mutations in ELA2, encoding neutrophil elastase, define a 21-day biological clock in cyclic haematopoiesis. *Nat. Genet.*, 1999, 23, 433-436.

[95] Belaaouaj. Neutrophil elastase-mediated killing of bacteria: lessons from targeted mutagenesis. Microbes. *Infect.*, 2002, 4, 1259-1264.

[96] Wiedow, O; Meyer-Hoffert, U. Neutrophil serine proteases: potential key regulators of cell signalling during inflammation. *J. Intern. Med.*, 2005, 257, 319-328.

[97] Gadher, SJ; Eyre, DR; Duance, VC; Wotton, SF; Heck, LW; Schmid, TM; Woolley, DE. Susceptibility of cartilage collagens type II. IX. X. and XI to human synovial collagenase and neutrophil elastase. *Eur. J. Biochem.*, 1988, 175, 1-7.

[98] Janusz, MJ; Doherty, NS. Degradation of cartilage matrix proteoglycan by human neutrophils involves both elastase and cathepsin G. *J. Immunol.*, 1991, 146, 3922-3928.

[99] Heck, LW; Blackburn, WD; Irwin MH; Abrahamson, DR. Degradation of basement membrane laminin by human neutrophil elastase and cathepsin G. *Am. J. Pathol.*, 1990, 136, 1267-1274.

[100] Suzuki, T; Moraes, TJ; Vachon, E; Ginzberg, HH; Huang, TT; Matthay, MA; Hollenberg, Marshall, J; McCulloch, CAG; Abreu, MTH; Chow, CW; Downey, GP. Proteinase-activated receptor-1 mediates elastase-induced apoptosis of human lung epithelial cells. *Am. J. Respir. Cell. Mol. Biol.*, 2005, 33, 231-247.

[101] Bank, U; Ansorge, S. More than destructive: neutrophil-derived serine proteases in cytokine bioactivity control. *J. Leukoc. Biol.*, 2001, 69, 197-206.

[102] Snider, GL; Stone, PJ; Lucey, EC; Breuer, R; Calore, JD; Seshadri, T; Catanese, A; Maschler, R; Schnebli, HP. Eglin C. a polypeptide derived from the medicinal leech prevents human neutrophil elastase induced emphysema and bronchial secretory cell metaplasia. *Am. Rev. Respir. Dis.*, 1985, 132, 1155-1161.

[103] Kao, RC; Wehner, NG; Skubitz, KM et al. Proteinase 3: a distinct human polymorphonuclear leukocyte proteinase that produced emphysema in hamsters. *J. Clin. Invest.*, 1988, 82, 1963-1973.

[104] Niehaus, GD; Reddan, WG. Development of a canine model of experimental emphysema by intratracheal instillation of elastase. *Chest,* 1980, 77, 276-278.

[105] Snider, GL. Chronic obstructive pulmonary disease: risk factors. pathophysiology and pathogenesis. *Annu. Rev. Med.*, 1989, 40, 411-429.

[106] Lee, WL; Downey, GP. Leukocyte elastase: physiological functions and role in acute lung injury. *Am. J. Respir. Crit. Care. Med.*, 2001, 164, 896-904.

[107] Kawabata, K; Hagio, T; Matsuoka, S. The role of neutrophil elastase in acute lung injury. *Eur. J. Pharmacol.*, 2002, 451, 1-10.

[108] Fischer, BM; Voynow, JA. Neutrophil elastase induces MUC5AC gene expression in airway epithelium via a pathway involving reactive oxygen species. *Am. J. Respir. Cell. Mol. Biol.*, 2002, 26, 447-452.

[109] Lee, WL; Downey, GP. Neutrophil activation and acute lung injury. *Curr. Opin. Crit. Care.*, 2001, 7, 1-7.

[110] Nathan, C. Points of control in inflammation. *Nature*, 2002, 420, 846-852.

[111] Hansen, G; Schuster, A; Zubrod, C; Wahn, V. Alpha 1-proteinase inhibitor abrogates proteolytic and secretagogue activity of cystic fibrosis sputum. *Respiration*, 1995, 62, 117-124.

[112] Nakajima, M; Chop, AM. Tumor invasion and extracellular matrix degradative enzymes: regulation of activity by organ factors. Seminars in Cancer Biology, 1991, 2, 115–127.

[113] Liotta, LA; Stetler-Stevenson, WG. Tumor invasion and metastasis: an imbalance of positive and negative regulation. *Cancer Research*, 1991, S5054-S5059.

[114] Nozawa, F; Hirota, M; Okabe, A; Shibata, M; Iwamura, T; Haga, Y; Ogawa, M. Elastase Activity Enhances the Adhesion of Neutrophil and Cancer Cells to Vascular Endothelial Cells. *J. Surg. Res.*, 2000, 94, 153-158.

[115] Sato, T; Takahashi, S; Mizumoto, T; Harao, M; Akizuki, M; Takasugi, M; Fukutomi, T; Yamashita, J. Neutrophil elastase and cancer. *Surgical Oncology*, 2006, 15, 217-222.

[116] Yamashita, J; Tashiro, K; Yoneda, S; Kawahara, K; Shirakusa, T. Local increase in polymorphonuclear leukocyte elastase is associated with tumor invasiveness in non-small cell lung cancer. *Chest*, 1996, 109, 1328-1334.

[117] Yamashita, J; Ogawa, M; Abe, M; Hayashi, N; Kurusu, Y; Kawahara, K; Shirakusa, T. Tumor Neutrophil Elastase Is Closely Associated With the Direct Extension of Non-small Cell LC Into the Aorta. *Chest*, 1997, 111, 885-890.

[118] Taniguchi, K; Yang, P; Jett, J; Bass, E; Meyer, R; Wang, Y; Deschamps, C; Liu W. Polymorphisms in the Promoter Region of the Neutrophil Elastase Gene Are Associated with LC Development. *Clin. Cancer. Res.*, 2002, 8, 1115-1120.

[119] Du Bois, RM; Bernaudin, JF; Paakko, P; Hubbard, R; Takahashi, H; Ferrans, V; Crystal RG. Human neutrophils express the alpha 1-antitrypsin gene and produce alpha 1-antitrypsin. *Blood*, 1991, 77, 2724 – 2730.

[120] Boudier, C; Pelletier, A; Gast, A; Tournier, JM; Pauli, G; Bieth, JG. The elastase inhibitory capacity and the α1-proteinase inhibitor and bronchial inhibitor content of bronchoalveolar lavage fluids from healthy subjects. *Biol. Chem.* Hoppe-Seyler, 1987, 368, 981-990.

[121] Nadziejko, C; Finkelstein, I; Balmes, JR. Contribution of secretory leukocyte proteinase inhibitor to the antiprotease defense system of the peripheral lung: effect of ozone-induced acute inflammation. *Am. J. Respir. Crit. Care Med.*, 1995, 152, 1592-1598.

[122] Frass, OM; Buhling, F; Tager, M; Frass, H; Ansorge, S; Huth, C; Welte, T. Antioxidant and antiprotease status in peripheral blood and BAL fluid after cardiopulmonary bypass. *Chest*, 2001, 120, 1599-1608.

[123] Owen, CA; Campbell, MA; Sannes, PL; Boukedes, SS; Campbell, EJ. Cell surface-bound elastase and cathepsin G on human neutrophils: a novel, non-oxidative mechanism by which neutrophils focus and preserve catalytic activity of serine proteinases. *J. Cell Biol.*, 1995, 131, 775-789.

[124] Korkmaz, B; Attucci, S; Jourdan, ML; Juliano, L; Gauthier, F. Inhibition of Neutrophil Elastase by α1-Protease Inhibitor at the Surface of Human Polymorphonuclear Neutrophils. *J. Immunology*, 2005, 175, 3329-3338.

[125] Tockman, MS; Anthonisen, NR; Wright, EC; Donithan, MG. Airways obstruction and the risk for lung cancer. *Ann. Intern. Med.*, 1987, 106, 512–518.

[126] Yang, P; Wentzlaff, KA; Katzmann, JA; Marks, RS; Allen, MS; Lesnick, TG; Lindor, NM; Myers, JL; Wiegert, E; Midthun, DE; Thibodeau, SN; Krowka, MJ. Alpha1-Antitrypsin Deficiency Allele Carriers among LC Patients. *Cancer. Epidemiol. Biomarkers. Prev.*, 1999, 8, 461-465.

[127] Yang, P; Bamlet, WR; Sun, Z; Ebbert, JO; Aubry, MC; Taylor, WR; Marks, RS; Deschamps, C; Swensen, SJ; Wieben, ED; Cunningham, JM; Melton, LJ; de Andrade, M. α1-Antitrypsin and Neutrophil Elastase Imbalance and Lung Cancer Risk. *Chest*, 2005, 128, 445-452.

[128] Topic, AS; Jelic-Ivanovic, ZD; Spasojevic-Kalimanovska, VV; Spasic, SM. Association of moderate alpha-1 antitrypsin deficiency with lung cancer in the Serbian population. *Arch. Med. Res.*, 2006, 37, 866-870.

[129] Yang, P; Schwartz, AG; Mc Allister, AE; Swanson, GM; Aston, CE. Lung cancer risk in families of nonsmoking probands: heterogeneity by age at diagnosis. *Genet Epidemiol*, 1999, 17, 253-273.

[130] Schwartz, AG; Ruckdeschel, JC. Familial Lung Cancer Genetic Susceptibility and Relationship to Chronic Obstructive Pulmonary Disease. *Am. J. Resp. Crital Care Medicine,* 2006, 173, 16-22.

[131] Sun, Z; Yang, P. Role of imbalance between neutrophil elastase and α1-antitrypsin in cancer development and progression. *Lancet Oncol.*,2004, 5, 182-190.

[132] Park, JY; Chen, L; Lee, J; Sellers, T; Tockman, MS. Polymorphisms in the promoter region of neutrophil elastase gene and lung cancer risk. *Lung Cancer*, 2005, 48, 315-321.

[133] Edgerton, ME; Fisher, DH; Tang, L; Frey LJ; Chen Z. Data mining for gene networks relevant to poor prognosis in lung cancer via Backward-Chaining Role Induction. *Cancer Informatics*, 2007, 2, 93-114.

[134] PubMed Central, a free archive of life science journals.

[135] URL: http://www.ncbi.nlm.nih.gov.

[136] Pruitt, KD; Katz, KS; Sicotte, H et al. Introducing RefSeq and LocusLink: curated human genome resources at the NCBI. Trends Genet, 200, 16, 44-47.

[137] URL: http//www.ncbi.nlm.nih.gov/project/LocusLink.

[138] Pruitt, KD; Maglott, DR. RefSeq and LocusLink: NCBI gene-centred resources. Nucleic Acids Res, 2001, 29, 137-140.

[139] URL: http//www.ncbi.nlm.nih.gov/project/LocusLink.

[140] Rebhan, M; Chalifa-Caspi, V; Prilusky J et al. GeneCards: encyclopedia for genes, proteins and diseases. Weizmann Institute of science, Bioinformatics Unit and Genome Center (Rehovot, Israel).

[141] URL:http://bioinformatics.weizmann.ac.il/cards.

[142] Higashiyama, M; Doi, O; Kodama, K. An evaluation of the prognostic significance of alpha-1-antitrypsin expression in adenocarcinomas of the lung: an immunohistochemical analysis. *Br. J. Cancer*, 1992, 65, 300-302.

In: Smoking and Lung Cancer
Editors: E. N. Powers and J. B. Cabbot
ISBN 978-1-60692-367-2

Chapter V

Increasing Trend of Lung Cancer in Serbia: The Prospectus of a Developing Country in Transition

Dragica P. Pesut[1], Ljudmila M. Nagorni-Obradovic[1], Tatjana N. Adzic[1], and Zorana A. Gledovic[2]

[1]University of Belgrade School of Medicine, Institute of Lung Disease and Tuberculosis, Research and Epidemiology Department, Belgrade, Serbia
[2]University of Belgrade School of Medicine, Institute of Epidemiology, Belgrade, Serbia

Abstract

Introduction: A new country-by-country report on tobacco use and control, co-published by the American Cancer Society, the World Health Organization and the International Union against Cancer, lends further support to the evidence that the tobacco industry is increasingly targeting women in developing countries, the largest remaining untapped market for cigarettes. Thus, tobacco's cancer burden is increasingly being shifted to developing countries. Serbia, a South East European country in transition, ranks among the top first several countries in Europe by tobacco use of its inhabitants: some 48% of the Serbian adult population smokes (men predominate), and in some urban areas this proportion is even higher, especially among women.

The aim of the chapter is to analyze the incidence rate and trend of lung cancer in Serbia in the period 1993-2005 with special regard to women and patients' tobacco smoking status.

Methods: In this descriptive study, annual collective data on newly- diagnosed cases of lung cancer, categorized by sex and tobacco smoking status (smokers, ex-smokers and non-smokers), have been analyzed for the 13-year period. The data represent a summary of all new cases of lung cancer in Serbia reported to the Research and Epidemiology Department of the Institute of Lung Diseases and Tuberculosis in Belgrade through the pulmonary facilities network. Population estimates were based on 1991 and 2002 census data with extrapolation.

Results: Total lung cancer incidence rate shows a slight increasing tendency (y=27.554+0.1473x) with a peak value of 33.8/100,000 population in the year 2003, and 26.7/100000 in the last year of analysis and significant differences among districts. Smokers, ex-smokers, and non-smokers account for 70.3%, 17% and 12.7%, respectively ($p<0.001$). Total number of lung cancer cases in women is doubled: a dramatic increase in tendency in smokers, but increase in former smokers, and even more in non smokers is found (y=4.0535+0.5182x). The male/female ratio in total was 4.25 but 6.9 in smokers, the latter showing a decreasing tendency in the observed period (y=9.1615-0.3758x).

Conclusion: Reducing smoking in the community will have a considerable positive effect on morbidity and mortality of lung cancer. As an example of a developing country in transition, Serbia needs urgent and continual increase of people's awareness towards tobacco smoking and other environmental harmful effects on human health, and health care workers' education on tobacco smoking as an addictive disease, its primary prevention and cessation. The relationship between tobacco smoking and lung cancer remains a challenge for further investigations that could lead to more effective therapy, and possibly a primary prevention of tobacco use.

Key words: tobacco smoking, lung cancer, risk factor, prevention, incidence, trend, women, Serbia

Introduction

During the second half of the 20th century, increasing lung cancer incidence and mortality trends have been observed globally [1,2]. Lung cancer is the most frequent type of cancer in the world in men (18% of newly diagnosed cases). In countries of the European Union it accounts for 21% of all cases of malignant diseases in men, and the cause of 29% of all malignancy-related death [3]. It usually appears in the sixth and seventh decade, but less frequently even in younger age [4-6].

Serbia is a South Eastern European country in transition, a former constituent of Yugoslavia. A study aimed to provide a comprehensive assessment of burden of selected cancers in Serbia by calculating disability adjusted life years (DALY) – the sum of the years of life lost from premature mortality and the years lived with disability– showed that the cancer burden was dominated by lung cancer in men and breast cancer in women [7].

Tobacco smoking is the most important risk factor for developing lung cancer and the changing epidemiology of this malignancy in many parts of the world is due to changing tobacco smoking prevalence [8,9]. While anti-tobacco polices over the last decades resulted in cancer decrease in the Western world, tobacco's cancer burden is increasingly being shifted to developing countries due to the tobacco smoking explosion in the developing world [10-13]. The recent trends in lung cancer mortality across Europe show decreased rates among men and increased rates in women [14].

Serbia ranks among the top several countries in Europe by tobacco use of its inhabitants: some 48% of the Serbian adult population smokes (men predominates), and in some urban areas this proportion is even higher, especially among women [15]. At the beginning of the 21st century, it is estimated that every second man and every third woman in Serbia smoke

[16]. The country is among the top in Europe in which passive smoking affects children [17]. The majority of former Yugoslav republics, together with some other countries of the Balkan region, share the same tobacco smoking prevalence problem. During the period of 1965-1990, the consumption of cigarettes increased by 98.2% (from 1.064 kg per capita in 1965 to 2.109 kg per capita in 1990), and a significant increasing tendency in cigarette consumption was registered in Montenegro [18].

A new country-by-country report on tobacco use and control, co-published by the American Cancer Society, the World Health Organization and the International Union against Cancer, lends further support to the evidence that the tobacco industry is increasingly targeting women in developing countries, the largest remaining untapped market for cigarettes [19]. Taking into account these data, a high proportion of smokers in Serbia and previous studies on lung cancer epidemiology in Serbia and Montenegro [15-18,20], we hypothesized that lung cancer in women in Serbia showed an increasing tendency at the turn of the century.

Aims and Methods

The aim of this chapter is to analyze the incidence rate and trend of lung cancer in Serbia in the 1994-2005 period with special regard to female patients and their distribution by tobacco smoking status.

In this descriptive study, annual collective data on newly-diagnosed cases of lung cancer, categorized by sex and tobacco smoking status (smokers, ex-smokers and non smokers), have been analyzed for the 13-year period. The data represent a summary of all new cases of lung cancer reported to Research and Epidemiology Department of the Institute of Lung Diseases and Tuberculosis in Belgrade, which is a national referral institution for lung diseases. Population estimates were based on 1991 and 2002 census data with extrapolation. Significant differences were assessed using the chi-squared test. $P<0.05$ was taken as the cut-off value for statistical significance.

Results

Total lung cancer incidence rate shows a slight increasing tendency ($y=27.554+0.1473x$) with a peak value of 33.8/100,000 population in the year 2003, and 26.7/100000 in the last year of analysis (Figure 1). We found significant differences in lung cancer incidence rates among districts varying from only 6.3-39.1/100000 in Moravicki and Jablanicki, respectively ($p<0.001$).

Smokers, ex-smokers, and non-smokers account for 70.3%, 17% and 12.6%, respectively ($p<0.001$). Total male:female ratio was 4.25 but 6.9 in smokers. Figure 2 shows a decreasing tendency of male/female ratio among lung cancer patient smokers.

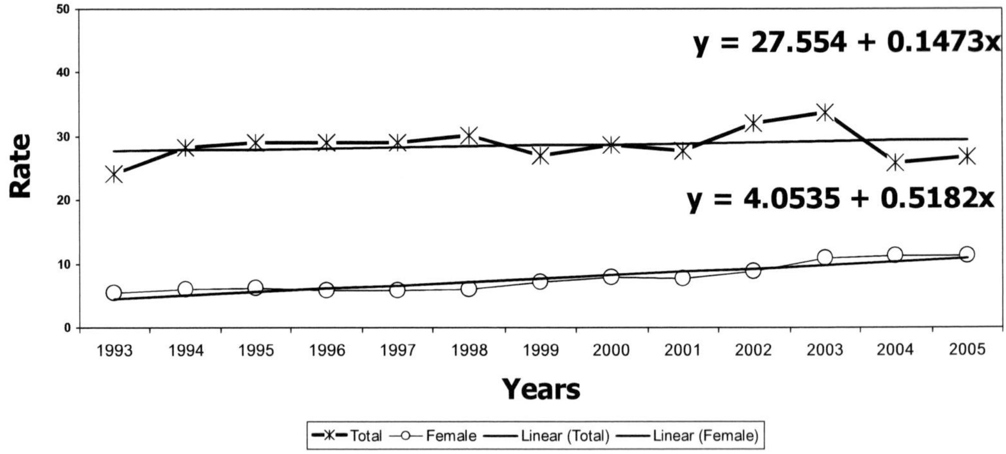

Figure 1. Time trends of lung cancer incidence rates, total and female, Serbia, 1993-2005, N^0/100,000 population.

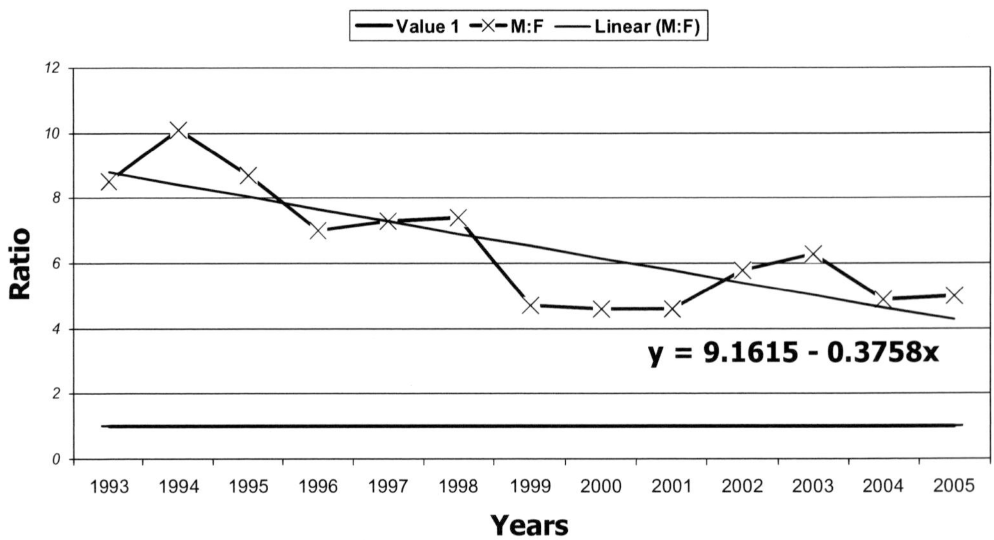

Figure 2. Male: Female ratio in lung cancer patients smokers, Serbia, 1993-2005.

Lung cancer in women is of dramatically increasing tendency (y=4.0535+0.5182x). The analysis by their tobacco smoking status showed not only increase in smokers (y=2.2415+0.2455x), but also in former smokers (y=1.7285+0.0929x), and even more in non smokers (y=0.3296+0.1012x) as it is shown at Figures 3 and 3a.

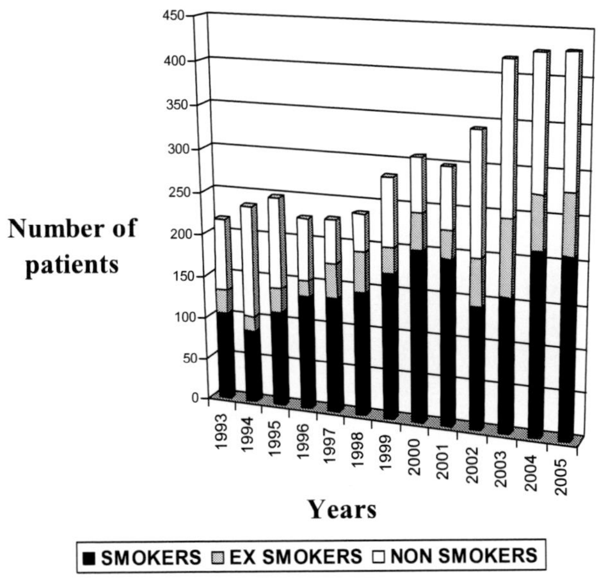

Figure 3. Tobacco smoking status of female lung cancer patients, Serbia, 1993-2005.

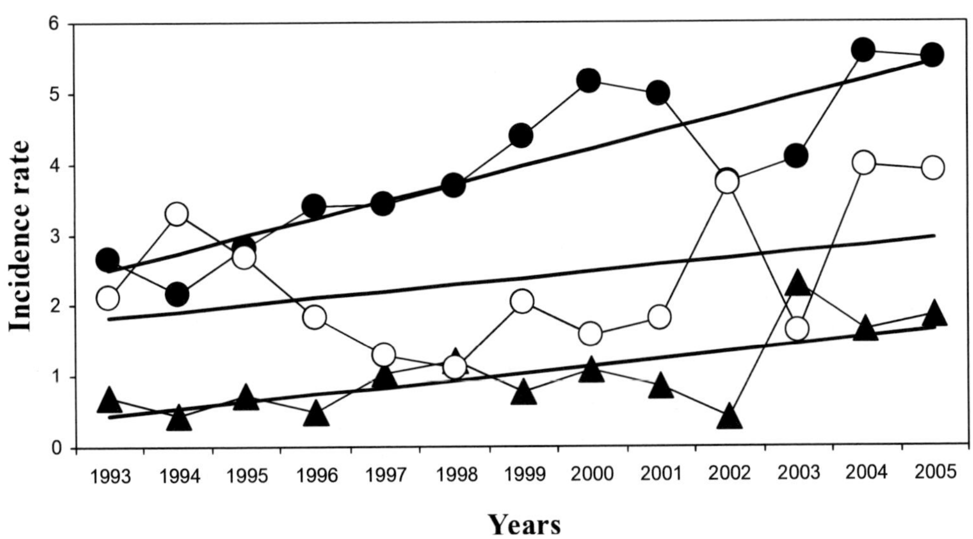

Figure 3 a. Incidence rate trends of lung cancer in women by tobacco smokink status. Serbia, 1993-2005 (N0/100,000 population).

Closed circles – smokers (y=2.2415+0.2455x)
Triangles – ex smokers (y=1.7285+0.0929x)
Open circles – non smokers (y=0.3296+0.1012x)

Lung Cancer in Smokers

Cigarette smoking is the leading cause of lung cancer and accounts for approximately 90 percent of all lung cancer cases in the USA. It was in 1950 when Wynder EL and Graham EA published the first paper linking cigarette smoking and lung cancer, which has been followed by their group's further experimental studies supporting the causative link between smoking and lung cancer formation [20]. However, it was not until 1964 that the first Surgeon General's report on smoking and health was issued concluding that cigarette smoking was the cause of lung cancer [21]. Both duration and smoking number of cigarettes per day are directly correlated with lung cancer risk [22]. Smokers who quit smoking decrease their lung cancer risk, although not to never-smoking levels. Although significantly lower than in active smokers, the risk remains several years after stopping smoking [23].

Although anti-tobacco polices over the last decades resulted in cancer decrease, lung cancer is still the leading cause of cancer mortality among both men and women in the USA, with over 170 000 new cases and over 150 000 deaths estimated in 2001 [24]. Age adjusted lung cancer incidence and mortality rates have decreased in men since 1990, reflecting the later birth cohorts' relative decline in smoking, while in women, for whom smoking behavior lagged a decade behind men, the rate is still increasing [25-27].

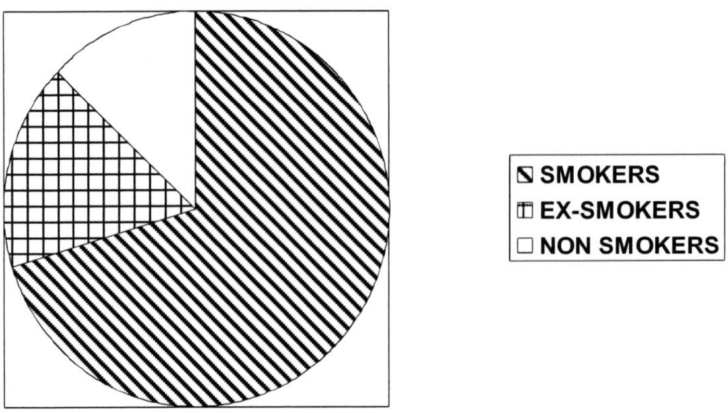

Figure 4. Tobacco smoking status of lung cancer patients in Serbia

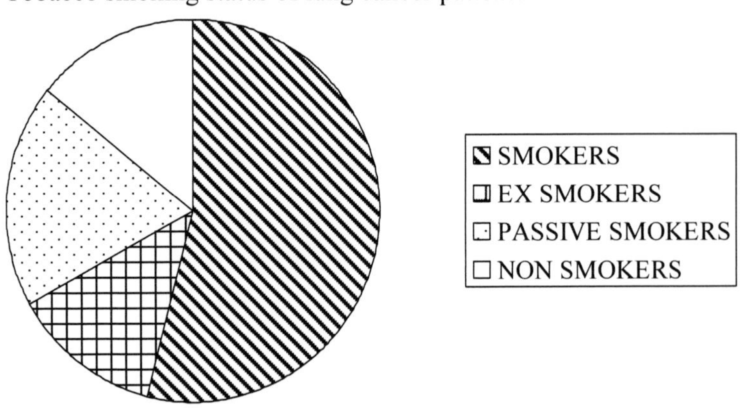

Figure 4a. Tobacco smoking status of female lung cancer patients - hospital based study

On the other hand, tobacco's cancer burden is increasingly being shifted to developing countries, which experienced tobacco smoking explosion [10-13,18]. Smoking is likely to have a particularly devastating effect on China, where smoking prevalence nowadays resembles that of America in the 1950s [13,28]. The annual death toll from smoking-related diseases in China already exceeds 1 million —2.5 times that in the United States — and is expected to double by 2025 if smoking rates are not reduced [13].

Serbia, a South Eastern European country, somewhere on the crossing between its developed West and the developing East is likely to fit tobacco smoking epidemiology of the other countries of Balkan region, where significant increasing tendency in cigarette consumption was registered. In Montenegro, a significant correlation between lung cancer mortality rates and cigarette consumption is also observed [18]. This latter Balkan-related study indicates that one can expect lung cancer mortality rates to continue to increase in men but even more so in women. The prediction is based on the fact that lung cancer morbidity and mortality reflects cigarette smoking patterns within a community, which existed 20 years ago. Cigarette smoking patterns vary by birth cohort, and lung cancer risk and mortality follow this trend [29].

Tobacco Smoke and Genetic Background Interplay

Although tobacco smoking is the major risk factor for developing lung cancer with more than 90% smokers in male and 50-70% in female lung cancer patients (women are more likely than men to have non-smoking-associated lung cancer), not all the smokers develop lung cancer but only 10% of them. This was possible to explain while taking into account human interindividual variation. It means that genetic factors may modify the influence of environmental factors, i.e. individual variation in susceptibility to harmful exogenous agents is innate - defined by genetic basis of an individual.

Iwasaki M, et al. investigated secular trends in cancer mortality among first-generation Japanese-Brazilians in the state of São Paulo between 1979 and 2001, and the results were compared with those for Japanese living in Japan and Brazilians living in the state of São Paulo. Standardized mortality ratios for liver and lung cancer increased in Japanese living in Japan over the last 20 years but no increasing trend was observed for Japanese-Brazilians [30]. Secular trends in mortality confirm the relative importance of environment in the development of cancer.

Cigarette smoking affects both early and late stages of the carcinogenic process. Suptile mechanisms of tobacco ingredients' action in step-by-step process of cancerogenesis have been a matter of particular analysis in many studies in 1970s and 1980s, these former predomnantly related to biochemical basis of susceptibility to lung cancer in humans [31-39], to be continued by investigation of dominant oncogenes and tumor supressor genes in 1980s [40-46]. Our population-genetic study based on the experience of Belgrade population-genetic school [47] showed significant difference in genetic structure of lung cancer patients when compared to health controls [48]. In 1994, Takahashi et al. showed the presence of p53 mutation in all the histological types of lung cancer. The results highlighted the role of p53 in pathogenesis of lung cancer and the fact that only one mutant allele is sufficient for malignant cell transformation.

Tobacco smoke is one of the well-known risk factors for oxidative stress, which plays important pathogenic role in appearance of lung cancer [49-53]. One of the most significant effects of oxygen radicals is DNA damage. Different compounds in tobacco smoke can react directly to form radicals, while other substances are pre-carcinogens and need to be activated by one or more of the P-450 cytochrome enzymes [50]. Human organisms defer by their DNA damage repair capacity. Research on genetic susceptibility to lung cancer showed high predisposition to cancer of individuals with germ-line mutations in DNA repair genes. A new approach based on the functional analysis of DNA repair enzymatic activity showed that reduced activity of 8-oxoguanine DNA glycosylase (OGG) is a risk factor in lung and head and neck cancers [54]. The combination of smoking and low OGG activity was associated with a higher risk, suggesting a potential strategy for risk assessment and prevention of lung cancer, as well as for other types of cancer.

Gender Differences

Some case-control studies suggest that, given equal smoking exposure, women may have a higher relative risk of developing lung cancer than men. According to the study of Bain C, et al, women do not appear to have a greater susceptibility to lung cancer than men, given equal smoking exposure [55]. Thus research should be focused on enhancing preventive interventions for all.

Lung Cancer in Non Smokers

Although smoking remains the predominant cause of lung cancer, lung cancer in never smokers is an increasingly prominent public health issue. Thus despite the clear casual connection between cigarette smoking and the vast majority of lung cancers, an increasing number of lung cancer in both men and women never smokers is observed in our 13-year analysis (Figures 5 and 5a). This suggest that both genetic and epigenetic phenomena have a role in the pathogenesis of lung cancer.

Wakelee HA, et al. recently reviewed the existing literature on lung cancer incidence and mortality rates among never smokers and presented new data regarding rates in never smokers from several large, prospective cohorts. The study supports earlier observations that women are more likely than men to have non-smoking-associated lung cancer. The distinct biology of lung cancer in never smokers is apparent in differential responses to epidermal growth factor receptor inhibitors and an increased prevalence of adenocarcinoma histology in never smokers [56].

The Influence of Passive Smoking

Apart from active smoking, passive smoking or so-called involuntary, second-hand or environmental tobacco smoking (ETS) increases the risk of developing lung cancer [57,58]. More than 50 studies of passive smoking and lung cancer risk in never smokers have been published over the past 25 years. The observations that non smokers exposed to ETS have elevated levels of tobacco smoke byproducts in biological samples alone are sufficient to identify tobacco smoke as an environmental carcinogen [57]. A study suggested that environmental exposure to tobacco smoke was associated weakly but consistently with increased risk of lung cancer [54]. According to the 2006 report of the Environmental Protection Agency (EPA), 40000 hours of passive smoking doubles the risk of lung cancer [58].

Recent legislation in many European countries related to smoking in the workplace is of great importance for prevention of many tobacco related diseases in passive smokers, but many of them stay unprotected in their households where tobacco smoke is a major source of indoor air pollution.

Almost a half of Serbian adult population smokes, and the country is among top countries in the world by passive smoking in children [17]. Our pilot one-year hospital based study on possible influence of exposure to ETS among adults in Serbia – female patients with lung cancer - showed that more than a half of those declared non smokers had long term exposure to ETS either at home or at working place [59] (Figure 4a). ETS is a major problem in China as well where 90% of the women are exposed to second-hand smoke at home [13,60]. Despite all the efforts in tobacco control during last few decades, cancer still kills 3000 people - passive smokers in the USA each year [58].

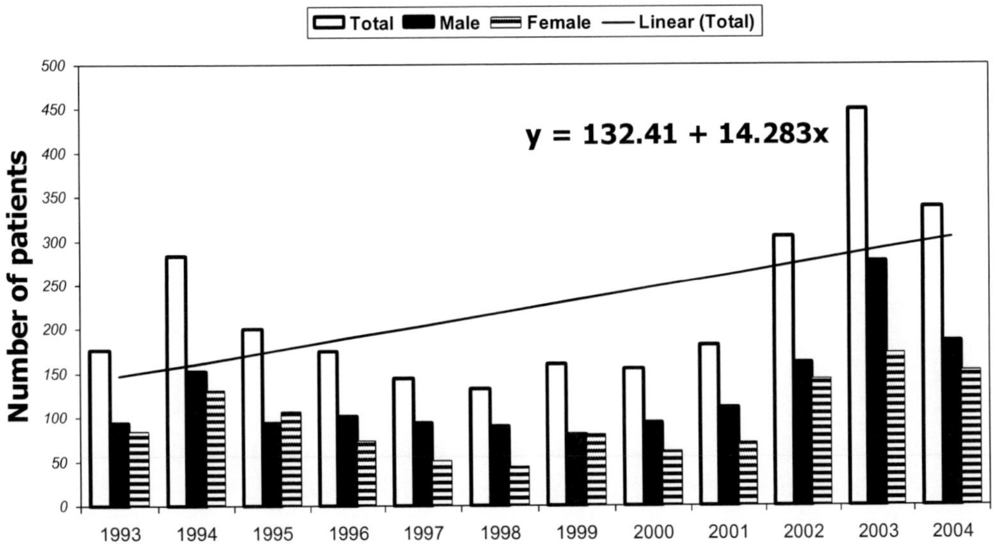

Figure 5. Distribution of lung cancer patients non smokers by sex Serbia, 1993-2004.

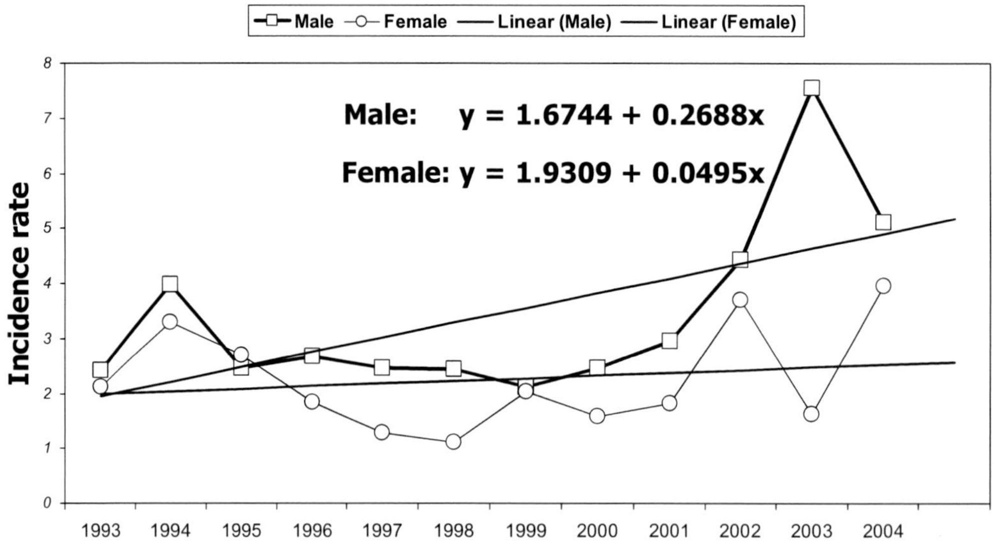

Figure 5a. Lung cancer incidence rate in non smokers by sex . Trend time, Serbia.

The Other Environmental Exposure

Environmental exposure including radiation, urban air pollution, professional exposure, fuel heating, together with genetic background, may contribute to lung cancer development. In a recent South African study, non-electric domestic fuel was associated with approximately 60% increase in the risk of smoking-related cancer. Risks were higher among smokers than former smokers, and all risk estimates increased with increasing levels of smoking duration and intensity [61]. Occupational exposures to tar and soot, asbestos, and metals such as arsenic, chromium, and nickel, have also been associated with increased lung cancer risk [22, 62]. Wood dust has been designated as a human carcinogen that can cause sino-nasal cancers. In the latest hospital based case-control study conducted at Roswell Park Cancer Institute, Buffalo, NY, USA, significant increase in risk of laryngeal and lung cancers was noted for subjects who were regularly exposed to wood dust for more than 20 years [63]. Descriptive epidemiologic data help generate the hypothesis that long-term exposure to low-dose of nitrogen oxides emissions may play a major role in causing adenocarcinoma of the lung. There is an urgent need to conduct further studies to determine whether the association is a causal one [64].

The exposure to traffic-related air pollution particles is associated with oxidative damage to DNA and this might be associated with increased risk of cancer. Humans exposed to urban air with vehicle emissions have elevated levels of oxidized guanine bases in blood cells and urine [65]. The results of a study of lung cancer risk from residential radon exposure and its radioactive progeny, performed with 200 cases were published recently. When the years of residency, smoking, education, income, and years of job exposure to known or potential carcinogens were all taken into consideration, college-educated subjects in comparison to high-school dropouts had a significant reduction in cancer risk [66].

The Role of Oxidative Stress

The human organism, which is constantly attacked by damaging compounds in the air, actuated mechanisms for defending and cleaning the lungs, which exert their action primarily against oxidant substances. Main natural antioxidants are tracheo – bronchial mucus, alveolar lining, endocellular enzymatic substances (superoxide – dismutase, catalase, glutatione peroxidase, glutatione reductase), membrane scarengers (vitamine E, beta carotene), extracellular antioxidants (plasma proteins – albumin, ceruloplasmin, transferrin, alfa 1 – antitrypsin; low molecular weight scavergens – bilirubin, methionine, uric acid; glutathione, catalase, superoxide – dismutase, vitamin C, vitamin E) [51]. When the natural antioxidants are ineffective, oxidative stress appears and it results in many respiratory disorders, including first and foremost cronic obstructive pulmonary disease (COPD), lung cancer and pulmonary fibrosis [52]. The role of underlying chronic lung diseases alone and, especially, COPD in development of lung cancer was a matter of discussion for few decades [67-69].

The administrative protective measures against air pollution are not applied enough on community level in many different urban settings and more systemic solutions are needed to protect population health. Thus a new research is particularly focused on the antioxidant potential of some food ingredients (e.g. capsaicin in red pepper) in mitigating the oxidative stress mediated damage produced during benzo(a)pyrene-induced lung cancer [70].

Constitutional Factors

It is already known that some constitutional factors also contribute to lung cancer appearance. Some of them are at least partially genetically influenced such as granulomatous and fibromatous disease [71,72]. Pulmonary fibrosis, either idiopathic or caused by chronic infection, might play a role in predisposition to lung adenocarcinoma [71,73]. It is also evidence based that connective tissue diseases (CTD) might be associated with various malignancies, and one of the most frequent is lung cancer. While tobacco smoking as the most significant risk factor for developing lung cancer, is especially considered risk factor in patients with rheumatoid arthritis and dermatomyositis [72], it seems that this malignancy is most frequent in non-smokers with systemic sclerosis [74, 75]. There are even studies that show higher risk for cancer occurrence in relatives of those who suffer from systemic sclerosis [76]. Despite the fact that the first case of cancer associated with CTD was published more than 50 years ago [77], our better understanding of pathogenesis in this association remains still unclear and risk factors for lung cancer development in CTD are still the subject of basic research. Those factors are defined as positive antricentromere antibody, presence of anti-tipoisomerase 1, and lung fibrosis in patients with systemic sclerosis [78-80].

Despite the fact that lung cancer more frequently occurs in men than in women, in our recent 10-year hospital based study on lung cancer in patients with CTD, the vast majority were women [81]. Apart from the previous epidemiological evidence that some CTDs are more frequent in women and only CTD pleuro-pulmonary complications are more frequent in men, it seems that female patients with CTD tend to develop lung cancer more frequently [71,73,82]. Thus relationship that exists between lung cancer and CTDs remains a challenge for further investigations that could make earlier detection, more effective therapy, better survival and, eventually, primary prevention of these diseases.

Dairy and Drugs Intake

Dairy consumption may affect biological pathways associated with carcinogenesis. Evidence for a link between cancer risk and dairy consumption in adulthood is increasing, but it seems that associations with childhood dairy consumption have not been studied adequately [83]. While high childhood total dairy intake was associated with a near-tripling in the odds of colorectal cancer in new Australian study, such dairy consumption association was not found for lung cancer; a positive association with lung cancer risk was confounded by tobacco smoking during adulthood [83].

Prior studies indicate that use of aspirin or other nonsteroidal anti-inflammatory drugs (NSAID) is associated with a decreased risk of non-small cell lung cancer (NSCLC). However, results have been contradictory in part because of variation in study design. The results of a new study suggest that long-term use of adult-strength aspirin may reduce the risk of NSCLC in women [84]. Prescription of non-aspirin NSAIDs for at least one year might be associated with a slightly reduced risk of lung cancer [85].

Smoking Prevention Programmes

The influences on tobacco smoking behavior are diverse, and these influences involve multiple cognitive, behavioral, and social systems. Relations between these influences may be reciprocal, and each may play a different role in the development of smoking [86]

Stopping smoking is concerned as one of the most efficient and most cost/effective measures for decreasing risk of developing a variety of smoking related diseases. It is evidence based that stopping smoking at any age is beneficial to ones health. Due to both pandemic character and harmful effects of tobacco use on human health, World Health Organization has prepared strategies for fight against tobacco smoking – smoking cessation methods and recommendations for professional help to smokers. Adolescent smoking prevention programs, beyond information giving, should include general competence skills training as well. Proper use of mass media when addressing adolescents or any target group is also very important in both effective primary prevention of tobacco smoking and cessation [86].

In smoking prevention programs, schools are a good channel to distribute the message through. In Serbia, an attendant of the forth year of primary school may find clear and concise information about harmful effects of both active and passive smoking in his/her Textbook of Science [15]. One of the key issues in fight against tobacco smoking among adolescents is the fight against positive image of smoker – an image that is in the focus of tobacco industry's advertising campaign. Skillfully created educational approach to preschool children and vulnerable group of adolescents should provoke them to develop the attitude that it is of utmost importance not to start smoking at all, to understand that tobacco smoking is a major risk factor for one's health. It includes not only proper information distributed at a proper moment, but also all the modern principles of the Information, Education, and Communication sciences, which makes it possible to reach the target group most effectively [86].

Conclusion

Reducing active smoking and passive smoking in the community will have a considerable positive effect on the morbidity and mortality of lung cancer. Although smoking remains the predominant cause of lung cancer, lung cancer in those who have never smoked is an increasingly prominent public health issue. Developing countries may need urgent and continual increasing people awareness among the public towards tobacco smoking's harmful effects on human health, and health care workers' education on tobacco smoking as an addictive disease, its prevention and cessation.

The relationship between tobacco smoking and lung cancer remains a challenge for further investigations that could make more effective primary prevention of tobacco use the best means for avoiding the morbidity and mortality of lung cancer.

References

[1] Davis L, Hoel D, Foks J, Lopez A. International trends in cancer mortality in France, West Germany, England and Wales, and the USA. *Lancet* 1990; 25: 8.

[2] Devesa SS, Blot WJ, Stone BJ, Miller BA, Tarone RE, Fraumeni JF Jr. Recent cancer trends in the United States. *JNCI* 1995; 87 (3): 175-82.

[3] Skuladottir H, Olsen JH. Epidemiology of lung cancer. *Eur. Respir. Mon.* 2001; 17 (6): 1-12.

[4] Wynder EL, Mobuchi K, Beatrie E. Jr. The epidemiology of inoperable lung cancer. Recent trends. *JAMA* 1970; 213: 2221-2228.

[5] Basara Z, Pesut D. Lung cancer in patients above the age of 46 years. Proceedings of Annual Meeting Pulmology Days in May, Banja Luka: Clinic of Lung Diseases, 2003, 49-51.

[6] Rosenberger A, Illig T, Korb K, Klopp N, Zietemann V, Woelke G, et al. Do genetic factors protected for early onset lung cancer? A case control study before the age of 50 years. *BMC Cancer* 2008 Feb 25; 8 (1): 60 [Epub ahead of print]

[7] Vlajinac H, Sipetic-Grujicic S, Jankovic S, Marinkovic J, Kocev N, Markovic-Denic L, Bjegovic V. Burden of Cancer in Serbia. *Croat. Med. J.* 2006; 47 (1): 134–41.

[8] Beckett WS. Epidemiology and aetiology of lung cancer. *Clin. Chest Med.* 1993; 14: 1-15.

[9] CDC. The health consequences of smoking: a report of the Surgeon General. Atlanta, GA: US Department of Health and Human Services, CDC, 2004.

[10] Patel JD, Bach PB, Kris MG. Lung Cancer in USA Women: A Contemporary Epidemic. *JAMA* 2004; 291: 1763-1768.

[11] Libby DM, Smith JP, Altorki NK, Pasmantier MW, Yankelevitz D, Henschke CI. Managing the Small Pulmonary Nodule Discovered by CT. *Chest* 2004; 125: 1522-1529.

[12] Wu W, Song S, Ashley DL, Watson CH. Assessment of tobacco-specific nitrosamines in the tobacco and mainstream smoke of Bidi cigarettes. *Carcinogenesis* 2004; 25: 283-287.

[13] Qin XJ, Shi HZ. Major causes of death during the past 25 years in China. *Chin. Med. J.* 2007; 120(24):2317-2320.

[14] Brennan P, Bray I. Recent trends and future directions for lung cancer mortality in Europe. *Br. J. Cancer* 2002; 87: 43-48.

[15] Pesut D, Basara Hadzi-Z. Tobacco smoking and lung cancer trend in Serbia – a 10-year analysis. *Med. Pregl.* 2006; 59 (5-6): 225-9.

[16] Danilovic M. Epidemiologic approach to tobacco smoking. In Pesut D. (Editor). Tobacco smoking and its prevention. Beograd: CIBID 2006; 7-9.

[17] Pesut DP. Passive smoking and professional assistance in smoking cessation. In: Milovanovic PD, Sakoman S, Micic VJ, Dimitrijevic I, editors. Addictive diseases, Monograph, European Centre for Peace and Development (ECPD) of the University for Peace of the United Nations (In Serbian). Beograd: 2004. Grafikom, p. 205-11.

[18] Gledovic Z, Bojovic O, Pekmezovic T. The pattern of lung cancer mortality in Montenegro. *Eur. J. Cancer Prev.* 2003;12 (5): 373-6.

[19] WHO. Tobacco Control Country Profiles. 2nd ed. 2003. Atlanta. Available from: http://www.wpro.who.int/nr/Rdoulyres/TCCP2.pdf

[20] Wynder EL, Graham EA. Tobacco smoking as a possible etiologic factor in bronchiogenic carcinoma; a study of 684 proved cases. *J. Am. Med. Assn.* 1950; 143: 329-36. (Reprinted as Landmark article *J. Am. Med. Assn.* 1985; 253: 2986-94)

[21] Wynder EL. Epidemiology of smoking and lung cancer: a historical perspective. *Lung Cancer* 1994; 11 (Suppl. 2): 1.

[22] Alberg AJ, Samet JM. Epidemiology of lung cancer. *Chest* 2003; 123: 21S-49S.

[23] Slama K. Current challenges in tobacco control. *Int. J. Tuberc. Lung Dis.* 2004; 8 (10): 1160-72.

[24] American Cancer Society. Cancer facts and figures 2003, http://www.cancer.org/docroot/STT/stt_0.aspp

[25] Wingo PA, Ries LA, Giovino GA, et al. Annual report to the nation on the status of cancer, 1973-1996, with a special section on lung cancer and smoking. *J. Natl. Cancer Inst.* 1999; 91: 675-90.

[26] Chu KC, Baker SG, Tarone RE. A method for identifying abrupt changes in US cancer mortality trends. *Cancer* 1999; 86: 157-69.

[27] Weir HK, Thun JM, Hankey BF, et. al. Annual report to the nation on the status of cancer, 1975-2000, featuring the uses of surveillance data for cancer prevention and control. *J. Natl. Cancer Inst.* 2003; 95: 1276-99.

[28] Smoking may kill 30% of China's middle-aged men by 2030. China Daily (Beijing), April 25, 2007. (Accessed June 28, 2007 at http://www.chinadaily.com.cn/china/2007-04/25/content_859410.htm)

[29] Jemal A, Chu KC, Tarone RE. Recent trends in lung cancer mortality in the United States. *J. Natl. Cancer Inst.* 2001; 93 (4): 277-83.

[30] Iwasaki M, Mameri CP, Hamada GS, Tsugane S. Secular trends in cancer mortality among Japanese immigrants in the state of São Paulo, Brazil, 1979-2001. *Eur. J. Cancer Prev.* 2008 Feb; 17 (1): 1-8.

[31] Kellermann G, Shaw CR, Lyten-Kellerman M. Aryl hydrocarbon hydroxylase inducibility and bronchogenic carcinoma. *New Engl. J. Med.* 1973; 289 (18): 934-7.

[32] Atlas SA, Vesell ES, Nebert DW. Genetic control of interindividual variationsin in the inducibility of aryl hydrocarbon hydroxylase in cultured human lymphocytes. *Cancer Res.* 1976; 36 (12): 4619-30.

[33] Emery AEH, Anand R, Danford N, Duncan W, Paton L. Aryl hydrocarbon hydroxylase inducibility in patients with cancer. *Lancet* 1978; 1 (8062): 470-2.

[34] Giurgis HA, Lynch HT, Mate T, Harris RE, Wells J, Anderson K, et al. Aryl hydrocarbon hydroxylase activity in lymphocytes from lung cancer patients and normal controls. *Oncology* 1976; 33 (3): 105-9.

[35] Conney AH. Induction of microsomal enzymes by foreign chemicals and carcinogenesis by polycyclic aromatic hydrocarbons: G. H. A. Clowes Memorial Lecture. *Cancer Res.* 1982; 42 (12): 4875-917.

[36] Harris CC, Autrup H, Connor R, Berret LA, McDowell EM, Trump BF. Interindividual variation in binding of benzo(a)pyrene to DNA in cultured human bronchi. *Science* 1976; 194 (4269): 1067-9.

[37] McLemore TL, Martin RR, Springer RR, Wray N, Cantrell ET, Busbee DL. Aryl hydrocarbon hydroxylase activity in pulmonary alveolar macrophages and lymphocytes from lung cancer and noncancer patients: correlation with family histories of cancer. *Biochem. Genet.* 1979; 17 (9-10): 795-806.

[38] Kouri RE, McKinney CE, Slomiany DJ, Snodgeass DR, Wray N, McLemore RL. Positive correlation between high aryl hydrocarbon hydroxylase activity and primary lung cancer in cryopreserved lymphocytes. *Cancer Res.* 1982; 42 (12): 5030-7.

[39] Korsgaard R, Trell E, Simonsson BG, Svensson G, Linden CJ. Genetically-induced lung cancer susceptibility in smokers (In German). *Prax. Clin. Pneumol.* 1983; 37 (Supl. 1): 679-81.

[40] Little CD, Nau MM, Carney DN, Gazdar AF, Minna JD. Amplification and expression of the c-myc oncogene in human lung cancer cell lines. *Nature* 1983; 306 (5939): 194-6.

[41] Saksela K, Bergh J, Lehto VP, Nilsson K, Alitalo K. Amplification of the c-myc oncogene in a subpopulation of human small-cell lung cancer. *Cancer Res.* 1985; 45 (4): 1823-7.

[42] Der DJ, Cooper GM. Altered gene products are associated with activtion of cellular ras k genes in human lung and colon carcinomas. *Cell* 1983; 32 (7): 201-8.

[43] Capon DJ, Seeburg PH, McGrath JP, Hayflick JS, Edman U, Levinson AD, Goeddel DV. Activation of Ki-ras2 gene in human colon and lung carcinomas by two different point mutations. *Nature* 1983; 304 (5926): 507-13.

[44] McCoy MS, Toole JJ, Cunningham JM, Chang EH, Lowry DR, Weinberg RA. Characterization of a human colon/lung carcinoma oncogene. *Nature* 1983; 302 (5903): 79-81.

[45] Santos E, Martin-Zanca D, Reddy EP, Pierotti MA, Della Porta G, Barbacid M. Malignant activation of a K-ras oncogene in lung carcinoma but not in normal tissue of the same patient. *Science* 1984; 223 (4637): 661-4.

[46] Bohmann D, Bos TJ, Admon A, Nishimura T, Vogt PK, Tijan R. Human Proto-Oncogene c-jun Encodes a DNA Binding Protein with Structural and Functional Properties of Transcription Factor AP-1. *Science* 1987; 238 (4832): 1386-92.

[47] Marinkovic D, Spremo B, Ilic M. Studies of human population-genetic variation. I. Comparisons of homozygous recessive traits in attendants of special and regular schools in SR Serbia. *Arh. Biol. Nauka* 1990; 42 (3): 11.

[48] Pesut D. Population-genetic approach in studying etiology of bronchogenic carcinoma and lung tuberculosis. PhD thesis, Belgrade: Univ. Belgrade, 1994.

[49] Van Zadwijk N. Antioxidants in the chemoprevention of lung cancer. *Lung Cancer* 1994; 11 (Suppl. 2): 96-7.

[50] Van Zandwijk N. N-acetylcysteine for lung cancer prevention. *Chest* 1995; 107 (5): 1437−41.

[51] Repine JE, Bast A, Lankhorst I. The Oxidative Stress Study Group: Oxidative stress in chronic obstructive pulmonary disease. *Am. J. Respir. Crit. Care. Med.* 1997; 156: 341 – 357.

[52] Halliwell B. Antioxidants in human health and disease. *Ann. Rev. Nutr.* 1996; 16: 33 – 50.

[53] Nagorni-Obradovic Lj, Pesut D, Skodric-Trifunovic V, Adzic T. Influence of tobacco smoke on the appearance of oxidative stress in patients with lung cancer and chronic obstructive pulmonary diseases. *Vojnosanit. Pregl.* 2006; 63 (10): 893-5.

[54] Paz-Elizur T, Sevilya Z, Leitner-Dagan Y, Elinger D, Roisman LC, Livneh Z. DNA repair of oxidative DNA damage in human carcinogenesis: Potential application for cancer risk assessment and prevention. *Cancer Lett.* 2008; [Epub ahead of print]

[55] Bain C, Feskanich D, Speizer FE, Thun M, Hertzmark E, Rosner BA, Colditz GA. Lung cancer rates in men and women with comparable histories of smoking. *J. Natl. Cancer Inst.* 2004; 96 (11): 826-34.

[56] Wakelee HA, Chang ET, Gomez SL, Keegan TH, Feskanich D, Clarke CA, et al. Lung cancer incidence in never smokers. *J. Clin. Oncol.* 2007; 25 (5): 472-8.

[57] Dockery DW, Trichopoulos D. Risk of lung cancer from environmental exposures to tobacco smoke. *Cancer Causes Control.* 1997; 8 (3): 333-45.

[58] The US Environmental Protection Agency (EPA). EPA report "Respiratory Health Effects of Passive Smoking. EPA/600/6-90/006F

[59] Pesut D, Adzic T, Nagorni-Obradovic Lj, Basara Z, Bozic D, Cvok T. Hospital based study of passive smoking in female lung cancer patients in Serbia and Montenegro. ERS Annual Congress 2006, Munich, Germany. *ERJ* 2006; Suppl, S1376.

[60] Second-hand smoke is a 'killer at large'. China Daily (Beijing), May 30, 2007. (Accessed June 28, 2007 at http://www.chinadaily.com.cn/cndy/2007-05/30/content_882976.htm)

[61] Stein L, Urban MI, Weber M, Ruff P, Hale M, Donde B, Patel M, Sitas F. Effects of tobacco smoking on cancer and cardiovascular disease in urban black South Africans. *British Journal of Cancer* advance online publication, 25 March 2008; doi:10.1038/sj.bjc.6604303 www.bjcancer.com

[62] Vineis P, Forastiere F, Hoek G, Lipsett M. Outdoor air pollution and lung cancer: recent epidemiologic evidence. *Int. J. Cancer* 2004;111 (5): 647-52.

[63] Jayaprakash V, Natarajan KK, Moysich KB, Rigual NR, Ramnath N, Natarajan N, Reid ME. Wood Dust Exposure and the Risk of Upper Aero-Digestive and Respiratory Cancers in Males. *Occup. Environ. Med.* 2008 Jan 8 [Epub ahead of print]

[64] Chen F, Cole P, Bina WF. Time trend and geographic patterns of lung adenocarcinoma in the United States, 1973-2002. *Cancer Epidemiol. Biomarkers Prev.* 2007;16 (12): 2724-9.

[65] Møller P, Folkmann JK, Forchhammer L, Bräuner EV, Danielsen PH, Risom L, Loft S. Air pollution, oxidative damage to DNA, and carcinogenesis. *Cancer Lett.* 2008 Mar 24; [Epub ahead of print]

[66] Thompson RE, Nelson DF, Popkin JH, Popkin Z. Case-control study of lung cancer risk from residential radon exposure in Worcester county, Massachusetts. *Health Phys.* 2008 Mar; 94 (3): 228-41.

[67] Davis AL. Bronchogenic carcinoma in chronic obstructive pulmonary disease. *JAMA* 1976; 235: 621-22.

[68] Samet MJ, Humble GC, Pathak RD. Personal and family history of respiratory disease and lung cancer risk. *Am. Rev. Respir. Dis.* 1986; 134: 466-70.

[69] Van der Wall AM, Huizinga E, Orie NGM, Sluiter HJ, Vrie, de K. Cancer and chronic non-specific lung disease. *Scand. J. Respir. Dis.* 1966; 47: 161-72.

[70] Anandakumar P, Kamaraj S, Jagan S, Ramakrishnan G, Vinodhkumar R, Devaki T. Capsaicin modulates pulmonary antioxidant defense system during benzo(a)pyrene-induced lung cancer in swiss albino mice. *Phytother. Res.* 2008 Apr; 22 (4): 529-33.

[71] Pesut D. Genetic factors in the predisposition for bronchogenic carcinoma. *Pluc. Bol.* 1989; 41:35-8.

[72] Yang Y, Fujita J, Tokuda M et al. Lung cancer associated with several connective tissue diseases: with a review of literature. *Rheumatol. Int.* 2001; 21:106-11.

[73] Bouros D, Hatzakis K, Labrakis H, Zeibecoglou K. Association of malignancy with diseases causing interstitial pulmonary changes. *Chest* 2002; 121:1278-89.

[74] Winkelmann K, Flach B, Unni K. Lung cancer and scleroderma. Arch. Dermatol. Res. 1988; 280:15-8.

[75] Hilli C, Nguyon A, Roder D, Robert-Thompson P. Risk of cancer in patients with scleroderma: a population based cohort study. *Ann. Rheum. Dis.* 2003; 62:72.

[76] Sakkas I, Moore F, Akritidis C. Cancer in families with systemic sclerosis. *Am. J. Med. Sci.* 1995; 310:223-5.

[77] Zatuchni J, Campbell N, Zorafonetis D. Pulmonary fibrosis and terminal bronchiolar carcinoma in scleroderma. *Cancer* 1953; 6:1147-58.

[78] Higuchi M, Horiuchi T, Ishibashi N, et al. Anticentromere antibody as a risk factor for cancer in patients with systemic sclerosis. *Clin. Rheumatol.* 2000; 19:123-6.

[79] Rothfield N, Kurtzman S, Vasques A et al. Association of anti-topoizomerase 1 with cancer. *Arthritis Rheum*. 1992; 35:724.
[80] Roumm D, Medsgar A. Cancer and systemic sclerosis-an epidemiologic study. *Arthritis Rheum*. 1985; 28:1336-40.
[81] Adzic T, Pesut D, Nagorni-Obradovic Lj, Stojsic J, Vasiljevic M, Bouros D. Clinical features of lung cancer in patients with connective tissue diseases: a 10-year hospital based study. *Respir. Med*. 2008; 102 (4):620-4.
[82] Bucca C, Rolla G. Women: lung and autoimmune disease. *Eur. Respir. Mon*. 2003; 25:190-203.
[83] Van der Pols JC, Bain C, Gunnell D, Smith GD, Frobisher C, Martin RM. Childhood dairy intake and adult cancer risk: 65-y follow-up of the Boyd Orr cohort. *Am. J. Clin. Nutr*. 2007 Dec; 86 (6): 1722-9.
[84] Van Dyke AL, Cote ML, Prysak G, Claeys GB, Wenzlaff AS, Schwartz AG. Regular adult aspirin use decreases the risk of non-small cell lung cancer among women. *Cancer Epidemiol. Biomarkers Prev*. 2008;17(1):148-57.
[85] Hernández-Díaz S, García Rodríguez LA. Nonsteroidal anti-inflammatory drugs and risk of lung cancer. *Int. J. Cancer* 2007 Apr 1;120(7):1565-72.
[86] Pesut DP, Maat MJ, Bursuc BN. Nicotiana tabacum – a Flower of Evil. In Lapointe MM. editor. Adolescent Smoking and Health Research. New York: Novapublishers 2008; 121-147.

This chapter is reviewed by

Slobodan S. Cikaric, MD, PhD
Professor School of Medicine University of Belgrade,
President of the Serbian Society against Cancer
Institute of Oncology and Radiology of the Republic of Serbia
11000 Belgrade, Pasterova 14, Serbia

Laura D. Ciobanu, MD, PhD, FERS
Assoc Professor School of Medicine&Pharmacy "Gr T. Popa"
University of Iasi
Clinical Hospital of Rehabilitation
700656 Iasi, Str. Pantelimon Halipa 14, Romania

In: Smoking and Lung Cancer
Editors: E. N. Powers and J. B. Cabbot

ISBN 978-1-60692-367-2

Chapter VI

Lung Cancer Screening: Rationale, Fundamental Principles for Interpretation, and Ethical Considerations

Idris Guessous[1,2,3], Fred Paccaud[3] and Jacques Cornuz[2,4]

1. Department of Epidemiology, Rollins School of Public Health, Emory University, Atlanta, USA
2. Department of Internal Medicine, Lausanne University Hospital, Lausanne, Switzerland
3. University Institute of Social and Preventive Medicine, Lausanne University, Lausanne, Switzerland
4. Department of Ambulatory Care and Community Medicine, Lausanne University, Lausanne, Switzerland

Abstract

In industrialized countries, lung cancer is among the most common cancers in both genders. In the US (2007), this cancer was diagnosed in 213,380 men and women, and 160,390 men and women are expected die of it. The highest rates are still observed in North America and Europe, but lung cancer is already the most common fatal cancer worldwide, with 1.04 million new cases and 921,000 deaths yearly. Lung cancer accounts for more deaths than breast and colon cancer combined. Unlike breast and colon cancers, there is currently no recommendation in favor of lung cancer screening.

The rationale of lung cancer screening is debated mostly because basic principles are misinterpreted. Thus, we first discuss the rationale for lung cancer screening by reviewing the fundamental conditions needed in order to propose a screening intervention. We will review fundamental concepts that are essential to appropriately design and interpret lung cancer screening studies, and will illustrate common systematic errors including lead time bias, length bias, and over-diagnosis.

We then review the available tools for lung cancer screening; we will show that, although each tool may detect lung cancer at an earlier stage compared with no intervention, all except low dose CT (LDCT) failed to reduce mortality. Screening studies from 1960 to now will be presented critically, including studies using LDCT, both and observational and experimental, in the US and Europe. Lastly, we will discuss lung cancer screening from ethical and social perspectives.

Since smoking is the major risk factor for lung cancer, some argue that the major intervention to decrease lung cancer is to prevent people from smoking or to make them quit, and have further argued that even if lung cancer screening trials report clear mortality reduction, resources should be allocated to smoking prevention rather than screening. We will argue that preventing tobacco use is the key element of lung cancer prevention, and must be therefore encouraged to reduce the incidence (primary prevention). However, this does not preclude the efforts to improve the treatment of lung cancer, and screening (secondary prevention) might be part of these efforts if effective.

1. Introduction

Worldwide, lung cancer is the most common cancer in terms of both incidence and mortality and this is true for both men and women [1,2]. Lung cancer is also the major cause of cancer-related mortality in men and women in industrialized countries [3,4]. In the US, it is estimated that lung and bronchus cancers will be diagnosed in 213,380 men and women and that 160,390 men and women will have died of it in 2007 [5]. The incidence and mortality rates are still higher for men than for women, although lung cancer mortality has increased markedly among women since 1960 [6]. Lung cancer accounts for more deaths than breast cancer and colon cancer combined [3,4]. But, contrary to breast and colon cancer, and despite the considerable amount of work that has been done, currently there is no recommendation in favor of lung cancer screening. Table 1 lists the clinical recommendations provided by various organizations [5,6,7]. None recommend screening. In this chapter, the rationale for lung cancer screening, the screening tools available for lung cancer, and the past, ongoing, and planned lung cancer screening studies will be presented. In addition, biased and unbiased measures of screening will be discussed. Finally, lung cancer screening will be considered from social and ethical standpoints. Because non-small cell lung cancer is the most frequently occurring type, the discussion will be limited to this entity.

2. Rationale for Lung Cancer Screening

2.1. Fundamental Conditions Needed in Order to Propose a Screening Program

Lung cancer mortality is high. Once diagnosed, the 5-year relative survival rate for lung cancer in the US varies between 2% and 47% [8]. The most important prognostic indicator in lung cancer is the extent of disease.

Table 1. Selected recommendations from health organizations

Organization	Recommendation
American Cancer Society, 2001 [5]	Recommends against routine screening of asymptomatic persons. Individuals interested in early detection should be encouraged to participate in trials.
American College of Chest Physicians, 2003 [6]	Recommends that individuals should only be screened in the context of well-designed clinical trials.
US Preventive Services Task Force, 2005 [7]	Evidence is insufficient to recommend for or against screening asymptomatic persons for lung cancer.

The Union Internationale Contre le Cancer and the American Joint Committee for Cancer Staging developed the tumor, node, and metastases (TNM) staging system which takes into account the degree of spread of the primary tumor, the extent of regional lymph node involvement, and the presence or absence of distant metastases.

The 5-year relative survival of TNM stage I, II, III, and IV lung cancer is 47%, 26%, 8%, and 2%, respectively [8]. Unfortunately, most cases of lung cancer are already advanced at diagnosis. Based on SEER data, only 16% of lung cancer cases are diagnosed while the cancer is still confined to the primary site (localized stage); 35% are diagnosed after the cancer has spread to regional lymph nodes or directly beyond the primary site; and 41% are diagnosed after the cancer has already metastasized (distant stage).

Given the dramatic morbidity and mortality of lung cancer and the positive correlation between disease stage and prognosis, interventions aimed at detecting lung cancer at an earlier stage have been pursued, notably through screening programs.

Several definitions for screening have been suggested. One of them defines screening as the examination of asymptomatic people in order to classify them as likely or unlikely to have the disease that is the object of screening (i.e., lung cancer). People more likely to have lung cancer are then investigated further to arrive at a final diagnosis. Thus, screening is a two-step process. The first step is to determine the likelihood of the disease, and the second step is to diagnose it (Figure 1). Screening is a secondary prevention and lung cancer screening may prevent disability or death, but not lung cancer itself. Often, the principles of screening are discussed through the ten criteria proposed 40-years ago by Wilson and Jungner in their report, "Principles and Practice of Screening for Disease" [9] (Table 2). Together, these criteria represent a useful check list, but do not provide a comprehensive overview of screening. Recognizing this, the fundamentals of screening will be presented in this chapter. This discussion is based on two textbooks [10, 11], and interested readers are invited to consult these references for further discussion.

Table 2. Conditions for screening (adapted from reference 9)

I. Important health problem	VI. Natural history/progression well understood
II. Recognizable at an early stage	VII. Acceptable to the population
III. Suitable test	VIII. Adequate facilities for the diagnosis and treatment of abnormalities
IV. Test repeated at regular interval for insidious onset	IX. Harm less than benefit
V. Cost of screening balanced against the benefit	X. Treatment at early stage offers more benefit

2.2. Fundamental Concepts about the Disease and the Screening Test

2.2.1. The Disease

The definition of screening is centered on people, and to be eligible for screening people must be *asymptomatic*. From a disease perspective, asymptomatic refers to preclinical phase. The preclinical phase of a disease is defined as the portion of the disease's natural history during which the disease is potentially detectable, but unrecognized [10,11]. In other words, the disease process has begun, but does not cause symptoms that bring it to medical attention. Virtually any disease presents with a preclinical phase. The goal of screening is to detect the disease during the preclinical phase. A diagnostic test is then perfomed only on the individual with a positive screening test. Cases diagnosed from the workup of positive screening tests are *screen-detected cases* [12]. Screen-detected cases cannot presume to be similar to symptom-detected cases. On the other hand, cases diagnosed after a patient seeks medical attention because of symptoms (clinical phase) are symptom-detected cases. The preclinical phase is related to two other important concepts: the lead time and the critical point.

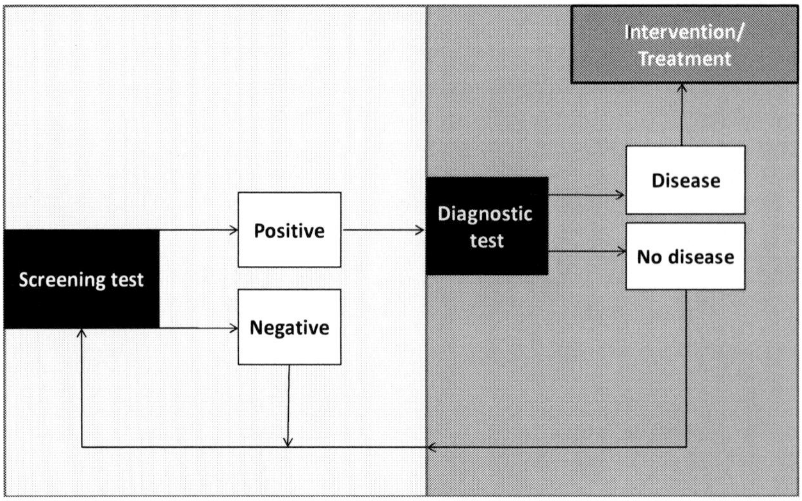

Figure 1. Screening: A two-step process.

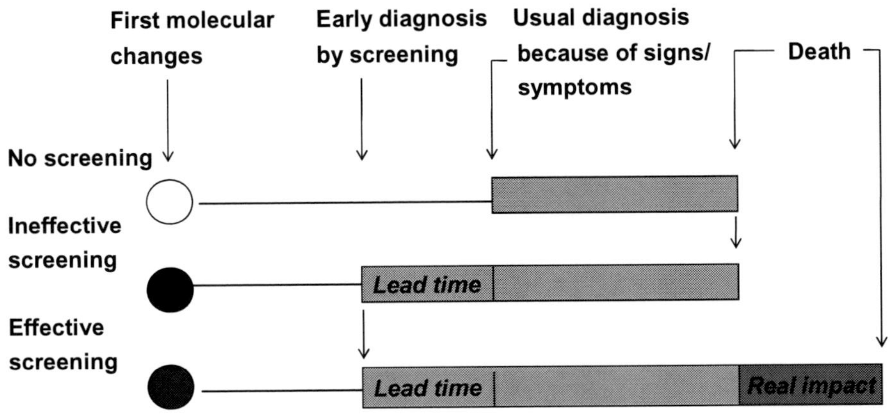

Figure 2. Lead time and lead time bias.

Lead Time

The lead time is the interval from detection to the time at which a diagnosis would have been made without screening [10]. In other words, lead time is the amount of time in which the diagnosis and, therefore, treatment are early [10]. Lead time is illustrated in Figure 2, and is a direct consequence of screening and should not be interpreted as the lead time bias, which is the systematic error in lead time interpretation. Lead time bias is discussed in the section, "Bias and Unbiased Measures of Efficacy in Screening and Lung Cancer Screening."

The lead time provided by a screening test can be calculated. For example, the lead time provided by computed tomography in lung cancer screening is about 4.5 years [12]. It means that, on average, lung cancer is diagnosed 4.5 years earlier in people screened for lung cancer with computed tomography compared with those not screened. While screened individuals are diagnosed earlier in their life, their disease also appears to be detected earlier in its phase of development. Because TNM classification is one measure of disease developement, screen-detected cases present at earlier TNM stages than symptom-detected cases. This stage-shift has been reported in most lung cancer screening trials where the proportion of stage I lung cancers detected varied between 60% and 100%. The proportion of individuals with lung cancer, but not invited for screening, that are diagnosed at stage I is dramatically less (around 16%) [6].

Critical Point

It is necessary that screened individuals present with a lead time compared with unscreened individuals. Some evidence suggests that once the disease has reached a certain threshold (e.g. metastasis), the lead time experienced by the individual would not improve his or her prognosis. For example, if a screening test detects lung cancer earlier, but after the cancer has metastased, the lead time gain is meaningless because the prognosis for screened individuals will not better than for unscreened individuals. More than providing lead time, a screening test should provide enough lead time to detect the disease before it reaches the threshold. The threshold is called the critical point or critical interval [10]. Although not a general rule, the critical point in cancer is often considered to be the point at which the cancer metastasizes. Based on the TNM lung cancer classification, only lung cancers with metastasis are stage IV. Thus, by shifting the stage distribution (decreasing the proportion of stage IV, increasing the proportion of earlier stages), lung cancer screening should increase the proportion of individuals whose lung cancer has not yet metastased. This relationship between the stage of the tumor and the presence of metastasis, which has been used since 1972, has been challenged by more recent biological and epidemiological findings. In 1996, Pantel et al. reported that more than half of patients with early stage lung cancer (stages I and II) actually presented with metastasis [13]. Early tumor cell dissemination appears to occur, and is underestimated by current staging procedures [14]. The identification of metastasis is subject to errors (failure to find metastasis when the cancer has actually metastased). Part of the reason is the sub-optimal performance of the available tools (e.g. imaging) to detect micrometastasis. Recent epidemiologic evidence also suggests a lack of correlation between TNM stage and survival in lung cancer patients [15].

To determine more accurately whether or not a disease has reached its critical point, better tools (e.g. biomarkers) and further epidemiological studies are needed.

2.2.2. The Test

In screening, the test's characteristics are as important as the disease's characteristics. Screening tests differ from diagnostic tests in many ways. First, the aim of a screening test is to determine the likelihood of a disease, not to determine whether the disease is present or not. The expectation of a screening test's performance will therefore be different (lower). A positive screening test is never definitive, and should almost always be followed by a diagnostic test (Abdominal aortic aneurysm and osteoporosis are exceptions). For example, the presence of atypical cells on sputum cytology (screening test) in a smoker must be followed by a histological examination (diagnostic test) of the pulmonary nodule. Second, screening tests are only performed on asymptomatic individuals; diagnostic tests can be performed on both asymptomatic and symptomatic individuals. The performance of screening tests, like that of diagnostic tests, is evaluated using the test's sensitivity, specificity, and predictive value. Sensitivity and specificity measure the ability of a test to correctly discriminate between diseased and nondiseased people. Sensitivity refers to the proportion of people with the disease who test positive. Specificity refers to the proportion of people without the disease who test negative. A test with poor sensitivity will miss people who have the disease (false negatives), and a test with poor specificity will falsely identify healthy people as being diseased (false positives). It is worth noting that the sensitivity and specificity are inversely related, so that an ideal test with 100% sensitivity and 100% specificity is rarely obtained. Both the sensitivity and the specificity are test-dependant and disease prevalence independent. That is, the sensitivity and specificity of a test in a given population (e.g. with a low prevalence of disease) will remain the same in another population (e.g. with a high prevalence of disease). In our example of lung cancer screening, the sensitivity and specificity of fluorescent bronchoscopy in smokers and never smokers will be the same, even though smokers have a higher prevalence of lung cancer. It is also important to realize the need for a gold standard to assess those classified as test-positive or test-negative. Often, the gold standard is the diagnostic test. Because the diagnostic test is also subject to error, Morrison stressed that any estimate of sensitivity should be regarded as the sensitivity (respectively specificity) of one test (the screening test) relative to another (the diagnostic test), rather than as a value with any absolute meaning [10].

Most of the time screening deals with the positive predictive value. The positive predictive value is the proportion of people with a positive screening test who are found by diagnostic evaluation to have the disease in question [10]. The predictive value is test and disease prevalence dependant. For example, the positive predictive value of a given fluorescent bronchoscopy screening test will be higher among smokers than non-smokers, because the prevalence of lung cancer is higher in the former population.

With few exeptions, including abdominal aortic aneurysm screening, screening must be repeated. For example, chest x-ray and computed tomography for lung cancer screening are evaluated bi-annually and annually, respectively. The main motivation is that, although the sensitivity of the test won't change, the sensitivity of the screening program will increase. Indeed, each time a screening test is repeated on a population, a proportion of false negative cases can be recaptured and correctly identified as positive cases. Thus, the overall sensitivity (the total number of people with lung cancer who tested positive / the total number of people with lung cancer) program will be higher compared with a unique screening test program.

2.3. Fundamental Concepts about Screening Organization and Interpretation

2.3.1. Screening Program

Another fundamental concept in screening is that in any population, screening should be considered as a screening *program (*other authors propose the term of *system* [16]). The screening program is neither a screening *test* only, nor only a combination of screening and diagnostic tests. This is fundamental for two reasons that are related: the effectiveness of screening and the optimal care of participants. To be effective, early detection of a disease must be followed by an effective intervention. To guarantee success, it is fundamental that screen-detected cases receive the intervention. Medical compliance is never total, even among symptomatic people who seek medical advice. Because screen-detected cases are asymptomatic, they might be even less likely to adhere to the intervention procedure. Providing a screening test without ensuring a maximum adherance will eventually be ineffective. Screening organized as a program should help achieve maximum adherence.

In addition to true positives and true negatives, there are inevitably two unfavourable outcomes of a screening test after diagnostic follow-up: false negatives and false positives. Because screening invites people who basically do not seek medical advice for a disease, it is the screening provider's responsibility to fully inform the participants about the risks and benefits of the program, to complete the follow-up of positive cases, and to support those who develop disease despite having been screened as well as those who end up as false positives [11].

A screening program should include at least the following components: defining and encouraging the participation of the target population; performing tests and interpreting test results; diagnostic follow-up of positive tests; intervention for diagnosed cases; and inviting negative test participants for regular screening. For each of these steps, the quality control and coordination between healthcare providers should be optimized.

Implementing a complete screening program will help to assess its efficacy. The efficacy of screening is estimated at a population level rather than at an individual level. For example, the efficacy of lung cancer screening depends on whether or not the rate of lung cancer mortality deacreases in the population screened. A program will provide better tools to estimate the effectiveness and impact of the screening on the health of the population.

2.3.2. Screening Depends on the the Success of Earlier Treatment

We previously mentioned that early intervention (generally a treatment) is a sine qua non part of the screening program. Actually, only effective intervention should be part of a screening program. The efficacy of an early intervention or set of interventions is generally assessed by comparing the outcome of people screened to those not screened, given that diagnosed cases from both groups receive the same intervention or set of interventions. In lung cancer screening, the disease-specific mortality rate after lobectomy and radiotherapy will be compared between people screened (with LDCT, for example) and people invited for usual care. If epidemiologic studies fail to demonstrate evidence of some benefit from early treatment, screening people is wrong.

In the previous example, we used mortality as the outcome of interest. Although it is the most serious outcome, other outcomes including morbidity, might be considered. Obviously, the outcome to be considered depends on the goal(s) of the screening program. For example, if the aim of a screening program is to reduce the cost of a disease, it would be appropriate to implement a screening program in which earlier treatment shows a significant cost reduction among those screened compared with those not screened, even if mortality is not reduced. It is therefore important to state initially the principal goal of a screening program to appropriately evaluate its efficacy. Although the morbidity due to lung cancer is important, the main purpose for a lung cancer screening program is to reduce mortality. Mortality should therefore be the outcome of interest to ultimately assess the efficacy of a lung cancer screening program.

2.3.3. The Risk of Screening is Not Intuitive

Finally, to fully capture the complexity of screening and lung cancer screening in particular, the way lay-persons and obviously some healthcare providers misinterpret screening must be discussed. Raffle et al. dedicated an entire chapter on how to prevent screening from starting when there is no sound evidence-base for it [11]. It is generally acknowledged that a treatment should not be prescribed when its benefit has not been demonstrated. In the same way, one would expect that screening programs should not take place when evidence of its benefit is lacking. Unfortunately, the prerequisite conditions needed in order for a screening program to be supported are less recognized. Differents reasons have been postulated to understand why people want screening, even though there is no evidence of a benefit. People may intuitively feel that screening is safe, simple, inexpensive, accurate, or at least that it is "better than doing nothing." Raffle et al. additionally presented the concept of "popularity paradox," which will be discussed later.

3. Screening Tools Available for Lung Cancer

Multiple screening tools for lung cancer have been evaluated. The principal and/or most promising tools will be discussed. An in depth description of biomarkers evaluated in early lung cancer detection is available elsewhere [17]

3.1. Chest Radiography

Chest radiography (CXR) was the first screening tool to be considered. CXR is a simple and inexpensive procedure. But the opportunity to detect suspicious nodules using CXR is compromised by the fact that one fourth of the lung parenchyma is hidden by mediastinal organs. Studies actually showed that CXR has a low sensitivity for detecting early lung cancer. Indeed, 90% of peripheral carcinomas and 75% of perihilar carcinomas were missed based on the results of a major screening trial using CXR as a screening tool [18, 19]. The low sensitivity of CXR, especially for lesions smaller than 2 cm, was confirmed in other studies [20, 21, 22]. Generally, the missed rate of detection of early lung cancer using CXR is assumed to be between 20% and 50%.

3.2. Sputum Cytology

Since 1960, sputum cytology has been proposed and used to look for dysplastic change as the preclinical marker for carcinoma in situ and invasive cancer [23]. The recent development of automated quantitative cytometry and molecular biomarkers has renewed the interest in sputum collection for lung cancer screening [24, 25]. Fluorescence in situ hybridization (FISH) and methylation are some other methods used to detect dysplasic modification in sputum [26, 27]. However, these methods have not consistently show better performance than sputum cytology.

3.3. Proteomics

Proteomics is the large-scale study of proteins, particularly their structure and function. The use of serum markers based on the proteomic pattern is under evaluation for several cancers and other chronic diseases [28, 29]. It has been suggested that the identification of specific polypeptides as biomarkers allows an earlier diagnosis of lung cancer. However, application of proteomics for lung cancer screening requires further investigation.

3.4. Fluorescent Bronchoscopy

Conventional bronchoscopy performed poorly as a screening method. Fluorescent bronchoscopy, using either drug-induced fluorescence or autofluorescence, has been proposed as a better tool for lung cancer screening [30]. Fluorescent bronchoscopy appeared to be more sensitive than conventional bronchoscopy, but its specificity remains low. Mortality reduction using fluorescent brochoscopy is currently lacking [30].

3.5. Low Dose Computed Tomography

The development of fast, high resolution CT scans (spiral or helical CT) allows the acquisition of multiple slice images within a single breath hold by the patient [3]. With multiple images, the 3-dimensional shape of small nodules can be characterized [31]. Diagnostic CT scan examination uses 200 milliampere seconds (mAs), but lower doses (around 60 mAs) can be used for screening purposes. Imaging with low-dose computed tomography (LDCT) is of lesser quality than the full dose CT, but is better than the one provided by CXR [32].

The first evaluation of LDCT as a screening tool was done in observational (i.e., non experimental) studies [33-40]. Results are presented in Table 2. LDCT appears to detect a larger number of lung cancers than CXR; for example, Henschke et al. reported 27 lung cancers by LDCT versus 7 by CXR [33]. Furthermore, the majority of lung cancers detected by LDCT were at stage I; e.g. 85% in the ELCAP study [33, 34]. Expectedly, the number of noncancerous lesions detected by LDCT largely exceeds the number of cancerous nodules, reflecting a low positive predictive value for LDCT. However, the proportion of patients finally undergoing a biopsy was low, and the proportion of cancers among those undergoing a biopsy was high, because non-invasive examinations carried out amongst positive screenees (such as high-resolution CT, serial CT scans, and 3-D reconstruction) strongly reduced the false positive rate. Overall, the biopsy rates after LDCT ranged between 4.8% and 14.5% of patients undergoing high-resolution CT, and 63% to 90% of these were diagnosed with cancer [7].

In 2006, authors from the International Early Lung Cancer Action Project (I-ELCAP) reported the 10-year outcome among patients with clinical stage I cancer detected on annual screening using LDCT. There were 31,567 asymptomatic persons at risk for lung cancer that were screened using LDCT from 1993 through 2005, and from 1994 through 2005, 27,456 repeated screenings were performed 7 to 18 months after the previous screening. Screening resulted in a diagnosis of lung cancer in 484 participants. Of the 484 participants diagnosed with lung cancer, 412 (85%) had clinical stage I lung cancer, and their estimated 10-year survival rate was 88% (95% confidence interval [CI], 84 to 91). Among the 302 participants with clinical stage I cancer who underwent surgical resection within 1 month after diagnosis, the survival rate was even greater at 92% (95% CI, 88 to 95) [41]. On the other hand, using the same study design (prospective screened-only study), Bach et al. found that screening for lung cancer with LDCT did not reduce the risk of death from lung cancer [42]. Indeed, among the 3246 asymptomatic current or former smokers screened, 38 deaths due to lung cancer were observed compared with the 38.8 expected deaths (risk ratio =1.0 95% CI, 0.7 to 1.3; P=0.90) [42]

Table 3. RCTs evaluating chest radiography and sputum cytology as a screening tool

Study	Intervention	Control	Lung cancer related mortality relative risk (95% CI)
Johns Hopkins Lung Project [45,46]	Annual CXR + 4 monthly SC	Annual CXR	0.80 (0.65-1.00)
Memorial-Sloan Kettering Lung Project [20,21]	Annual CXR + 4 monthly SC	Annual CXR	0.98 (0.76-1.26)
Mayo Lung Project [18,19]	4 monthly CXR/SC	Advised to have CXR/SC annually	1.03 (0.93-1.14)
Czechoslovak Lung Study [47,48]	6 monthly CXR/SC the 3 first years + annual CXR for 3 more years	CXR at baseline + CXR/SC after 3 years + annual CXR for 3 more years	1.16 (1.00-1.35)

[CXR: chest radiography; SC: sputum cytology; CXR/SC: both].

Table 4. Observational studies evaluating LDCT as a screening tool [NR: not reported]

Study, Year, Location	Number of participants	Sex	Age (Median)	Exposure (Median) [Former smokers proportion]	Noncalcified pulmonary nodule N(%)	Lung cancer N(%)	Stage I disease N(%)
Henschke, 1999, USA [33,34] (ELCAP)	1,000	M=540 F=460	≥60(67)	Only smokers ≥10 pack-yr (45)	233(23.3%)	27(2.7%)	23 (85%)
Sone, 2001, Japan [35]	5,483	M=2,971 F=2,512	≥40(64)	Smokers or former smokers [46.1%] ≥1 pack-yr (NR)	279 (5.1%)	22(0.4%)	22 (100%)
Diederich, 2002, Germany [36]	817	M=588 F=229	≥40(53)	Only smokers ≥20 pack-yr (45)	409 (50.1%)	11 (1.35%)	6 (58%)
Nawa, 2002, Japan [37]	7,956	M=6,319 F=1,637	≥50(NR)	Smokers or former smokers [62.1%] (NR)	2,099 (26.4%)	36 (0.45%)	31 (86%)
Sobue, 2002, Japan [38] (ALCA)	1,611	M=1,415 F=196	≥40(NR)	Smokers or former smokers [86%]	186 (11.5%)	13 (0.81%)	10 (77%)
Swenson, 2002, USA [39,40] (Mayo Clinic)	1,520	M=785 F=735	≥50(59)	Only smokers ≥20 pack-yr (45)	782 (51.4%)	21 (1.38%)	14 (66%)

4. Lung Cancer Screening Studies, from 1950 to the Present

4.1. Past and Ongoing Lung Cancer Screening Studies

Since the 1950s, six nonrandomized screening studies and four randomized clinical trials (RCTs) have been performed using CXR with or without sputum cytological examination. Overall, the non randomized screening studies suggested a lower case fatality rate, but no clear reduction in mortality from lung cancer [43]. The RCTs suggest no effect of CXR screening, with or without sputum cytological examination, on lung cancer mortality as recently confirmed by a meta-analysis [44]. Results are summarized in Table 4 [18,19,20,21, 45,46,47,48].

From the perspective of large-scale screening trials (i.e. to assess the feasibility of enrollment, randomisation, and follow-up) using LDCT, several pilot RCTs have been conducted. Included are the Lung Screening Study (LSS) [3], the Garg and colleagues study [49], and the French Depiscan [50]. An Israeli RCT has been reported by others, but the results are unpublished (or untraced) [32].

The Lung Screening Study (LSS) [3] is a 1-year sub-project of the US Prostate, Lung, Colorectal, and Ovarian Cancer Screening trial. There were 3,318 participants who were randomised into a LDCT arm (N=1,660) and a CXR arm (N=1,658). The evaluation is related to prevalent cases (and not to incident cases when several screening waves are taken into account). The proportion of screenees with a positive test was 20.5% in the LDCT arm and 9.8% in the CXR arm. The detection rates of cancer were 1.9% for LDCT and 0.45% for CXR.

The study conducted by Garg and colleagues [49] was a small single wave study with a LDCT arm (N=92) compared with a no-screen group (N=98) arm. Thirty-three percent of screenees in the LDCT arm presented with a positive test, defined as the presence of one to six noncalcified nodules.

DEPISCAN [50] is a RCT which was conducted in the perspective of the GRANDEPISCAN. Among the 744 participants recruited, 678 were finally included for randomization. Seventy percent of them were male, the mean age was 57 years [range, 47 to 77 years], and the proportion of ex-smokers was 32.5%. CXR was used as the screening tool in the control group (N=339) and LDCT in the experimental group (N=339). During the intermediary analysis, nodules (one or more) were detected in 51.8% of the LDCT screenees (N=216). Six were diagnosed as cancer. Among the CXR screenees (N=209), nodules (one or more) were detected in 7.4%, and one was diagnosed as cancer.

Table 3 presents the three ongoing RCTs [51-53]. The National Lung Screening Trial (NLST) [51] combines several initiatives from the US National Cancer Institute and the American College of Radiology Imaging Network. Here, 50,000 participants were randomised to a LDCT arm (N=25,000) and a CXR arm (N=25,000). The study is designed to have a statistical power of 90% to detect a 21% mortality reduction. The end of follow-up is expected in 2009.

Table 5. Ongoing and planned RCTs for lung cancer screening with LDCT

LDCT	Ongoing RCTs			Planned RCTs	
Trial name	NLST [51]	Nelson [52]	DLCG [53]	Grandepiscan [54]	Norway [55]
Country	USA	Netherlands + Belgium	Denmark	France	Norway
Start	2002	2003	2004	2006	Not reported
Number of years of screening	3	3	5	5	5
Frequency of screening	Annual	Years 1, 2, 4	Annual	Annual	Annual
Total duration (screening + follow-up)	5	7	National registery	10	7
Cancer-related mortality endpoint	Yes	Yes	Yes	Yes	Yes
Age inclusion criteria	55-74	50-75	50-65	50-70	57-71
Pack-year inclusion criteria	≥30	≥20	≥20	≥22.5	≥20
Ex-smokers included	Yes	Yes	Yes	Yes	No
Number of participants	50,000	16,000	4,000	40,000	23,000
Randomization	1:1	1:1	1:1	1:1	1:1
Multicenter	Yes	Yes	Yes	Yes	Yes
Screening procedures in control group	Chest x-ray	None	None	Chest x-ray	None
Smoking cessation program	No	Yes	Yes	No	Yes

The Nederlands-Leuvens Longkanker Screenings Onderzoek (NELSON) trial is a Dutch-Belgian study which began in April 2003, and 16,000 participants are expected to enroll in the trial [52].

The Danish Lung Cancer Group (DLCG) trial began in November 2004 in close collaboration with the Danish Institute of data security and the Danish National Cancers Central Registries (for the annual followup). The study will enroll 4,000 participants. The Danish data are expected to be pooled with those of the NELSON trial [53].

Both the NELSON and the DLCG trials compare LDCT to usual care (i.e. exclude a CXR or any other screening in the control group as was done in the NLST trial).

4.2. Planned Lung Cancer Screening Studies

Table 3 describes the characteristics of planned RCTs [54, 55]. Two large RCTs for lung cancer screening with LDCT (the LUCAS project in the UK and a German project) were unable to get the required funding [56,57].

Finally, there are other observational, single-arm studies, both ongoing and planned [58-61].

To summarize, there may be five RCTs evaluating LDCT as a screening tool for lung cancer, with a total of 133,000 subjects. The control groups include either a non-screen or chest X-ray to screen participants, and all trials except one include ex-smokers as participants.

A major point to be discussed is related to the heterogeneity between the different trials regarding the inclusion criteria, therapeutic procedures, and control group. This reflects different practicalities and resources between countries, but these circumstances may limit the pooling of data. Most of the large RCTs protocols are based on the International Early Lung Cancer Action Project (I-ELCAP) [62]. This project provides practical recommendations that are related to, for example, the production and reading of images, or to the screening frequency. However, despite this coordinated effort, there are differences among RCTs, both planned and ongoing, in terms of the age of the participants, definition of the target population (e.g. the number of pack-years), screening frequency, duration of follow-up, etc.

A major difference between the trials is the presence or absence of screening in the control group. The most appropriate control should be a no-screen group, because there is currently no evidence based strategy with an impact on lung cancer mortality. This was the choice made by the NELSON and Danish RCTs. On the contrary, the NLST and the GRANDEPISCAN use a CXR screened group as a control. The argument is that the efficacy of CXR screening is still under evaluation within the framework of the Prostate, Lung, Colorectal and Ovarian Cancer Screening trial [63]. This two-arm project (2 x 74,000 subjects) is currently ongoing, offering the intervention arm a CXR screening (one at entry and then annually for 5 years) and no screening to the control arm: thus, if the result is positive, CXR would become the new standard against which LDCT should be evaluated. The argument against the use of CXR is that its efficacy has not been proven, resulting in unnecessary irradiation in the control group.

A further point is a matter of decision making in public health; how many RCTs are needed to provide conclusive evidence for a sound decision? As a matter of fact, the effectiveness of mammography among women older than 50 years was recognized after the completion of eight RCTs (N=212,000). The effectiveness of fecal occult blood testing was recognized after four RCTs (N=330,000). This question is related to the power of the studies.

The power of a study is defined as the probability of detecting a difference between two interventions when a difference does exist [64]. Eliciting the power of a comparative study is a controversial matter after the negative results of RCTs on CXR screening. Several authors consider that the targeted reduction of mortality (30%) was too large, and that more modest gains (e.g. 15%) should be considered as sufficient. For example, two widely accepted screening strategies achieve mortality reductions between 22% to 28% for breast cancer, and between 16% to 23% in colorectal cancer. However, decreasing the targeted reduction of mortality means a substantial increase in the study population.

Another way to increase the power of a comparative study is to select a study population at higher risk for the disease, i.e. to increase the probable number of events in each arm available for the analysis. There is of course a trade-off between increasing power of the study and the decreasing generalizability of the results when populations at extremely high risks are considered.

Van Klaveren and colleagues[65] have listed useful recommendations on the way the study population should be selected to evaluate lung cancer screening: smokers with a smoking history of at least 30 years, average consumption of at least 20 cigarettes a day (≥30 pack-years), and ex-smokers within 5 years of quitting. Considering the current trend of increased smoking among teenagers, people should be invited for screening once they have reached 30 pack-years, regardless of age. For the upper age cut-off, Van Klaveren and colleagues recommend the age at which the life-expectancy of the population drops below 10 years, i.e. 70 and 75 years for males and females, respectively [65].

5. Bias and Unbiased Measures of Efficacy in Screening and Lung Cancer Screening

Most studies have shown that 1) LDCT screening detects a significant number lung cancers, 2) that the majority of lung cancers detected by screening are stage I, and 3) that in some cases, the 10-year survival rate appeared to be as high as 90% if the lung cancer is detected by screening. Still, there is currently no scientific evidence for recommending systematic lung cancer screening. We will now discuss some fundamental concepts of screening that explain why the efficacy of lung cancer screening is actually still lacking. Bias will be covered first. Then, the need for randomized controlled trials using mortality as the primary endpoint will be discussed.

5.1. Bias in Screening

Although largely discussed in Morrison's 1982 texbook, "Screening in chronic disease" [10], the impact of bias in screening has only recently received full attention. Indeed, after the spectacular results reported by the I-ELCAP investigators, numerous letters to the editor [66] as well as special articles [67, 68, 69] immediately stressed that this result was misleading because it was biased.

The authors referred to three major biases that are specifically encountered in screening studies: lead-time bias, length-time bias, and overdiagnosis.

5.1.1. Lead-time Bias

We previously defined lead-time as the interval from detection to the time at which a diagnosis would have been made without screening. Futhermore, we mentioned the necessity for a screening program to offer some lead-time. Although necessary, this measure says nothing about the efficacy of a screening program when the endpoint is mortality. Indeed, even an ineffective screening program will advance the time of diagnosis (Figure 2). The time from diagnosis is a biased measure of survival.

The third observation that the 10-year survival rate appeared to be as high as 90% in some cases, if lung cancer is detected by screening, might be a simple consequence of lead-time bias.

5.1.2. Length–time Bias

Length–time bias refers to the fact that screening preferentially detects disease with a long preclinical phase (prognostic selection). Diseases with long preclinical phases tend to be less aggressive and more favorable in terms of lethality. For example, a retrospective study using DNA flow cytometry showed that screen-detected tumors were less aggressive than symptom-detected tumors [70].

5.1.3. Overdiagnosis

Screening tests asymptomatic individuals and treats the positive cases. However, some lesions that become known as a result of screening would never have progressed to a symptomatic state. Because each positive cases is treated, there is no way to know which lesions would have remained asymptomatic. As a consequence, a proportion of individuals are unnecessarily treated because they were overdiagnosed. For years, the debate turned around whether overdiagnosis can be associated with lung cancer, a highly fatal cancer when symptom-detected. Currently, there is strong evidence that some lung cancers, like any other cancers [71, 72] may remain asymptomatic [73]. The question arises as to what proportion will remain asymptomatic, and how often screening programs detect lesions which would not affect survival. Data are still conflicting. In an autopsy study, 28% of lung cancers identified were not diagnosed during life [74]. On the other hand, there are data showing that patients with screen-detected, early-stage cancers suffered a high lethality if left untreated [75].

The two first observations, that LDCT screening detects a significant number of lung cancers and that the majority of lung cancers detected by screening are at stage I, might simply be the consequence of length-time bias and overdiagnosis.

We previously mentioned "popularity paradox" as one reason why people misinterpret screening. To illustrate the "popularity paradox," we will use lung cancer screening as an example. Imagine that a lung cancer screening program using CXR is proposed annually to smokers aged 40 to 59 years. Assume that the performance of the test is as follows: sensitivity 80%, specificity 70%. Also, assume that the rate of overdiagnosis is 10%. Thus, if 2000 smokers are screened, 800 will be true positives, 200 false negatives, 700 true negatives, and 300 false positives. Given the rate of overdiagnosis, 80 true positives would actually present with disease that would never progress to a symptomatic state. Imagine now that the overdiagnosis rate increases from 10% to 50%. The performance of the test being equal, 400 of the 800 true positives would never have progressed to a symptomatic state. Because every true positive is treated, there is no way to know who presented with disease that would never progress to a symptomatic state. On the other hand, all will think their lives had been saved by the screening program. As shown from this example, as the rate of overdiagnosis increases (from 10% to 50%), the more people (80 to 400) incorrectly believe they owe their life to the screening program (popularity paradox) [11].

To evaluate the efficacy of screening to reduce lung cancer morbidity and/or mortality, one should consider measures that are independent of early diagnosis. Two rates are independent and appropriate measures: the overall mortality rate and the disease-specific mortality rate. Often, even a meaningful reduction in disease mortality will only have a small nonstatistically significant effect on overall mortality. Evaluating the overall mortality rate only could lead one to incorrectly reject the efficacy of a screening program. Disease-specific mortality rate is more sensitive and is therefore more frequently used.

Although the advantages of observational designs compared with randomized controlled trials are debatable in some situations [76], when assessing the efficacy of a screening program, randomized controlled trials remain the most robust design, notably because both known and unknown potentials confounders are, on average, equally distributed between screenees and controls. In other words, the randomization tends to avoid the possibility that one group (e.g. screenees) represent a factor (e.g. health awareness) associated with both the exposure (e.g. screening) and the outcome (e.g. mortality) more or less than the other group (e.g. controls).

To summarize, the best approach to assess the efficacy of lung cancer screening to reduce lung cancer mortality is a randomized controlled trial with lung cancer mortality as the endpoint.

6. Why Isn't Primary Prevention Enough for Lung Cancer? Beyond Evidence, an Ethical Consideration

A key feature of lung cancer is the availability of a primary prevention, since smoking is related to 90% of lung cancer cases [3]. Accordingly, some argue that the major intervention to decrease lung cancer rate is to prevent people from smoking or to make them quit. This intervention seems to be effective. For example, lung cancer mortality has effectively decreased in the UK with the decrease in smoking prevalence [77]. Some further argue that even if screening trials report a clear reduction in mortality, resources should be allocated to tobacco prevention rather than to screening. Although preventing tobacco consumption must be encouraged and supported to reduce the lung cancer incidence (primary prevention), it is necessary but not sufficient, and secondary prevention of lung cancer should be supported if it is effective. Three major arguments may be presented: first, the prevalence of smoking is only beginning to decrease, and only in men and in the US. Millions of individuals have already been exposed and have an increased lifetime risk of lung cancer. Second, the lung cancer risk reduction after smoking cessation is very different from the cardiovascular risk reduction observed in exsmokers. Indeed, 8-years after quitting, the risk ratio of cardiovascular events for an exsmoker compared to a person who had never smoked decreases from 1.9 to 1.2. On the other hand, the risk ratio for lung cancer decreases from 18 to 16, and remains two-fold greater after 20 years [78]. Therefore, the effect of smoking will be observable for decades and for millions of people, even with effective tobacco prevention programs. Finally, because most smokers are willing to quit but cannot, smokers should be considered as suffering from smoking as from any other addiction. Over decades, Western society has exposed people to tobacco and facilitated tobacco consumption, and smokers have been condemned to smoke. If the ongoing trials reveal robust evidence of efficacy and cost-effectiveness, then it will be an ethical obligation to offer smokers and exsmokers early diagnosis of this otherwise highly fatal cancer, since smokers and exsmokers should not be sentenced twice.

Additionally, there are worrying signs that lung cancer may become a "cancer of the poor." Although it has been known for years that tobacco use is highest among those with the lowest socioeconomic status (SES), differences in tobacco control policies across SES strata are only starting to be considered. For example, while individuals with higher SES may be offered pharmacological therapy for smoking cessation and/or have enough resources to live smoke free, individuals of the lowest SES may not. Recently, the lower socioeconomic group has been shown to run an increased risk of lung cancer compared with the higher status group [79].].

The aggregation of lung cancers among the poorest adds some pros and cons in support of lung cancer screening programs. On one hand, it has been reported that individuals with lower SES tend to use screening less frequently [80]. In addition, recent evidence suggests that smokers are also less likely to frequent screening programs independently of their SES. In 2007, Silvestri et al. reported the results of a survey assessing the attitudes towards screening for lung cancer among smokers and their non-smoking counterparts. The investigators surveyed more than 2,000 people. They found that smokers were less likely to have access to health care, less willing to pay for a screening test, less willing to undergo an appropriate treatment for a screen-detected cancer, and less likely than non-smokers to consider CT screening for lung cancer [81]. Such attitudes would reduce the effectiveness of lung cancer screening. If proven effective, interventions that can modify these negatives attitudes towards lung cancer screening should be implemented as well. On the other hand, a major pro for offering effective secondary prevention is related to health disparities. If effective, lung cancer screening may be offered to the poorest for whom tobacco control policies are less effective, such that they have a better chance of surviving lung cancer. This is true worldwide, since lung cancer is no longer a rare disease in most developing countries in the world. Indeed. according to a report published in 2002, just over half of lung cancer cases (50.1%) occur in developed countries [82].

Conclusion

Taking care of lung cancer patients will remain a daily task for many years to come. This is true worldwide, not only because of the grim prevision in developing countries [83], but for current and former smokers in the developed world. The incidence of lung cancer is increasing among women, and is only beginning to decrease among men. Furthermore, there are worrying signs of increasing tobacco consumption among adolescents. Even though primary prevention is available, the evaluation of early diagnosis for lung cancer is a sound project. While non experimental studies are of some interest, only well-conducted, randomized, controlled trials with mortality as an endpoint will lead to a definitive recommendation for or against lung cancer screening.

References

[1] van Klaveren RJ, Habbema JDF, Pedersen JH, de Koning HJ, Oudkerk M, Hoogsteden HC. Lung cancer screening by low-dose spiral computed tomography. *Eur. Respir. J.* 2001;18:857-66.

[2] Parkin DM, Pisani P, Ferlay J. Global cancer statistics. CA *Cancer J. Cli*n. 1999;49:33-64.

[3] Gohagan J, Marcus P, Fagerstrom R, Pinsky P, Kramer B, Prorok P. Writing Committee, Lung Screening Study Research Group. Baseline findings of a randomized feasibility trial of lung cancer screening with spiral CT scan vs chest radiograph: the Lung Screening Study of the National Cancer Institute. *Chest* 2004;126:114-21.

[4] Jett JR, Midthun DE. Screening for lung cancer: current status and future directions: Thomas A. Neff lecture. *Chest* 2004;125:158S-62S.

[5] American Cancer Society 2008. Cancer facts and figures: 1999. Atlanta, GA: American Cancer Society, 1999; 1-36.

[6] Bach PB, Niewoehner DE, Black WC. American College of Chest Physicians. Screening for lung cancer: the guidelines. *Chest* 2003; 123:83S-88S.

[7] Humphrey LL, Teutsch S, Johnson M; U.S. Preventive Services Task Force. Lung cancer screening with sputum cytologic examination, chest radiography, and computed tomography: an update for the U.S. Preventive Services Task Force. *Ann. Intern. Med.* 2004; 140:740-53.

[8] SEER. Available at http://seer.cancer.gov/statfacts/html/lungb.html.

[9] Wilson JMP, Jungner G. Principles and Practice of Screening for Disease. Geneva, Switzerland, World Health Organization, 1968. Public Health Papers, number 39.

[10] Morrison SA. Introduction, In: Screening in Chronic Disease. 2nd edition; Oxford University Press, 1992, pp 3-20.

[11] Morrison SA. Screening in Chronic Disease. 2nd edition Oxford University Press, 1992.

[12] Raffle AE, Gray MJA. Screening: evidence and practice. Oxford University Press, 2007

[13] Henschke CI, Yankelevitz DF. CT screening for lung cancer: update 2007. *Oncologist* 2008;13:65-78.

[14] Pantle K, Izbicki J, Passlick B et al. Frequency and prognostic significance of isolated tumour cells in bone marrow of patients with non-small-cell lung cancer without overt metastasis. *Lancet* 1996; 347:649.

[15] Passlick B. Micrometastases in non-small cell lung cancer (NSCLC). *Lung Cancer* 2001; 34 Suppl 3:S25-9.

[16] Patz EF, Jr, Rossi S, Harpole DH, Jr, Herndon JE, Goodman PC. Correlation of tumor size and survival in patients with stage IA non-small cell lung cancer. *Chest* 2000; 117:1568-71.

[17] Raffle AE, Gray MJA. What screening is, and is not. In: Screening: evidence and practice. Oxford University Press, 2007, pp 33-59.

[18] Brambilla C, Fievet F, Jeanmart M, de Fraipont F, Lantuejoul S, Frappat V, Ferretti G, Brichon PY, Moro-Sibilot D. Early detection of lung cancer: role of biomarkers. *Eur. Respir. J. Suppl.* 2003 Jan;39:36s-44s.]

[19] Fontana RS, Sanderson DR, Taylor WF, Woolner LB, Miller WE, et al. Early lung cancer detection: results of the initial (prevalence) radiologic and cytologic screening in the Mayo Clinic study. *Am. Rev. Respir. Dis.* 1984; 130:561-5.

[20] Flehinger BJ, Kimmel M, Polyak T, Melamed MR. Screening for lung cancer. The Mayo Lung Project revisited. *Cancer* 1993; 72:1573-80.

[21] Melamed MR, Flehinger BJ, Zaman MB, Heelan RT, Perchick WA, Martini N. Screening for early lung cancer. Results of the Memorial Sloan-Kettering study in New York. *Chest* 1984;86:44-53.

[22] Flehinger BJ, Melamed MR, Zaman MB, Heelan RT, Perchick WB, Martini N. Early lung cancer detection: results of the initial (prevalence) radiologic and cytologic screening in the Memorial Sloan-Kettering study. *Am. Rev. Respir. Dis.* 1984;130:555-60.

[23] Queckel Quekel LG, Kessels AG, Goei R, van Engelshoven JM. Miss rate of lung cancer on the chest radiograph in clinical practice. *Chest* 1999; 115:720-4.

[24] Petty TL. Sputum cytology for the detection of early lung cancer. *Curr. Opin. Pulm. Med.* 2003; 9:309-12.

[25] McWilliams A, Mayo J, MacDonald S, leRiche JC, Palcic B, Szabo E, et al. Lung cancer screening: a different paradigm. *Am. J. Respir. Crit. Care Med.* 2003; 168:1167-73.

[26] Dalrymple-Hay MJ, Drury NE. Screening for lung cancer. *J. R Soc. Med.* 2001; 94:2-5.

[27] Romeo MS, Sokolova IA, Morrison LE, Zeng C, Barón AE, Hirsch FR, Miller YE, Franklin WA, Varella-Garcia M. Chromosomal abnormalities in non-small cell lung carcinomas and in bronchial epithelia of high-risk smokers detected by multi-target interphase fluorescence in situ hybridization. *J. Mol. Diagn.* 2003;5:103-12.

[28] Kettunen E, Salmenkivi K, Vuopala K, Toljamo T, Kuosma E, Norppa H, Knuutila S, Kaleva S, Huuskonen MS, Anttila S. Copy number gains on 5p15, 6p11-q11, 7p12, and 8q24 are rare in sputum cells of individuals at high risk of lung cancer. *Lung Cancer* 2006; 54:169-76.

[29] Petricoin EF, Ardekani AM, Hitt BA, Levine PJ, Fusaro VA, Steinberg SM, et al. Use of proteomic patterns in serum to identify ovarian cancer. *Lancet* 2002; 359:572-7.

[30] Petricoin EF 3rd, Ornstein DK, Paweletz CP, Ardekani A, Hackett PS, Hitt BA, et al. Serum proteomic patterns for detection of prostate cancer. *J. Natl. Cancer Inst.* 2002; 94:1576-8.

[31] Stanzel F. Fluorescent bronchoscopy: contribution for lung cancer screening? *Lung Cancer* 2004; 45 Suppl 2:S29-37

[32] Mulshine JL, Smith RA. Lung cancer. 2: screening and early diagnosis of lung cancer. *Thorax* 2002; 57:1071-8.

[33] Marcus PM, Fagerstrom RM, Prorok PC, Gohagan JK, Kramer BS. Screening for Lung Cancer with helical CT Scanning. *Clin. Pulm. Med.* 2002; 9:323-329.

[34] Henschke CI, McCauley DI, Yankelevitz DF, Naidich DP, McGuinness G, Miettinen OS, et al. Early Lung Cancer Action Project: overall design and findings from baseline screening. *Lancet* 1999; 354:99-105.

[35] Henschke CI, Yankelevitz DF, Libby DM, McCauley D, Pasmantier M, Altorki NK, et al. Early lung cancer action project: annual screening using single-slice helical CT. *Ann. N Y Acad. Sci.* 2000; 952:124-34.

[36] Sone S, Li F, Yang ZG, Honda T, Maruyama Y, Takashima S, et al. Results of three-year mass screening programme for lung cancer using mobile low-dose spiral computed tomography scanner. *Br. J. Cancer* 2001; 84:25-32.

[37] Diederich S, Wormanns D, Semik M, Thomas M, Lenzen H, Roos N, et al. Screening for early lung cancer with low-dose spiral CT: prevalence in 817 asymptomatic smokers. *Radiology* 2002; 222:773-81.

[38] Nawa T, Nakagawa T, Kusano S, Kawasaki Y, Sugawara Y, Nakata H. Lung cancer screening using low-dose spiral CT: results of baseline and 1-year follow-up studies. *Chest* 2002;122:15-20.

[39] Sobue T, Moriyama N, Kaneko M, Kusumoto M, Kobayashi T, Tsuchiya R, et al. Screening for lung cancer with low-dose helical computed tomography: anti-lung cancer association project. *J. Clin. Oncol.* 2002; 20:911-20.

[40] Swensen SJ, Jett JR, Sloan JA, Midthun DE, Hartman TE, Sykes AM, et al. Screening for lung cancer with low-dose spiral computed tomography. *Am. J. Respir. Crit. Care Med.* 2002;165:508-13.

[41] Swensen SJ, Jett JR, Hartman TE, Midthun DE, Sloan JA, Sykes AM, et al. Lung cancer screening with CT: Mayo Clinic experience. *Radiology* 2003; 226:756-61.

[42] International Early Lung Cancer Action Program Investigators, Henschke CI, Yankelevitz DF, Libby DM, Pasmantier MW, Smith JP, Miettinen OS. Survival of patients with stage I lung cancer detected on CT screening. *N Engl. J. Med.* 2006; 355: 1763-71.

[43] Bach PB, Jett JR, Pastorino U, Tockman MS, Swensen SJ, Begg CB. Computed tomography screening and lung cancer outcomes. *JAMA* 2007; 297:953-61.

[44] Patz EF Jr, Goodman PC, Bepler G. Screening for lung cancer. *N Engl. J. Med.* 2000; 343:1627-33.

[45] Manser RL, Irving LB, Byrnes G, Abramson MJ, Stone CA, Campbell DA. Screening for lung cancer: a systematic review and meta-analysis of controlled trials. *Thorax* 2003; 58:784-9.

[46] Frost JK, Ball WC Jr, Levin ML, Tockman MS, Baker RR, Carter D, et al. Early lung cancer detection: results of the initial (prevalence) radiologic and cytologic screening in the Johns Hopkins study. *Am. Rev. Respir. Dis.* 1984; 130:549-54.

[47] Tockman M. Survival and mortality from lung cancer in a screened population: The Johns Hopkins study. *Chest* 1986; 89:325s-326s.

[48] Kubik A, Polak J. Lung cancer detection. Results of a randomized prospective study in Czechoslovakia. *Cancer* 1986; 57:2427-37.

[49] Kubik AK, Parkin DM, Zatloukal P. Czech Study on Lung Cancer Screening: post-trial follow-up of lung cancer deaths up to year 15 since enrollment. *Cancer* 2000; 89:2363-8.

[50] Garg K, Keith RL, Byers T, Kelly K, Kerzner AL, Lynch DA, et al. Randomized controlled trial with low-dose spiral CT for lung cancer screening: feasibility study and preliminary results. *Radiology* 2002; 225:506-10.

[51] Blanchon T, Lukasiewicz-Hajage E, Lemarie E, Milleron B, Brechot JM, Flahault A; Groupe Depiscan. DEPISCAN--a pilot study to evaluate low dose spiral CT scanning as a screening method for bronchial carcinoma. *Rev. Mal. Respir.* 2002; 19:701-5.

[52] The National Lung Screening Trial (NLST), available at: http://cancer.gov/clinicaltrials/view_clinicaltrials.aspx?version=healthprofessionalandcdrid=257938andprotocolsearchid=451616.

[53] The Nederlands-Leuvens Longkanker Screenings Onderzoek (Nelson), trial design and first screening results the NEderlands-Leuvens Longkanker Screenings Onderzoek (Nelson), a prospective randomised clinical trial on lung cancer screening by spiral CT, poster session 2, P-259, Early Detection and Chemoprevention.

[54] The Danish Lung Cancer Group, protocol, screening for lung cancer, a randomised controlled screening trial of low-dose CT-scanning, September 2004.

[55] Flahault A, Grandépiscan: Evaluation de l'impact d'une stratégie de dépistage du cancer bronchique par le scanner hélicoïdal à faible dose, sur la mortalité spécifique par cancer bronchique, available at : http://www.u444.jussieu.fr/depiscan

[56] Norstein J, Cancer Registry of Norway, International Cancer Screening Conference, Oslo, Norway-December 2004.

[57] Dobson R. Screening trial for lung cancer planned for UK. BMJ 2000; 320:270

[58] National Cancer Research Network. Available at: http://www.ncrn.org.uk/csg/groups.asp?groupID=8

[59] Zulueta JF. Proyecto europeo de la deteccion precoz de cancer de pulmon, Clinica Universitaria de Navarra, Pamplona, Spain.

[60] Shaham D. Hadassah Medical Organization, Israel.Available at: http://www.hadassah.org.il/English

[61] Giunta S. Screening sul tumore del polmone. La TC-spirale "low-dose" nella diagnosi precoce del cancro del polmone in soggetti a rischio. Available at: http://www.ifo.it/ifo.3B023B0c.run

[62] New York Early Lung Cancer Action Program (NY-ELCAP). Available at: http://www.nyelcap.org

[63] Henschke CI. International Early Lung Cancer Action Program: Protocol. Available at: http://icscreen.med.cornell.edu/ielcap.pdf

[64] Prorok PC, Andriole GL, Bresalier RS, Buys SS, Chia D, Crawford ED, et al.; Prostate, Lung, Colorectal and Ovarian Cancer Screening Trial Project Team. Design of the Prostate, Lung, Colorectal and Ovarian (PLCO) Cancer Screening Trial. *Control Clin. Trials* 2000; 21:273S-309S.

[65] Fletcher RH, Fletcher SW, Wagner EH. Clinical epidemiology: the essentials, 3rd ed. Lippincott Williams and Wilkins, 1996.

[66] van Klaveren RJ, de Koning HJ, Mulshine J, Hirsch FR. Lung cancer screening by spiral CT. What is the optimal target population for screening trials? *Lung Cancer* 2002; 38:243-52.

[67] Correspondance. *N Engl. J. Med.* 2007 Feb 15;356(7):743-7

[68] Lock M, Rodrigues G. Computed tomographic screening for lung cancer. *Can. Fam. Physician* 2007; 53:1334-6;

[69] Pastorino U. Does screening for stage I lung cancer improve survival in a high-risk population? *Nat. Clin. Pract. Oncol.* 2007; 4:218-9.

[70] Welch HG, Woloshin S, Schwartz LM, Gordis L, Gøtzsche PC, Harris R, Kramer BS, Ransohoff DF. Overstating the evidence for lung cancer screening: the International Early Lung Cancer Action Program (I-ELCAP) study. *Arch Intern. Med.* 2007; 167:2289-95.

[71] Hakama M, Holli K, Visakorpi T, Pekola M, Kallioniemi OP. Low biological aggressiveness of screen-detected lung cancers may indicate over-diagnosis. *Int. J. Cancer* 1996; 66:6-10.

[72] Bangma CH, Roemeling S, Schröder FH. Overdiagnosis and overtreatment of early detected prostate cancer. *World J. Urol.* 2007;25:3-9,

[73] Jones JL. Overdiagnosis and overtreatment of breast cancer: progression of ductal carcinoma in situ: the pathological perspective. *Breast Cancer Res.* 2006; 8:204.

[74] Black WC. Overdiagnosis: An underrecognized cause of confusion and harm in cancer screening. *J. Natl. Cancer Inst.* 2000; 92:1280-2

[75] McFarlane MJ, Feinstein AR, Wells CK. Clinical features of lung cancers discovered as a postmortem "surprise". *Chest* 1986; 90:520-3.

[76] Sobue T, Suzuki T, Matsuda M, Kuroishi T, Ikeda S, Naruke T. Survival for clinical stage I lung cancer not surgically treated. Comparison between screen-detected and symptom-detected cases. The Japanese Lung Cancer Screening Research Group. *Cancer* 1992; 69:685-92.

[77] Ioannidis JP, Haidich AB, Pappa M, et al. Comparison of evidence of treatment effects in randomized and nonrandomized studies. *JAMA* 2001; 286:821–30.

[78] 77 Peto R, Darby S, Deo H, Silcocks P, Whitley E, Doll R. Smoking, smoking cessation, and lung cancer in the UK since 1950: combination of national statistics with two case-control studies. *BMJ* 2000 Aug 5;321(7257):323-9.

[79] Humair JP, Cornuz J. Desaccoutumance au tabac. Document de référence pour les médecins 2005

[80] Ekberg-Aronsson M, Nilsson PM, Nilsson JA, Pehrsson K, Löfdahl CG. Socio-economic status and lung cancer risk including histologic subtyping--a longitudinal study. *Lung Cancer* 2006; 51:21-9.

[81] Schwartz KL, Crossley-May H, Vigneau FD, Brown K, Banerjee M. Race, socioeconomic status and stage at diagnosis for five common malignancies. *Cancer Causes Control* 2003;14:761-6.

[82] Silvestri GA, Nietert PJ, Zoller J, Carter C, Bradford D. Attitudes towards screening for lung cancer among smokers and their non-smoking counterparts. *Thorax* 2007; 62:126-30.

[83] Parkin DM, Bray F, Ferlay J, Pisani P. Global cancer statistics, 2002. CA Cancer J Clin 2005; 55:74-108.

[84] Jha P, Chaloupka F. Economics of Tobacco control. London: Oxford University Press, 2000.

Reviewed by Prof. Jack Mandel, chair of the Department of Epidemiology, Rollins School of Public Health, Emory University, Atlanta.

All authors declare no competing interest and therefore have nothing to declare.
Date of Draft:
March 2008

In: Smoking and Lung Cancer
Editors: E. N. Powers and J. B. Cabbot
ISBN 978-1-60692-367-2

Chapter VII

Genetic Susceptibility to Second-Hand Smoke

Yen-Ching Chen[1,3], Jen-Hau Chen[2] and David C. Christiani[3,4]
[1] Channing Laboratory, Department of Medicine, Brigham and Women's Hospital, Harvard Medical School, Boston, MA, USA
[2] Department of Internal Medicine, National Taiwan University Hospital, Taipei, Taiwan
[3] Occupational Health Program, Department of Environmental Health, Harvard School of Public Health, Boston, MA, USA
[4] Pulmonary and Critical Care Unit, Department of Medicine, Massachusetts General Hospital, Harvard Medical School, Boston, MA, USA

Abstract

Second-hand smoke (SHS) is also referred as passive smoke, involuntary smoke, environmental tobacco smoke, and environmental cigarette smoke. The sources of SHS include exposure from relatives at home, work place, and in public. Experimental and epidemiologic studies have observed the intake and metabolism of SHS (National Research Council (U.S.).

Part of the importance of SHS stems from the fact that the levels of some carcinogens, e.g., polycyclic aromatic hydrocarbon (PAH), benzo(a)pyrene (BP) and 4-aminobiphenyl (4-ABP, an arylamine), are actually higher in undiluted SHS than in mainstream smoke (i.e., active smoke) (National Research Council 1986). In addition, the size of the particles in SHS is smaller than those in mainstream smoke and, therefore, these particles are more likely to be deposited in the lung (Dockery and Trichopoulos 1997; Hecht 1999). The association between SHS and lung cancer or childhood asthma has been studied extensively. While it is well-recognized that 80-90% of all lung cancer is attributable to cigarette smoking, only 15% of all smokers develop this disease and about 10% of all diagnosed lung cancers are never smokers (Hammond and Seidman 1980).

In summary, for different health effects, significant associations have been observed in genetic markers, including risk modification by germline polymorphisms, gene expression changes, and somatic alterations.

Some gaps in our knowledge of SHS health effects remain. The associations between sequence variants of genes involved in phase I and II metabolism and cell cycle pathways and the risk of lung cancer have been widely explored for SHS exposure and conclusive findings are not yet available.

Keywords: Second-hand smoke, genetic susceptibility, biomarkers.

Introduction

Second-hand smoke (SHS) is also referred as passive smoke, involuntary smoke, environmental tobacco smoke, and environmental cigarette smoke. The sources of SHS include exposure from relatives at home, work place, and in public. Experimental and epidemiologic studies have observed the intake and metabolism of SHS (National Research Council, U.S., Committee on Passive Smoking, 1986; Hecht, Carmella et al. 1993; Hackshaw, Law et al. 1997; Parsons, Carmella et al. 1998; Repace, Jinot et al. 1998). Part of the importance of SHS stems from the fact that the levels of some carcinogens, e.g., polycyclic aromatic hydrocarbon (PAH), benzo(a)pyrene (BP) and 4-aminobiphenyl (4-ABP, an arylamine), are actually higher in undiluted SHS than in mainstream smoke (i.e., active smoke) (National Research Council 1986). In addition, the size of the particles in SHS is smaller than those in mainstream smoke and, therefore, these particles are more likely to be deposited in the lung (Dockery and Trichopoulos 1997; Hecht 1999). The association between SHS and lung cancer or childhood asthma has been studied extensively. While it is well-recognized that 80-90% of all lung cancer is attributable to cigarette smoking, only 15% of all smokers develop this disease and about 10% of all diagnosed lung cancers are never smokers (Hammond and Seidman 1980) (Figure 1A). Epidemiological investigations have found 1.6- and 1.2-fold increased risk of lung cancer among non-smokers exposed to SHS based on data from the USA and Europe, respectively (1992; Boffetta, Agudo et al. 1998), and a risk of 1.3 was reported by the Surgeon General and National academy of Sciences (1986; 1986). Since the completion of Human Genome Project in the early 2000s, abundant genome data allow us to explore the association between SHS exposure and human health effects at the genetic level. Unlike phenotypic markers, genetic markers are stable over time and are easy to measure. Therefore, it is possible to assess variations in genes involved in xenobiotic detoxification, metabolism, DNA repairs, apoptosis, cell cycle control, angiogenesis, tumor suppressor, and other cellular responses related to SHS exposure.

Some polymorphisms (see Table 1-3, later in text), sequence variants of *GSTP1, GSTM1, CYP1A 1, CYP1B1, p53, NAT2, NAD(P)H:quinone oxidoredictase 1 (NQO1), O6-alkylguanine DNA alkyltransferase (AGT), alpha1-antitrypsin (α1-AT)*, expression of *K-ras, Bax,* or *Nrf2*-dependent antioxidant and cytoprotective genes, and hypermethylation of *MGMT*, have been related to exposure to SHS. However, previous studies have been restricted to Caucasians. Studies that compare different ethnic groups are important for a more complete understanding of variations of genetic profiles and risk related to SHS.

Moreover, it is important to consider other environmental or occupational exposures, e.g. arsenic, asbestos (Amos, Xu et al. 1999; Nelson, Christiani et al. 1999), chromium (VI) (Hu, Feng et al. 2004), nickel and vinyl chloride (Williams and Sandler 2001), cadmium (Yang, Julan et al. 2006), UV radiation, and dietary aflatoxin (Dogliotti, Hainaut et al. 1998), smoked meat, cheese, and fish (Whyatt, Garte et al. 1995), which may interact with SHS and lead to more severe or complicated health effects. Large regions of the human genome have not been explored for SHS-related health effects. Besides association studies, linkage analyses and microarray studies are useful approaches to narrow and identify the susceptibility genes related to SHS exposure. Once susceptibility genes are identified, genes involved in the same molecular or biological pathway could be analyzed together to comprehensively assess the effect of SHS. This article includes a review of existing literature addressing genetic susceptibility to SHS and presents perspectives for future studies in this field.

Carcinogens in Second-Hand Smoke

SHS contains over 4,000 compounds (2005), 69 of which are known carcinogens and could be divided into: PAH, heterocyclic compounds, nitrosamines, aromatic amines, N-heterocyclic amines, aldehydes, volatile hydrocarbons, miscellaneous organic compounds, and inorganic compounds (Hoffmann and Hoffmann 2001). Some are more commonly reported, including PAH, 4-ABP (Schonberger and Van Schayck 1998; Faraglia, Chen et al. 2003), BP (Merlo, Andreassen et al. 1998; London, Smart et al. 2000; De Flora, Balansky et al. 2003; Wolf, Kutz et al. 2005), BP diol-epoxide (BPDE) (Stierum, Hageman et al. 1997; Song, Lippman et al. 2005), benzene, 4-(methylnitrosoamino)-1-(3-pyridyl)-butanone (NNK) (National Research Council 1986; Abdel-Rahman and El-Zein 2000; De Flora, Balansky et al. 2003), 7H-dibenzo[c,g]carbazole (DBC) (Mitchell and Warshawsky 1999), acetaldehyde (Matsuda, Kawanishi et al. 1998), 1,3-butadiene (Norppa 2004), styrene (Norppa 2004), acrolein (Borchers, Carty et al. 1999; Borchers, Wesselkamper et al. 1999), cadmium (Yang, Julan et al. 2006), and arsenic (Chen, Su et al. 2005), etc. In addition, the ratio of levels of BP in SHS to the mainstream has been used as a good surrogate of BP exposure and has been reported to be 2.5-3.5 (Hecht 1999). The details of 69 carcinogens in cigarette smoke are available in Monograph 13. Risks associated with smoking cigarettes with low machine-measured yields of tar and nicotine, National Cancer Institute (Hoffmann and Hoffmann 2001) on the website (http://cancercontrol.cancer.gov/tcrb/monographs/13/). Among these carcinogens, 11, 8 and 47 are confirmed, probably, and possibly human carcinogens.

Health Effects Related to Second-Hand Smoke

Several health effects have been linked to SHS and can be divided into (1) respiratory health effects: lung cancer (Malats, Camus-Radon et al. 2000; Hou, Falt et al. 2002; Hung, Boffetta et al. 2003), asthma (Colilla, Nicolae et al. 2003; Raherison, Taytard et al. 2003; Kurz and Ober 2004; Choudhry, Avila et al. 2005; Meyers, Postma et al. 2005), chronic obstructive pulmonary disease (COPD) (Silverman and Speizer 1996; Borchers, Wert et al. 1998; Walter, Gottlieb et al. 2000; Mayer and Newman 2001; Girod and King 2005), mucus hypersecretion, inflammation, airway hyperreactivity (Borchers, Wert et al. 1998; Borchers, Wesselkamper et al. 1999), and lung function changes (von Ehrenstein, von Mutius et al. 2002), (2) reproductive and developmental effects: oral cleft (Little, Cardy et al. 2004) and low birth weight (Martin and Bracken 1986), (3) cardiovascular effects: atherosclerosis (Heeschen, Jang et al. 2001), cardiovascular disease (myocardial infarction, cerebral stoke, and sudden cardiac death) and cardiovascular function (e.g., blood pressure and heart rate) (Humble, Croft et al. 1990; Stoney, Lentino et al. 1998; Dautzenberg 2004), (4) other cancers: cancers of nasal sinus, cervix, breast, bladder, and ovary (1999; IARC 2004; Reynolds, Hurley et al. 2004; 2005; Chen, Su et al. 2005; Baker, Odunuga et al. 2006), and (5) eye and nose irritation (1999), angiogenesis (Heeschen, Jang et al. 2001; Zhu, Heeschen et al. 2003), worsening of cystic fibrosis (1999), and diabetes (Houston, Houston et al. 2006). Other diseases like Parkinson's disease, chronic pancreatitis, pancreatic cancer, cancers of liver, kidney, oral and nasal cavities, esophagus, larynx, pharynx, stomach, urinary tract, and cervix (Talamini, Bassi et al. 1999; Phillips 2002; Parain, Hapdey et al. 2003; Dautzenberg 2004) have been explored among smokers. However, the association between SHS exposure and these health effects are unclear.

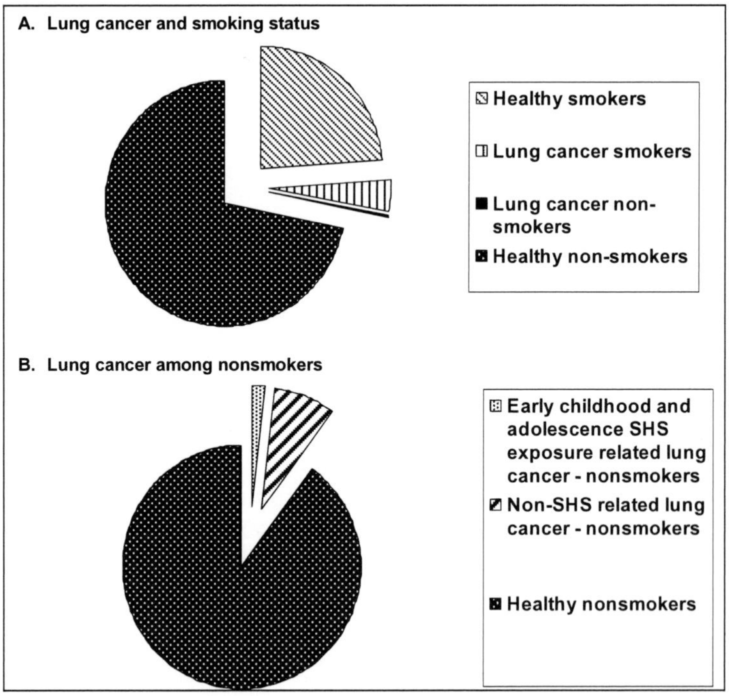

Figure 1. Second-hand smoke, active smoke and lung cancer (Hammond and Seidman 1980; Janerich, Thompson et al. 1990; Weiss 1997; Samet, Brenner et al. 1998).

Females are more commonly affected. Most women are non-smokers and thus more likely to expose to SHS containing higher levels of some carcinogens than those in the mainstream smoke. The number of lung cancer cases among non-smokers is increasing, and a large proportion of them are female adenocarcinoma (Harris, Zang et al. 1993; Kabat 1996; Chen, Chen et al. 2004). In the USA, adenocarcinoma is the most common subtype of lung cancer, accounting for 40% and 50-80% of lung cancer in smokers and never-smokers, respectively (Pulling, Divine et al. 2003). Besides adenocarcinoma, ovarian damage (Matikainen, Perez et al. 2001), complicated pregnancy (e.g., placenta praevia, placental abnormalities) (Martin and Bracken 1986; Kukla, Hruba et al. 2001), and spontaneous abortion (1999) are also related to SHS exposure among women. The high smoking rate among males makes it difficult to assess the health effects resulting from SHS exposure among men. Therefore, the female populations have been frequently selected as the group among which to assess the relationship between genetic susceptibility and SHS exposure to reach statistical power (Schonberger and Van Schayck 1998; Gealy, Zhang et al. 1999; Vahakangas, Bennett et al. 2001; Kiyohara, Wakai et al. 2003; Ng, Tan et al. 2005; Yang and Pyo 2005). For example, the overall smoking prevalence in Chinese women in Singapore has been 3% since the 1980s (1993), but the incidence of lung cancer in the 1980s was comparable with that among women in Canada and the UK, where smoking prevalence was much higher (Parkin, Muir et al. 1992; Burns 1994). Lung cancer incidence for female smokers was 2.3 in a meta-analysis including 8 studies in China (Liu 1992). Because of the significant difference in smoking rates between Chinese females and women in the West (MacLennan, Da Costa et al. 1977; Koo and Ho 1990), further studies are needed to elaborate the ethnic and geographic differences.

Children are another subpopulation susceptible to SHS because they have higher chance of SHS exposure, immature metabolic system, and higher levels of cell division and growth (Perera 1997; Krajinovic, Sinnett et al. 2002). About 17% of lung cancers among nonsmokers are attributable to high levels of SHS exposure during early childhood and adolescence (Janerich, Thompson et al. 1990; National Research Council 1993; Perera 1997) (Figure 1B). Exposure *in utero* to active maternal cigarette smoking and passive maternal cigarette exposure are two routes by which a fetus can be exposed to SHS (Byrd and Howard 1995). According to the Third National Health and Nutrition Examination Survey, 43% of children (age 4-11) were exposed to SHS at home (Pirkle, Flegal et al. 1996). About 10% of current smokers had a child at home, and the state-specific prevalence ranged from 12.3% in California to 34.2% in Kentucky (1997) for children (age<18) exposed to SHS. The perinatal and childhood health effects related to maternal SHS exposure include (1) fetal growth: behavior problems, decreased intellectual achievement (Martin and Bracken 1986; Olds, Henderson et al. 1994; Streissguth, Sampson et al. 1994), lower neonatal birth weight, small-for-gestational age, and premature delivery (Martin and Bracken 1986; Mainous and Hueston 1994; Dejin-Karlsson, Hanson et al. 1998; Hanke, Kalinka et al. 1999; Wu, Zhang et al. 2001; Hong, Lee et al. 2003; Yang, Julan et al. 2006), (2) congenital malformation: oral cleft palate (Little, Cardy et al. 2004), and (3) fetal loss: infant mortality (Kharrazi, DeLorenze et al. 2004) and sudden infant death (1999; Adgent 2006),(4) cancer: hematopoietic malignancies (e.g., acute lymphoblastic leukemia) (Shu, Ross et al. 1996; Ji, Shu et al. 1997; Sorahan, Prior et al. 1997; Finette, O'Neill et al. 1998; Canalle, Burim et al. 2004) and brain tumor (Baldwin and Preston-Martin 2004), and (5) allergic and respiratory effects: asthma (Casimir 1996; Lorente, Romo et al. 1998; Bjorksten 1999; de Blic 1999; Ronmark, Jonsson et al. 1999; Chan-Yeung, Manfreda et al. 2000; Gilliland, Li et al. 2002; Peden 2002; Kurz and Ober 2004; Arruda, Sole et al. 2005; Bener, Janahi et al. 2005; Wenten, Berhane et al. 2005; Li, Romieu et al. 2006), wheezing, cough, phlegm, chronic bronchitis, pneumonia, middle ear infection (General 1986; National Research Council 1986; 1992; 1997; Cook and Strachan 1997; 1998; Chen, Rennie et al. 1998; Gergen, Fowler et al. 1998; Strachan and Cook 1998; 1999; Gilliland, Li et al. 2002; Arshad, Kurukulaaratchy et al. 2005), and atopic eczema (Kramer, Lemmen et al. 2004). However, some studies suggested that children whose mothers smoked during their pregnancy were not at an increased risk of cancer (Pershagen, Ericson et al. 1992; Klebanoff, Clemens et al. 1996; Sorahan, Prior et al. 1997). It is more difficult to recruit children than adults, but it is important to do research on them, because early SHS exposure figures greatly in predicting disease risk in later life.

Lung Cancer

Lung cancer is the most well-known disease related to SHS and is the 1st and 2nd cause of death in the USA for men and women, respectively (Parkin, Pisani et al. 1999; 2003). The American Cancer Society reported the incidence rate of cancer of the lung and bronchus (Jemal, Siegel et al. 2006) in males as 77.8, 76.7, 113.9, 59.4, 42.6, and 44.6 per 100,000 and age-adjusted to the 2000 US standard population for all races, whites, African Americans, Asian Americans/Pacific Islanders, American Indians/Alaska Natives, and Hispanic Latinos, respectively. For females, the incidence rates were 48.9, 51.1, 55.2, 28.3, 23.6, and 23.3 per 100,000 for the same standard population and ethnic groups above. In the USA, tobacco use increased from 1915 (Sellers, Potter et al. 1992) and lung cancer risk from SHS increased approximately 1.6-fold (1992; Fontham, Correa et al. 1994; Cardenas, Thun et al. 1997; Boffetta, Agudo et al. 1998). A meta-analysis of 37 studies reported the excess risk of lung cancer increased 24% among nonsmokers live with smokers (Hackshaw, Law et al. 1997). A large case-control study (Boffetta, Agudo et al. 1998) including 7 European countries found that a 1.16- and 1.15-fold increased, but not significant, risk of lung cancer among individuals exposed to SHS from the spouse and at the workplace, respectively. The cessation of exposure from both sources decreases the excess risk (Boffetta, Agudo et al. 1998). Active smoking accounted for 90% of lung cancer deaths, and lung cancer in lifelong never smokers accounted for 11,000 deaths in 1995 (Samet, Brenner et al. 1998). Among adult nonsmokers, SHS exposure lead to about 3,000 lung cancer death and 35,000 deaths from ischemic heart disease each year (2006).

Besides passive and active smoking, several other factors have been reported to modify the risk of lung cancer. These include diet (Fontham 1990; Alavanja, Brownson et al. 1992; Ko, Lee et al. 1997), occupational exposure (Boffetta 1993; Collier and Pritsos 2003), prior lung disease (Alavanja, Brownson et al. 1992; Gao 1996; Ko, Lee et al. 1997), and indoor air pollutants (e.g., fumes from cooking oils) (Gao 1996; Wang, Zhou et al. 1996; Ko, Lee et al. 1997), coal or wood combustion (Gao 1996; Ko, Lee et al. 1997), and family history of lung cancer (Wang, Zhou et al. 1996). Comprehensive inclusion of various risk factors could provide better prediction of lung cancer risk.

Asthma

Asthma has become an important public health problem. Recent studies suggest that maternal smoke exposure during pregnancy is an important risk factor for childhood asthma and wheezing (Martinez, Cline et al. 1992; Gilliland, Li et al. 2001; von Mutius 2002). However, this association was not found by others (1992; 1997; Cook and Strachan 1997; 1998; Strachan and Cook 1998; 1999; 2000). In addition, some studies have suggested that an interaction between family history of asthma or atopy and exposure to tobacco smoke in early childhood, but not *in utero,* influences the risk of asthma (Ronmark, Jonsson et al. 1999; Jaakkola, Nafstad et al. 2001; Larsson, Frisk et al. 2001; von Mutius 2002). Besides SHS exposure, factors like air pollution from traffic or industries, dust mite, pet allergens, cold air, respiratory infections, medication, and exercise can exacerbate asthma symptoms (1992; 1997; Cook and Strachan 1997; 1998; Strachan and Cook 1998; 1999; Barnes 1999; Jordaan, Ehrlich et al. 1999; Gold 2000; Ehrlich, Jordaan et al. 2001; Thorn, Brisman et al. 2001). The population-attributable risk for SHS exposure in children has been estimated to range from 9% for asthma prevalence to 25% for hospital admissions due to lower respiratory symptoms (Rushton, Courage et al. 2003).

Chronic Obstructive Pulmonary Disease (COPD)

Chronic obstructive pulmonary disease (COPD) is a disease with permanent narrowing of small bronchi, or destruction of acini (emphysema); chronic bronchitis and emphysema are related diseases. Some irritants in cigarette smoke (e.g., aluminum silicate and kaolinite) have been related to COPD (Girod and King 2005). Indians have a higher incidence rate of COPD than other ethnic groups: it has been diagnosed in 4.1% of subjects, with a male-to-female ratio of 1.56:1 and a smoker-to-nonsmoker ratio of 2.65: 1 (Jindal, Aggarwal et al. 2006). In this population, nonsmokers with SHS exposure had a 1.4-fold risk of COPD (95% CI=1.21-1.61) as compare to those without SHS exposure. Individuals with exposure to both SHS and solid fuel combustion had a higher risk of COPD than those with SHS exposure alone (Jindal, Aggarwal et al. 2006). The gender differences on COPD risk reflect that smoking is an important risk factor for men who have higher smoking rate. Like lung cancer, other environmental factors may lead to synergistic effects. This is possibly a result of combination of environmental exposure and genetic susceptibility.

Acute Lymphoblastic Leukemia (ALL)

Acute lymphoblastic leukemia (ALL) is the most common malignancy affecting children and accounts for 30% of all childhood cancers (Canalle, Burim et al. 2004). Accumulating evidence shows that either maternal exposure to SHS or a history of paternal, but not maternal, smoking was associated with an increase risk of leukemia and lymphoma in children under 5 years of age (Shu, Ross et al. 1996; Ji, Shu et al. 1997; Sorahan, Prior et al.

1997). However, very few studies have explored the association between SHS exposure and the risk of ALL.

Diabetes

Smoking has been linked to impaired response to glucose tolerance tests and insulin resistance (Janzon, Berntorp et al. 1983; Attvall, Fowelin et al. 1993) and increased incidence of diabetes (Rimm, Manson et al. 1993; Rimm, Chan et al. 1995; Kawakami, Takatsuka et al. 1997; Wannamethee, Shaper et al. 2001; Will, Galuska et al. 2001), but this result was not replicated in other studies (Wannamethee, Shaper et al. 2001). The role of SHS exposure to diabetes has not been explored until very recently (Houston, Houston et al. 2006). In a population composed of Caucasians and African Americans, the 15-year incidence of glucose intolerance was highest among smokers (21.8%), followed by never smokers with SHS exposure (17.2%), former smokers (14.4%), and lowest among never smokers without SHS exposure (11.5%) (Houston, Houston et al. 2006). Some studies have shown a dose-response association between smoking and incidence of diabetes (Rimm, Manson et al. 1993; Kawakami, Takatsuka et al. 1997).

Intermediate Biomarkers for Second-Hand Smoke Exposure

Intermediate biomarkers are very useful in predicting the internal dose of tobacco smoke exposure, the degree of metabolism and activation/deactivation of carcinogens, angiogenesis, cell cycle, and immune response. Examples include urinary tobacco-specific N-nitroso compounds (Hecht 2002), cytogenetic endpoints in pulmonary alveolar macrophages, bone marrow and peripheral blood erythrocytes, apoptosis and proliferating cell nuclear antigen, DNA adducts (e.g., 8-hydroxy-2-deoxyguanosine (8-OHdG), BPDE-DNA adducts, ^{32}P-postlabelled bulky adduct, oxidative damage to DNA) (Hong, Kim et al. 2001; Phillips 2002; Georgiadis, Demopoulos et al. 2004; IARC 2004), protein adducts formed by 4-ABP and PAH (Maclure, Katz et al. 1989; Hammond, Coghlin et al. 1993; Hecht 1998), sequence variants (detailed later in text), gene expression (e.g., *p53* and *K-ras*), thiobarbituric acid-reactive substances (index of lipid peroxidation and oxidative stress) (De Flora, Izzotti et al. 2005), aplasia of the chest wall muscles, ipsilateral anomalies of upper extremity due to maternal cigarette smoking (Slezak and Sasiadek 2000), deficiency of α1-antitrypsin (Silverman and Speizer 1996), cotinine (a metabolite of nicotine); vascular endothelial growth factor (VEGF), monocyte chemoattractant protein 1 (MCP-1) levels, and circulating endothelial progenitor cells (EPC) related to tumor angiogenesis (Zhu, Heeschen et al. 2003); sister chromatid exchanges (SCEs) (Vineis, Bartsch et al. 1994; Tang, Warburton et al. 1999); levels of oxidative stress measured by proinflammatory nuclear transcription factor-kappa B, activator protein-s (mouse brain) (Manna, Rangasamy et al. 2006); and activation of COX-2, mitogen activated protein kinase and c-Jun N-terminal kinase (Manna, Rangasamy et al. 2006).

Some biomarkers can indicate the site where carcinogens were ingested into body. For example, BP and NNK accumulated in the central and peripheral lung, respectively, which is due to different lipid solubilities (Gerde, Muggenburg et al. 1997; Gerde, Muggenburg et al. 1998; Pulling, Divine et al. 2003). The half-life of the cytogenetic markers differ greatly and can therefore reflect various lengths of SHS exposure. Cotinine has a plasma half-life of 21 to 48 hour in nonsmokers (Sepkovic, Haley et al. 1986; Ahijevych, Tyndale et al. 2002). PAH-albumin has a half-life of 21 days (Tang, Warburton et al. 1999). SCEs in lymphocytes can reflect SHS exposure in previous years (Tang, Warburton et al. 1999).

Biomarkers related to active smoking may not be useful for SHS exposure and related health effects. For example, single-strand DNA breaks were increased among smokers but not among SHS-exposed nonsmokers (Holz, Meissner et al. 1993). Some DNA adducts, e.g., BPDE-DNA, bulky DNA and 8-OHdG, were significantly associated with SHS exposure in some studies (Mooney, Santella et al. 1995; Zenzes, Puy et al. 1998; Georgiadis, Topinka et al. 2001) but not in others (Holz, Meissner et al. 1993; Daube, Scherer et al. 1997; Petruzzelli, Celi et al. 1998; Besaratinia, Maas et al. 2002). In addition, elevation of SCEs is not common in passive smokers (Sorsa, Husgafvel-Pursiainen et al. 1989; Sardas, Karahalil et al. 1995). On the contrary, hemoglobin adducts of 4-ABP and adducts of 3-ABP found in nonsmokers exposed to SHS were similar to adducts found in smokers, but the levels were significantly higher among individuals heavily exposed than those with undetectable SHS exposure (Maclure, Katz et al. 1989; Hammond, Coghlin et al. 1993; Hecht 1998). Elevated levels of some adducts have been observed in SHS-exposed non-smoking women and children compared to unexposed ones, e.g., PAH-DNA, PAH-albumin, and 4-ABP-hemoglobin adducts (Crawford, Mayer et al. 1994; Whyatt, Santella et al. 1998; Tang, Warburton et al. 1999). Therefore, key features of ideal biomarkers for SHS exposure would be (1) changes in the markers are significantly different between smokers and SHS-exposed nonsmokers, (2) the markers are sensitive to SHS exposure, and (3) the markers can be easily detected among SHS-exposed individuals. In addition, there are also ethnic differences among children. A US study found that African–American children had higher levels of cotinine and PAG-albumin than Hispanic children after controlling for SHS exposure (Tang, Warburton et al. 1999).

Biomarkers of Biologically Effective Dose/ Early Effect

Several markers (e.g., carcinogen metabolites and DNA and protein adducts) were used to estimate the biological effective dose. Findings from association studies using this type of biomarker were summarized in Table 1.

Table 1. Association studies use biomarkers of biologically effective does/early effect.

Gene	Genotype	Study population	Outcome	Findings	Reference
1-OHP					
CYP1A1 GSTT1 GSTM1	MspI Null Null	Italian nonsmokers	Urinary 1-hydroxyperene	NS	(Merlo, Andreassen et al. 1998)
DNA adduct					
CYP1A1	CYP1A1*4 (C2453A) CYP1A1*2A (MspI) CYP1A1*2B (A2455G)	Greek nonsmokers	DNA adducts	NS NS NS	(Georgiadis, Topinka et al. 2005)
	MspI MspI+GSTM1 null MspI +GSTP1 (Ile/Val) MspI +EPHX slow	Greek with significant SHS exposure	DNA adducts	S S S S	(Georgiadis, Demopoulos et al. 2004)
	MspI Ile462Val	Korean women and their newborns	Neonatal 8-hydroxy-deoxyguanosine and malondialdehyde	NS NS	(Hong, Kim et al. 2001)
CYP1B1	Leu432Val	Workers in a Hungarian alumina plant	DNA adducts	S	(Schoket, Papp et al. 2001)
	Arg48Gly + Ala119Ser Leu432Val Asn453Ser	Greek with negligible SHS exposure	DNA adducts	S S S	(Georgiadis, Demopoulos et al. 2004)
CYP2E1	Maternal PstI (G-1259C)	Korean women and their newborns	Neonatal 8-hydroxy-deoxyguanosine and malondialdehyde	NS	(Hong, Kim et al. 2001)
EPHX	His139Arg Tyr113His	Greek nonsmokers	DNA adducts	S S	(Georgiadis, Demopoulos et al. 2004)
GSTT1	Null Null+CYP1A1 MspI	Greek nonsmokers	DNA adducts	NS	(Georgiadis, Demopoulos et al. 2004)
	Null	Korean women and their newborns	Neonatal 8-hydroxy-deoxyguanosine and malondialdehyde	NS	(Hong, Kim et al. 2001)
GSTM1	Null+CYP1A1 MspI	Greek nonsmokers	DNA adducts	S	(Georgiadis, Demopoulos et al. 2004)
	Null Null+GSTP1 AG orGG	Polish nonsmokers	PAH-DNA adducts in human mononuclear white blood cells	NS	(Butkiewicz, Grzybowska et al. 2000)
	Null	Korean women and their newborns	Neonatal 8-hydroxy-deoxyguanosine and malondialdehyde	S (8-OHdG) NS(MDA)	(Hong, Kim et al. 2001)

Gene	Genotype	Study population	Outcome	Findings	Reference
GSTP1	Ile/Val Ile/Val + GSTM1 null	Polish nonsmokers	PAH-DNA adducts in human mononuclear white blood cells	NS	(Butkiewicz, Grzybowska et al. 2000)
	Ile/Val +CYP1A1 MspI	Greek nonsmokers	DNA adducts	S	(Georgiadis, Demopoulos et al. 2004)
EPHX	Tyr113His His139Arg	Greek	DNA adducts	NS	(Georgiadis, Demopoulos et al. 2004)
NAT2	Slow acetylator	Males with low or null nicotine-cotinine levels	DNA adducts (4-ABP)	S	(Vineis, Bartsch et al. 1994)
XPD	Exon 10 Exon 23 Exon 10 AA+exon23GG	Swedish nonsmoking populaton	DNA adducts	S S S	(Hou, Falt et al. 2002)
IgE					
CD14	+1437 -159 TT	Latinos (Puertp Ricans, Mexicans, and African Americans)	IgE levels	S	(Choudhry, Avila et al. 2005)

Carcinogen Metabolites

Cotinine is a metabolite of nicotine, which is highly specific for tobacco smoke, and its level can be measured in the blood, saliva, or urine (2006). In the USA, cotinine could be detected in 70% to 43% of population from 1988-91 to 2002 (2006). About 20% of children have been exposed to SHS at home and their cotinine levels are 2-fold higher than those in adults (2006). In a study composed of African-American and Hispanic children, cotinine level was significantly elevated among the SHS exposed children ($P<0.05$) (Tang, Warburton et al. 1999). However, no studies have evaluated how genetic changes affect the association between these markers and SHS-related health effects.

Urinary 1-hydroxyperene (1-OHP) is the metabolite of pyrene. *CYP1A1* MspI, *GSTM1, or GSTT1* null genotypes were not associated with urinary 1-OHP levels among Italian police officers exposed to PAHs (Merlo, Andreassen et al. 1998). The level of hair nicotine, which is one of the main components in tobacco smoke, from people working in the bars or restaurants (Al-Delaimy, Fraser et al. 2001); urinary 4-Methylnitrosamino-1-(3-pyridyl)-1-butanol (NNAL), which is a metabolite of tobacco-specific carcinogen 4-(methylnitrosamino)-1-(3-pyridyl)-1-butanone (NNK) from infants to estimate SHS exposure from their family members (Hecht, Carmella et al. 2006).

DNA Adducts

Several studies have investigated how genetic polymorphisms modify the association between SHS exposure and the levels of DNA adducts. Below are detailed by genes.

CYPs

Cytochrome P450 (CYPs) are drug-metabolizing enzymes involved in phase I activation. Because of their role in activation of toxicants taken into the human body, genes encoding these enzymes have been more widely explored for SHS exposure than genes involved in other pathways. *CYP1A1* MspI, C2453A, and A2455G variant carriers showed a higher, but not significant, level of PAH-DNA adducts and aberrant chromosome after SHS exposure (Georgiadis, Topinka et al. 2005). Significantly higher level of DNA adducts was observed for *CYP1A1* MspI (Georgiadis, Topinka et al. 2005), combination of *CYP1A1* MspI/*GSTM1* null, *CYP1A1* MspI /*GSTP1* (Ile/Val), and *CYP1A1* MspI /*EPHX* slow polymorphism but not for *CYP1A1**4 (C2453A) (Georgiadis, Demopoulos et al. 2004). As a whole, the levels of DNA adducts were not modified by *CYP1A1* genotypes and SHS exposure. On the contrary, the genetic polymorphism of *CYP1B1,* Leu432Val, was related to elevated levels of DNA adducts in white blood cells of workers in a Hungarian aluminum plant who were exposed to PAH (Schoket, Papp et al. 2001). In addition, among Greek nonsmokers, *CYP1B1* variant carriers (Arg486Gly+Ala119Ser, Leu432Val, or Asn453Ser) with significant SHS exposure had significantly higher PAH-DNA adduct levels and aberrant chromosomes (Georgiadis, Demopoulos et al. 2004).

GSTs

Glutathione S-transferase (GSTs) are phase II detoxification enzymes encoded by four classes of polymorphic genes: alpha, mu, pi, and theta (Daniel 1993; Awasthi, Sharma et al. 1994; Wilce and Parker 1994). Alteration in the mu and theta class genes have been linked to tobacco-associated lung cancer (Bennett, Alavanja et al. 1999). Enzyme activity reach saturation with high-level carcinogen exposure among individuals who had either high or low GST activity, but this phenomenon was not observed with low-level exposure (Kiyohara, Wakai et al. 2003). Therefore, genetic polymorphisms of these genes may be ideal to assess the effects of low-level tobacco exposure, SHS.

In a Greek nonsmoking population, the DNA adduct level was highest among individuals carrying *GSTM1* null and *CYP1A1* MspI variant (1.27 ± 1.15 adducts per 108 nucleotides), and lowest among individuals with the *CYP1A1* and *GSTM1* wild type (0.83 ± 1.08 adducts per 108 nucleotides) ($P = 0.006$) (Georgiadis, Demopoulos et al. 2004). However, DNA adduct levels were not significantly elevated among nonsmokers carrying *GSTM1* null or the combination of *GSTM1* null/*CYP1A1* MspI and *GSTP1* (Ile/Val)/*GSTM1* null (Georgiadis, Demopoulos et al. 2004). In a Polish nonsmoking population, the levels of PAH-DNA adducts in white blood cells were not modified by *GSTM1* null, *GSTP1* Val, the combination of *GSTM1* null and *GSTP1* AG or GG genotypes, or the combination of genotypes of *GSTM1* and *GSTP1,* but the adduct levels were significantly higher in summer among smokers carrying *GSTP1* AG or GG genotype (Butkiewicz, Grzybowska et al. 2000).

NAT2

NAT2 (N-acetyltransferase 2) is expressed in the liver and in the mucus of colon and bladder (Hein 1988; Hayes, Bi et al. 1993; Frederickson, Messing et al. 1994). NAT2 activates and deactivates hydrazine drugs, carcinogens, and arylamine, which widely exist in industry, cooked food and environmental contaminants (Hein 1988; Hein, Doll et al. 1993; Vatsis, Weber et al. 1995). Its polymorphisms can be categorized into three phenotypes: rapid, intermediate, and slow acetylator, which were determined by mutations at positions 481 (NAT2*5A), 590 (NAT2*6A) and 857 (NAT2*7A), respectively (Blum, Demierre et al. 1991). The cutpoint to differentiate slow and rapid acetylator is 0.6 for the ratio of 5-acetylamino-6-formylamino-3-methyluracil to 1-methylxanthine (Bartsch, Caporaso et al. 1990; Butler, Lang et al. 1992; Cribb, Isbrucker et al. 1994). The 4-ABP adducts were significantly higher among *NAT2* slow acetylators than rapid acetylators at low or null nicotine-cotinine levels, and this phenomenon was not observed at higher nicotine-cotinine levels (Vineis, Bartsch et al. 1994).

EPHX

EPHX (Microsomal epoxide hydrolase) is an important phase I gene, because of its ability to hydrolate PAH epoxy metabolites to the carcinogenic form. The two polymorphic variants in exons 3 (Tyr113His) and 4 (His139Arg) were found to confer lower and higher activity, respectively (Hassett, Aicher et al. 1994). However, the association between genetic polymorphisms of *EPHX* and the risk of lung cancer has not been established. Nonsmokers with the *EPHX* "fast" phenotype (Arg139Arg) had lower DNA adduct levels than those with the "slow" phenotype (His139His), therefore sequence variants of *EPHX* also plays a role in phase II detoxification (Georgiadis, Demopoulos et al. 2004). Individuals carrying *CYP1A1* MspI variant and *EPHX* "slow" polymorphisms had significantly higher DNA adduct levels (Georgiadis, Demopoulos et al. 2004).

XPD

The XPD (Xeroderma pigmentosum complementation group D) protein is involved in transcription-coupled nucleotide excision repair (NER) and forms a complex with the basal transcription factor IIH polypeptide 2 (TFIIH) during transcription-coupled repair. NER consists of global genome repair and transcription-coupled repair pathways, both of which repair bulky DNA adducts and UV-induced DNA damage (Bohr, Smith et al. 1985; Hou, Falt et al. 2002). Mutations in *XPD* cause a severe depression of NER and some cancer-prone effects (de Boer and Hoeijmakers 2000). In a Swedish nonsmoking population, there was a significant trend of increasing adduct level when the number of *XPD* variant allele in exon 10 (p=0.02) or exon 23 increased (p=0.001). The trend increased further when individuals carry the combination of exon 10 AA and exon 23 GG genotype (p=0.02) (Hou, Falt et al. 2002).

MDA, 8-OHdG

In a Korean population, neonatal malondialdehyde (MDA, an index of lipid peroxidation) and 8-OHdG were not affected by maternal SHS exposure and genotypes of *CYP1A1 MspI* and Ile462Val, *CYP2E1 PstI,* and *GSTT1 null* (Hong, Kim et al. 2001). However, maternal *GSTM1* null genotype and SHS exposure was associated with an increasing neonatal oxidative damage (8-OHdG) (P=0.007) but not significant for MDA (Hong, Kim et al. 2001).

Besides the examples above, BPDE-DNA adducts, ^{32}P-postlabelled bulky adduct, urinary 5'-Hydroxymethyluracil, and 8-Oxo-7,8-dihydroguanine are also DNA adducts. Among them the last two markers are oxidative DNA damage and repair (Bianchini, Donato et al. 1998) and.

Protein Adducts

Protein adducts formed by 4-ABP and PAH (Maclure, Katz et al. 1989; Hammond, Coghlin et al. 1993; Hecht 1998) have been used for estimate exposure to tobacco smoke. In a study composed of African-American and Hispanic children, 4-ABP-hemoglobin adducts and PAH-albumin were significantly higher ($P < 0.05$) among SHS-exposed children as compare to those without exposure (Tang, Warburton et al. 1999). In a study composed of Caucasians and Asians, the 4-ABP adducts (DNA adducts in bladder cells) were significantly higher among *NAT2* slow acetylators than rapid acetylators at low or null nicotine-cotinine levels, and this phenomenon was not observed at higher nicotine-cotinine levels (Vineis, Bartsch et al. 1994).

IgE, Eosinophils

CD14 is involved in modulating plasma IgE levels (Holt, Sly et al. 1997; O'Donnell, Toelle et al. 2004) and is part of the receptor complex for endotoxin, which has been found in cigarette smoke particles (Hasday, Bascom et al. 1999; Larsson, Szponar et al. 2004; Vercelli 2004). Endotoxin has been reported as a risk factor of respiratory disease among smokers or SHS-exposed nonsmokers (Hasday, Bascom et al. 1999; Larsson, Szponar et al. 2004). Linkage studies showed that human chromosome 5q31, where *CD14* is located, is the region linked to asthma and its related phenotypes (e.g., atopy and airway hyperresponsiveness) (Hoffjan and Ober 2002; Hoffjan, Nicolae et al. 2003). In a Latino population, there was a significant interaction between plasma IgE levels, *CD14* -159 genotypes, and SHS exposure (p= 0.0002) (Choudhry, Avila et al. 2005). SHS-exposed individuals with *CD14* -159 TT genotype showed the lowest IgE levels regardless of ethnicity (Choudhry, Avila et al. 2005). In a Dutch population, elevated IgE+ cells and eosinophils were observed in the nasal mucosa for children exposed to SHS, but the levels were not elevated for Langerhans cells, T cells, B cells and granulocytes, macrophages, and mast cells, (Vinke, KleinJan et al. 1999),

VEGF, MCP-1, ECP

In a Lewis lung cancer model, SHS exposure significantly increased levels of vascular endothelial growth factor (VEGF), monocyte chemoattractant protein 1 (MCP-1), and circulating endothelial progenitor cells (EPC), which were related to tumor angiogenesis

(Zhu, Heeschen et al. 2003). Though angiogenesis is considered an important process related to carcinogenesis, its role in SHS-related health effects is unclear.

Biomarkers of Second-Hand Smoke Genetic Effects

Biomarkers discussed in this section include change of gene expression, somatic alterations in tissue, post-translational changes (e.g., SCEs and CAs) and epigenetic modification (e.g., DNA methylation). These studies are mainly experimental or functional studies. The advantages of experimental and functional studies as compare to association studies include that (1) easy to adjust or change the experiment status, (2) studies performed in a well controlled environment and therefore less interferences, (3) small sample size, and (4) easy to observe the physiological changes resulting from SHS exposure. Association study is an approach commonly used to explore the relationship between sequence variants of genes and SHS related health effects. This approach is important because (1) many factors could be included, but not necessary controlled, in the study, therefore the findings are close to the real world, (2) large sample size could reach enough statistical power, and (3) collection and determination of genetic polymorphic markers are relatively stable, easier, faster, and cheaper than performing experimental studies. Therefore, these markers could be widely applied in large studies. Because of the large number of experimental studies, Table 2 only listed the findings from human *in vivo* studies.

Table 2. Association studies use biomarkers of second-hand smoke genetic effects

Gene	Genotype/genetic changes	Study population	Outcome	Findings	Reference
Gene expression					
CYP1A1		Polish	Placental mRNA expression levels	NS	(Whyatt, Garte et al. 1995)
CYP1B1		Taiwanese nonsmokers	Expression levels	S	(Wu, Wu et al. 2004)
AhR		Taiwanese nonsmokers	Expression levels in the peripheral leukocytes	NS	(Wu, Wu et al. 2004)
Somatic mutation					
p53	G:C to A:T transitions (mutations in exons 4-8)	European Caucasian nonsmokers without SHS exposure	Lung cancer tumors	S	(Husgafvel-Pursiainen, Boffetta et al. 2000)
	G:C to A:T transitions	Caucasian nonsmoking females with SHS exposure	Lung cancer tumors	S	(Vahakangas, Bennett et al. 2001)
	G:C to A:T transitions	American nonsmoking women	Carcinoid lung tumors	S	(Gealy, Zhang et al. 1999)

Table 2. (Continued)

Gene	Genotype/genetic changes	Study population	Outcome	Findings	Reference
	G→ T transversion (lung cancers) G→A transition (non-lung cancer)	European nonsmokers	Lung cancer tumors	S (smokers vs. nonsmokers) S (lung cancer vs. non-lung cancers)	(Hainaut and Pfeifer 2001)
K-ras	Mutations on codon 12 or 13	Caucasian ex- and nonsmoking females	Lung cancer tumors	NS	(Vahakangas, Bennett et al. 2001)
	Mutations in exon 1	American nonsmoking females	Carcinoid lung tumors	NS	(Gealy, Zhang et al. 1999)
	Mutation in codon 12 (transition vs. transversion)	Never smokers (99 Whites and 44 Hispanics)	Lung adenocarcinom a	NS	(Pulling, Divine et al. 2003)
HPRT	Exon2-3 genomic HPRT deletions	Maternal SHS exposure and their newborns	HPRT mutational spectrum in newborns	S (SHS exposed vs. non-exposed)	(Finette, O'Neill et al. 1998)
Chromosome aberrations					
CYP1B 1	Arg48Gly + Ala119Ser Leu432Val Asn453Ser	Greek with negligible SHS exposure	Chromosome aberrations	NS NS NS	(Georgiadis, Demopoulos et al. 2004)
CYP1 A1	MspI MspI+GSTM1 null MspI +GSTP1 (Ile/Val) MspI +mEH	Greek with significant SHS exposure	Chromosome aberrations	S NS NS NS	(Georgiadis, Demopoulos et al. 2004)
	CYP1A1*4 (C2453A) CYP1A1*2A (MspI) CYP1A1*2B (A2455G)	Greek nonsmokers	Chromosome aberrations	NS NS NS	(Georgiadis, Topinka et al. 2005)
GSTT1	Null Null+CYP1A1 MspI	Greek nonsmokers	Chromosome aberrations	NS	(Georgiadis, Demopoulos et al. 2004)
GSTM 1	Null+CYP1A1 MspI	Greek nonsmokers	Chromosome aberrations	NS	(Georgiadis, Demopoulos et al. 2004)
GSTP1	Ile/Val +CYP1A1 MspI	Greek nonsmokers	Chromosome aberrations	NS	(Georgiadis, Demopoulos et al. 2004)
Post-translational changes					
Chrom osomal aberrat ions		Caucasian-predominant population (71%)	Chromosomal aberrations in newborns umbilical cord blood	S (in utero exposure, yes vs. no)	(Pluth, Ramsey et al. 2000)

Gene	Genotype/genetic changes	Study population	Outcome	Findings	Reference
Epigenetic effects					
p16, DAPK, RASS F1A	Promoter methylation	Caucasians : 82% Others : 18%	K-ras mutation spectrum	NS (smokers vs. nonsmokers)	(Divine, Pulling et al. 2005)
MGM T/AGT	Methylation	Never smoker (99 Whites and 44 Hispanics)	Methylation	S (Never-smokers: 66% vs. smoker: 47%)	(Pulling, Divine et al. 2003)

Gene Expression

CYPs (Cytochrome P450)

In Sprague-Dawley rats, the *in utero* SHS exposure induces pulmonary *CYP1A1* in the first day of life, but not fetal *CYPs* genes (Lee, Royce et al. 2000). Compared to placentas from nonsmoking women, *CYP1A 1* mRNA levels were significantly increased in placentas from current smokers *(P* < 0.001) and ex-smokers *(P* < 0.01) but were marginal increased for placentas from those with SHS exposure (Whyatt, Garte et al. 1995). In a Polish population, the *CYP1A 1 Mspl* RFLP was not a significant determinant of *CYP1A 1* mRNA levels among nonsmokers (Whyatt, Garte et al. 1995). In a Taiwanese population, expression levels of *CYP1B1,* but not *CYP1A1,* were significantly increased in peripheral leukocytes when non-smoking cases were compared to controls (Wu, Wu et al. 2004).

AhR (Aryl Hydrocarbon Receptor)

Aryl hydrocarbon receptor (AhR) regulates xenobiotic-metabolizing enzymes (e.g., CYPs) and its ligand includes various aromatic hydrocarbons (e.g., PAH). In C57BL/6N and DBA/2N mice study, compounds in SHS binds to the AhR and stimulates its transformation, nuclear localization, dioxin responsive element binding, and activation of *CYP1A1* gene transcription (Gebremichael, Tullis et al. 1996). In a Taiwanese population, there was no significant elevation of expression of *AhR* in the peripheral leukocytes when non-smoking lung cancer cases were compared to controls (Wu, Wu et al. 2004). No other association studies have been performed so far.

11β-HSD2 (11β-Hydroxysteroid Dehydrogenase Type 2)

The enzyme encoded by *11β-hydroxysteroid dehydrogenase type 2 (11β-HSD2)* plays a role in fetal development, especially fetal birth weight (Stewart, Rogerson et al. 1995; Murphy, Zakar et al. 2002). This gene may play a role in maternal SHS exposure and the fetal health effects. A human tophoblast cell model showed that exposure to cadmium, a component in tobacco smoke, led to decrease in levels of 11β-HSD2 protein and mRNA, *11β-HSD2* promoter activity, and repression of *11β-HSD2* transcription (Yang, Julan et al. 2006). This gene may play a role in the fetal health effects of maternal SHS exposure, but no association studies have been performed.

COX-2

COX-2, also called prostaglandin-endoperoxide synthase 2 (PTGS2) is expressed in a limited number of cell types and is responsible for the prostanoid biosynthesis involved in inflammation and mitogenesis. The expression of this gene is deregulated in epithelial tumors (Kurie and Dubois 2001). In a mice study, SHS exposure led to increased levels of reactive oxygen species, which lead to increase of nuclear transcription factor-kappa B (NF-kB) activation, higher levels of proinflammatory NF-kB and activator protein-1, activation of mitogen-activated protein kinase and c-Jun N-terminal kinase in different regions of the brain, and activation of COX-2 in all the regions of the brain (Manna, Rangasamy et al. 2006). Because COX-2 plays a role in the innate immune response, its genetic polymorphisms may be associated with SHS-related health effects.

CXCR1 (CXC Chemokine Receptors 1)

The protein encoded by CXC chemokine receptors 1 *(CXCR1),* a receptor for interleukin 8 (IL8), is a member of the G-protein-coupled receptor family. CXCR1 binds to IL8 with high affinity and transduces the signal through a G-protein activated second messenger system. CXCR1 and CXCR2 mediate neutrophil recruitment to inflammatory sites (Catusse, Liotard et al. 2003). Therefore, SHS exposure may regulate the chemokines (IL-8) and their receptors (CXCR1), and then the following tumorigenesis. An animal study indicated that chicken exposed to SHS differentially stimulated the CXCR1 isoform I in primary fibroblast (Li, Lu et al. 2000).

NK-1R (Neurokinin-1 Receptor)

Neurokinin-1 receptor (NK-1R) is a receptor for neurokinin substance P, which is released from sensory C-fiber terminals and immunoinflammatory cells (Wong, Sun et al. 2002). An *in situ* hybridization study found 2-fold increase of *NK-1R* expression among lung samples from nonsmokers as compare to those from smokers (Bai, Zhou et al. 1995). The different sensitivity of *NK-1R* expression makes it an ideal marker to differentiate SHS exposure. In C57BL/6 mice, SHS exposure was related to downregulation of NK-1R mRNA in heart tissue, upregulation in the liver and kidney, but the *NK-1R* expression was not significantly change in the lungs and spleen tissues (Wong, Sun et al. 2002). However, no association studies has been reported.

Muc2 and Muc5ac

Mucin glycoproteins are adhesive, viscous, and elastic, they could trap objects enter airway and remove them through mucociliary movement (Borchers, Wert et al. 1998). Rats and mice exposed to acrolein, a compound in photochemical smog and tobacco smoke, showed increasing mucus hypersecretion, as a result of elevation of expression of *MUC5ac* and levels of macrophages and neutrophils (Borchers, Wert et al. 1998). However, this phenomenon was not observed for *MUC2* gene (Borchers, Wert et al. 1998; Borchers, Wesselkamper et al. 1999). Therefore, chronic inflammation plays a role in mucus hypersecretion, a characteristic of COPD.

Ki-67, PCNA, p21, cyclin D1, p53, filaggrin, loricin, and cytokeratins 1 and 10

Cell cycle and cell differentiation have been known to play a role in carcinogenesis. Exposure of mice and rat oral keratinocytes to nicotine changed of the mRNA and protein levels of nicotinic acetylcholine receptors and the cell cycle and cell differentiation markers Ki-67, PCNA, p21, cyclin D1, p53, filaggrin, loricrin, and cytokeratins 1 and 10, which may lead to some pathobiologic effects of tobacco products in oral tissues (Arredondo, Nguyen et al. 2001).

Bax

The protein encoded by *BCL2-associated X protein (BAX)* belongs to the BCL2 protein family, members of which act as anti- or pro-apoptotic regulators in a wide variety of cellular activities. The expression of *BAX* is regulated by the tumor suppressor *p53* and has been shown to be involved in p53-mediated apoptosis. An animal study found that PAH exposed mice showed an induction of the expression of *Bax* in oocytes, followed by apoptosis (Matikainen, Perez et al. 2001). No association studies have been performed.

Antioxidant Enzymes

Tobacco smoke increases oxidative stress and thus slightly increased gene expression of protein disulfide isomerase (PDI) and catalase in a rat model as below. Administered high dose of ascorbic acid (vitamin C) to osteogenic disorder Shionogi (ODS) rat, which lacks ascorbic acid synthesis enzyme, significantly decreased of the expression of genes encode antioxidant enzymes (e.g., CuZn-superoxide dismutase (SOD), MnSOD, catalase and PDI) and xenobiotic metabolizing enzymes (e.g., CYP1A2) (Ueta, Tadokoro et al. 2003). The reduction of expression of plasma glutathione peroxidase was not significant (Ueta, Tadokoro et al. 2003). Therefore, vitamin C intake may reduce the oxidative stress resulting from cigarette smoking.

Ribosomal Protein L31 and Zis

Injection BP into male Sprague–Dawley rats, increasing growth and proliferation rate (athrogenic phenotype), suppression of mRNA level for *ribosomal protein L31* and *Zis* genes, overexpression of gas-5 and mitochondrial mRNAs were observed in the cultured vascular smooth muscle cells (Lu, Alejandro et al. 2002). In the same study, these findings were confirmed by in situ hybridization experiments *in vivo*.

Somatic Mutations

p53

p53 is a tumor suppressor gene involved in cell growth and proliferation. Some studies found that *p53* mutation occurs more frequently in smokers (26%) and former smokers (67%) than never-smokers exposed to spousal SHS (13%) and lifetime never-smokers (10-19%) (Husgafvel-Pursiainen, Boffetta et al. 2000; Vahakangas, Bennett et al. 2001). However, another study found that *p53* mutation frequency was similar between smokers and nonsmokers (Gealy, Zhang et al. 1999). These disparities may result from different *p53* mutations, study population, and small sample size used in the latter studies. The type and spectra of *p53* mutation were consistently and significantly different between smokers and nonsmokers (Gealy, Zhang et al. 1999). For example, G:C to T:A transversions and some mutational hotspots in codon 157-158, 179, 245-249, 273 and 282 (Cherpillod and Amstad 1995; Denissenko, Pao et al. 1996; Hernandez-Boussard and Hainaut 1998) were more frequently observed among smokers (19-31%) as compared to G:C to A:T transitions, which were more common among never smokers (22-57%) (Gealy, Zhang et al. 1999; Husgafvel-Pursiainen, Boffetta et al. 2000; Hainaut and Pfeifer 2001; Vahakangas, Bennett et al. 2001). In a European Caucasian population, G:C to T:A transversions were associated with elevated risk of lung cancer when compared ever-smokers to never smokers with SHS exposure (OR=2.9, 95% CI=1.2-7.2) or compared ever-smokers to never smokers without SHS exposure (OR=4.4, 95% CI=1.2-16.2) (Husgafvel-Pursiainen, Boffetta et al. 2000). In summary, G:C to A:T transitions in *p53* are markers observed among nonsmokers and thus may be useful markers for predicting SHS-related effects.

K-ras

Kirsten ras (K-ras) is an oncogene and encodes a protein belongs to small GTPas superfamily. It has two isoforms different in the C-terminal region as a result of alternative splicing. A mice study showed that *K-ras* mutation in exon 2 maybe a specific target for SHS (Witschi, Oreffo et al. 1995). For *p53* mutant mice, the *K-ras* mutation spectrum was similar in tumors from the different groups (group a: 5 months SHS exposure+4.5 months recover period, group b: 9.5 months continuative SHS exposure) (Yao, Wang et al. 2005). In one study, the mutations in *K-ras* codon 12 accounted for 30-40% of lung adenocarcinoma among smokers and former uranium miners; less than 11% of adenocarcinoma cases were found among nonsmokers (Vahakangas, Bennett et al. 2001). In a Caucasian female nonsmoking population, mutations on *K-ras* codon 12 and 13 were not associated with lung cancer risk (Vahakangas, Bennett et al. 2001). Similar findings were observed in an American nonsmoking female population for mutation in exon 1 for the risk of carcinoid lung tumors (Gealy, Zhang et al. 1999) and in another Caucasian-predominant population for mutations in codon 12 and the risk of lung adenocarcinoma (Pulling, Divine et al. 2003). The difference in frequencies of *K-ras* mutation between smokers and nonsmokers were not sufficient to make them ideal markers for SHS exposure. This may explain the null findings between smokers and nonsmokers in prior studies.

P16, DAPK, RASSF1A

P16, located in chromosome 9p21, is involved chromosomal inversions, translocations, heterozygous deletions, and homozygous deletions in malignant cell lines from various tumors (Liggett and Sidransky 1998). *Death-associated protein kinase 1 (DAPK1)* is a tumor suppressor gene and is a positive mediator of interferon induced programmed cell death (Lee, Rho et al. 2005). *Ras effector homolog 1 (RASSF1A)* is a tumor suppressor gene and encodes a protein similar to the RAS effector proteins. Loss or altered expression of *RASSF1A* has been associated with the pathogenesis of a variety of cancers (Byun, Lee et al. 2001). The inactivation of this gene was found to be correlated with the hypermethylation of its CpG-island promoter region (Liu, Yoon et al. 2002). SHS-related adenocarcinoma was partly induced through cell cycle control by *p16* (Jarmalaite, Kannio et al. 2003), signal transduction by *RASSF1A*, and apoptosis via *DAPK* and *RASSF1A* (Tang, Khuri et al. 2000; Dammann, Schagdarsurengin et al. 2003). In an animal study, an additive effect was observed in SHS-exposed mice with a mutant *p53* transgene and *p16* deletion (Wang, Zhang et al. 2005). Possible associations between genetic polymorphisms of these genes and SHS-related health effects have not been assessed.

HPRT

Hypoxanthine–guanine phosphoriboslytransferase (HPRT) is involved in the purine salvage pathway, which phosphoribosylates purine analogs and leads to cytotoxicity (Finette, O'Neill et al. 1998). Among SHS-exposed newborns, a significant difference in *HPRT* mutational spectra, increasing genomic deletions mediated by V(D) recombinase, was observed in those exposed *in utero* to cigarette smoke (Finette, O'Neill et al. 1998). Therefore, the sequence variants in *HPRT* may serve as a good indicator for fetal SHS exposure.

Post-Translational Changes

Sister Chromatid Exchanges (SCEs)

Sister chromatid exchanges (SCE) is a marker reflect the genetic damages resulting from exposure to carcinogens (Tucker, Eastmond et al. 1997). SCEs were correlated with DNA adducts and somatic mutations (Carrano 1986) and were related to SHS-exposure previously (Morimoto, Miura et al. 1984). Because of the long half-life, SCEs in lymphocytes can reflect SHS exposure in past years (Tang, Warburton et al. 1999). However, elevation of SCEs is not common in passive smokers (Sorsa, Husgafvel-Pursiainen et al. 1989; Sardas, Karahalil et al. 1995). In a population composed of Hispanic and African-American children, the SCE level was marginally increased when compared SHS-exposed children to those without exposure (P=0.076) (Tang, Warburton et al. 1999). The SCE level was higher among African-American children than the level among Hispanic children after controlling for SHS exposure (P=0.059).

Chromosomal Aberrations (CAs)

Chromosomal aberrations (CAs) are structural aberrations comprising chromosome-type and chromatid-type breaks and rearrangements (Norppa 2004). CAs can predict cancer risk among nonsmokers but not depend on the time between the chromosome analysis and cancer diagnosis (Bonassi, Hagmar et al. 2000), this could be explained by individual susceptibility (Norppa 2004). *CYP1A1* MspI, C2453A, and A2455G variant carriers showed a higher, but not significant, level of aberrant chromosome after SHS exposure (Georgiadis, Topinka et al. 2005). In a Caucasian-predominant population, a significant association between the newborn *CYP1A1 Msp*I polymorphism and CA frequencies was observed in the newborns umbilical cord blood (heterozygotes vs. wild type: p=0.02), but not for other genes (*CYP2D6* and *CYP1A1,* and phase II genes: *NAT1, NAT2, GSTT1, GSTM1, GSTP1*, and *epoxide hydrolase*) (Pluth, Ramsey et al. 2000). Exposure to tobacco smoke *in utero* also appeared to increase fetal translocation frequencies (maternal smoking status, yes vs. no: $p=0.045$) (Pluth, Ramsey et al. 2000).

Epigenetic Effects

Promoter Methylation

In a Caucasian-predominant population, the prevalence of methylation of the *p16, DAPK,* and *RASSF1A* genes were similar between adenocarcinomas from smokers and nonsmoker and were also independent of *K-ras* mutation (Divine, Pulling et al. 2005). *O6-methylguanine-DNA methyltransferase (MGMT)* or *O6-alkylguanine DNA alkyltransferase (AGT)* encodes a DNA repair enzyme that removes the guanine at the O6 position and transfers the alkyl group to an internal cysteine acceptor site (Cohet, Borel et al. 2004) to protect carcinogenesis from alkylating agents (Pulling, Divine et al. 2003). For example, the adduct *O*6-alkylguanine, which is the metabolite of *N*-nitroso compounds (IARC 2004), can be inactivated by MGMT. When DNA repair by MGMT failed, transition mutation in *K-ras* may take place (Pulling, Divine et al. 2003). *MGMT* methylation was more frequent in tumors from never-smokers than from smokers (66 vs. 47%) (Pulling, Divine et al. 2003). Transcriptional silencing may occur when methylation of a CpG island in the *MGMT* promoter region is affected (Esteller, Hamilton et al. 1999; Esteller, Toyota et al. 2000). Because the methylation of *MGMT* was more frequent in tumors from never-smokers, it might be a good marker for SHS related health effects.

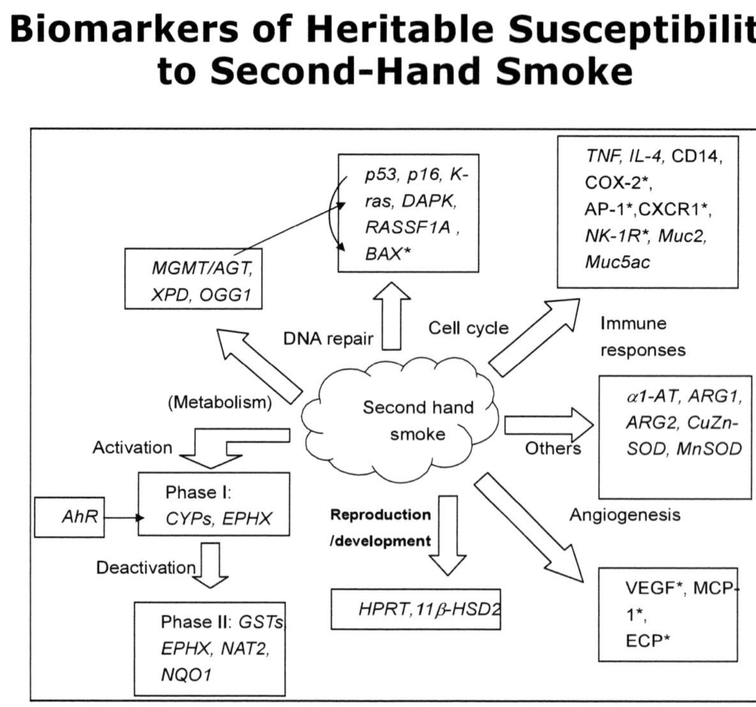

Figure 2. Genes and enzymes involved in pathways related to second-hand smoke exposure. *Association studies were not available.

There is abundant evidence of the association between active tobacco smoke and various ill effects on health. A great deal of genetic data has been generated since the completion of Human Genome Project. However, few studies have assessed genetic susceptibility and the risk of SHS-related health effects. To date, associations between genetic polymorphisms and the risk of some SHS-related health effects or intermediate status have been assessed for *GSTP1* (Miller, De Vivo et al. 2003; Canalle, Burim et al. 2004), *GSTT1* (Hong, Lee et al. 2003), *GSTM1* (Nyberg, Hou et al. 1998; Bennett, Alavanja et al. 1999; Kiyohara, Wakai et al. 2003; Wenzlaff, Cote et al. 2005), *NAT2* (Vineis, Bartsch et al. 1994; Nyberg, Hou et al. 1998; Schonberger and Van Schayck 1998), *CYP1A1* (Merlo, Andreassen et al. 1998; Hung, Boffetta et al. 2003; Georgiadis, Topinka et al. 2005; Ng, Tan et al. 2005), *CYP1B1* (Wenzlaff, Cote et al. 2005), *p53* (mice and human) (Gealy, Zhang et al. 1999; Husgafvel-Pursiainen, Boffetta et al. 2000; Vahakangas, Bennett et al. 2001; De Flora, Balansky et al. 2003; Yao, Wang et al. 2005), *NAD(P)H:quinone oxidoredictase 1 (NQO1)* (Bock, Wenzlaff et al. 2005), *O(6)-alkylguanine DNA alkyltransferase (AGT)* (Cohet, Borel et al. 2004), *xeroderma pigmentosium complementation group D (XPD)* (Hou, Falt et al. 2002), *tumor necrosis factor (TNF)* (Wenten, Berhane et al. 2005), *CD14* (Choudhry, Avila et al. 2005), *8-oxoguanine DNA glycosylase (OGG1)* (Sunaga, Kohno et al. 2002), *alpha1-antitrypsin (α1-AT)* (children) (von Ehrenstein, von Mutius et al. 2002), *Arginase II (ARG2)* (Li, Romieu et al. 2006), *epoxide hydrolase (EPHX1)* (Wu, Zhang et al. 2001), and *supF (E. coli)* (Matsuda, Kawanishi et al. 1998).

Based on the existing studies, the genetic markers listed above and discussed in earlier sections could be categorized into different biological pathways: (1) metabolism (activation/deactivation), (2) DNA repair, (3) cell cycle, (4) immune response, (5) reproduction/development, (6) angiogenesis, and (7) others (Figure 2). The findings regarding of genetic polymorphisms of individual genes or their joint effects are detailed below. Findings from association studies are summarized in Table 3.

Table 3. Association studies use biomarkers of heritable susceptibility to second-hand smoke

Gene	Genotype	Study population	Outcome	Findings	Reference
Metabolism (Activation)					
CYP1A1	Msp I (T6235C)	Chinese nonsmokers	Lung cancer	S	(Song, Tan et al. 2001)
	Msp I Ile462Val	Japanese nonsmokers	Lung adenocarcinoma	NS NS	(Sunaga, Kohno et al. 2002)
	Msp I	Lifetime nonsmoking Japanese women	Lung cancer	NS	(Kiyohara, Wakai et al. 2003)
	Msp I Ile462Val (A4889G) Msp I+GSTM1 null Msp I+GSTT1 null	Lifetime Chinese female nonsmokers	Lung cancer	S S NS NS	(Ng, Tan et al. 2005)
	Ile462Val Ile462Val + GSTM1 null	Caucasians nonsmokers (pooled analysis)	Lung cancer	S S	(Hung, Boffetta et al. 2003)

Table 3. (Continued)

Gene	Genotype	Study population	Outcome	Findings	Reference
	MspI	Never smokers	Lung cancer	NS	(Wenzlaff, Cote
	Ile462Val	(Caucasians: 82%,		NS	et al. 2005)
		African Americans:			
		18%)			
	Msp I	Caucasian-predominant population (68%)	Lung cancer	NS	(Vineis, Veglia et al. 2003)
	Ile462Val	Caucasian female never-smokers	Lung cancer	NS	(Bennett, Alavanja et al. 1999)
	MspI	Italian traffic police officers	Lung Cancer	NS	(Merlo, Andreassen et al. 1998)
	Msp I	Children with SHS	Childhood acute	NS	(Infante-Rivard,
	C2453A	exposure	lymphoblastic	NS	Krajinovic et al.
	A2455G	(Caucasians: 95%)	leukemia	NS	2000)
CYP1B	Leu432Val	Never smokers	Lung cancer	S	(Wenzlaff, Cote
1	Leu432Val + NQO1	(Caucasians: 82%,		S	et al. 2005)
	C609T	African Americans:		S	
	Leu432Val +	18%)		S	
	GSTM1null				
	Leu432Val + GSTP1				
	Ile105Val				
Metabolism (Deactivation)					
GSTT1	Null	European nonsmoking Caucasians	Lung cancer	NS	(Malats, Camus-Radon et al. 2000)
	Null	Caucasian female never-smokers	Lung cancer	NS	(Bennett, Alavanja et al. 1999)
	Null	Nonsmokers (Caucasian: 95%)	Lung cancer (all, adenocarcinoma, non small cell lung cancer)	NS	(Nazar-Stewart, Vaughan et al. 2003)
	Null	Never smokers (Caucasians: 82%, African Americans: 18%)	Lung cancer	NS	(Wenzlaff, Cote et al. 2005)
	Null	Caucasians nonsmokers (pooled analysis)	Lung cancer	NS	(Hung, Boffetta et al. 2003)
	Null	Japanese nonsmokers	Lung adenocarcinoma	NS	(Sunaga, Kohno et al. 2002)
	Null	Greek nonsmokers	Lung cancer	NS	(Georgiadis,
	Null+CYP1A1			NS	Demo-poulos et
	Ile462Val				al. 2004)
	Null	Chinese female lifetime	Lung cancer	NS	(Ng, Tan et al.
	Null+CYP1A1 MspI	nonsmokers		S	2005)
	Null+CYP1A1			NS	
	Ile462Val				

Gene	Genotype	Study population	Outcome	Findings	Reference
GST M1	Null	Caucasian female never-smokers	Lung cancer	S	(Bennett, Alavanja et al. 1999)
	Null	Japanese nonsmokers	Lung adenocarcinoma	S	(Sunaga, Kohno et al. 2002)
	Null	Lifetime non-smoking Japanese women	Lung Cancer	S	(Kiyohara, Wakai et al. 2003)
	Null Null+ GSTP1 Val	Never smokers (Caucasians: 82%, African Americans: 18%)	Lung cancer	S S	(Wenzlaff, Cote et al. 2005)
	Null Null +CYP1A1 MspI Null +CYP1A1 Ile462Val	Lifetime Chinese female non-smokers	Lung cancer	NS NS NS	(Ng, Tan et al. 2005)
	Null Null + NAT2 slow acetylator	Swedish never smokers	Lung cancer	NS S	(Nyberg, Hou et al. 1998)
	Null	European nonsmoking Caucasians	Lung cancer	NS	(Malats, Camus-Radon et al. 2000)
	Null	Nonsmokers (Caucasians: 62%)	Lung cancer	NS	(Tang, Rundle et al. 1998)
	Null	Nonsmokers (Caucasian: 95%)	Lung cancer (all types, adenocarcinoma, non small cell lung cancer)	NS	(Nazar-Stewart, Vaughan et al. 2003)
	Null+CYP1A1 Ile462Val	Caucasians non-smokers (pooled analysis)	Lung cancer	S	(Hung, Boffetta et al. 2003)
	Null	Caucasian: 61% Hispanics: 24.5% African Americans: 4% Asians: 5%	Asthma and wheezing in children (in utero SHS exposure)	S	(Gilliland, Li et al. 2002)
GSTP 1	Ile/Val (A→G)	US Caucasians	Lung cancer	NS	(Miller, De Vivo et al. 2003)
	Ile/Val +GSTM1 Null	Never smokers (Caucasians: 82%, African Americans: 18%)	Lung cancer	S	(Wenzlaff, Cote et al. 2005)
NOQ 1	Ser187Pro (T allele)	Nonsmokers (Caucasians, 77% African Americans, 23%)	Lung cancer	NS	(Bock, Wenzlaff et al. 2005)
	Ser187Pro Pro/Pro + GSTT1 null	Japanese nonsmokers	Lung adenocarcinoma	NS NS	(Sunaga, Kohno et al. 2002)

Table 3. (Continued)

Gene	Genotype	Study population	Outcome	Findings	Reference
NAT2	Slow acetylator	Non-smoking Chinese females	Lung cancer	S	(Seow, Zhao et al. 1999)
	Slow acetylator Slow acetylator + GSTM1 null	Swedish never smokers	Lung cancer	NS S	(Nyberg, Hou et al. 1998)
DNA repair					
MGMT /AGT	143Val + 178Arg	Caucasians	Adenocarcinoma Small cell carcinoma Squamous cell carcinoma	S NS NS	(Cohet, Borel et al. 2004)
XPD	Exon 10 and 23	Swedish never smoker (<1 cigarette/day during a year)	Lung cancer	S	(Hou, Falt et al. 2002)
OGG1	Ser326Cys	Japanese nonsmokers	Lung adenocarcinoma	NS	(Sunaga, Kohno et al. 2002)
Immune response					
TNF	TNF G-308	Children Caucasian: 54% Hispanic: 32% Others: 14%	Respiratory illness-related school absences	S	(Wenten, Berhane et al. 2005)
IL-1	IL-1A -889, IL-1B -511, IL-1A +3954	German nonsmokers	Periodontal disease	NS	(Meisel, Schwahn et al. 2004)
CD14	+1437 -159 -810	Latinos (Puertp Ricans, Mexicans, and African Americans)	Asthma severity and lung functions	S (asthma severity, FEV1) S (asthma severity, IgE) S (IgE)	(Choudhry, Avila et al. 2005)
Others					
α1-AT	PiMS	German children with SHS exposure	Lung function	S	(von Ehrenstein, von Mutius et al. 2002)
ARG1 ARG2	A/G, T/A, C/T, T/C G/C, T/C G/A, T/C	Mexican children	Childhood asthma and atopy	NS S NS	(Li, Romieu et al. 2006)

Metabolism (Activation/Deactivation)

CYPs (Cytochrome P450)

CYP1A1

CYP1A1 MspI and Ile462Val are two SNPs commonly studied and are in high linkage disequilibirum with each other (Hayashi, Watanabe et al. 1991). However, both variant alleles are rare in Caucasians and African Americans (Kiyohara 2000; Georgiadis, Demopoulos et al. 2004). For *CYP1A1* MspI, significant elevated risk of lung cancer was observed among nonsmokers in a Chinese population (odds ratio (OR)=3.2, 95% confidence interval (CI)=1.5-6.7) (Song, Tan et al. 2001). An insignificant association was found in two Japanese nonsmoking populations (Sunaga, Kohno et al. 2002; Kiyohara, Wakai et al. 2003), a Chinese lifetime nonsmoking female population (Ng, Tan et al. 2005), two Caucasian nonsmoking populations (Hung, Boffetta et al. 2003; Wenzlaff, Cote et al. 2005), a pooled population composed of Caucasian and Asian non-smokers (Vineis, Veglia et al. 2003), and an Italian nonsmoking population (Merlo, Andreassen et al. 1998). For joint effects, Chinese female nonsmokers carrying MspI CC genotype showed a two-fold increased risk of lung cancer when they were also null for *GSTT1* (OR=2.7, 95 CI=1.1-6.9) as compare to other genotype combinations combined (Ng, Tan et al. 2005). But an increased lung cancer risk was found for the combination of MspI CC genotype and *GSTM1* null (Ng, Tan et al. 2005). The vast majority of prior studies showed null associations; therefore, the MspI polymorphism may not be an important risk factor for SHS-related lung cancer.

The sequence variant *CYP1A1* Ile462Val was significantly associated with lung cancer in a pooled Caucasian nonsmoking population including 14 case-control studies (all lung cancer: OR=2.99, 95% CI=1.51-5.91; adenocarcinoma: OR=4.85, 95% CI=2.03-11.6) (Hung, Boffetta et al. 2003) and a Chinese female nonsmoking population (OR=2.8, 95% CI=1.1-7.6) (Ng, Tan et al. 2005). A null association was reported in a US Caucasian female never-smoking population (Bennett, Alavanja et al. 1999), and a Japanese population (Sunaga, Kohno et al. 2002). Regarding joint effects, Caucasian non-smokers with combined *CYP1A1* Ile462Val variant and *GSTM1* null genotype showed a 4.67-fold increased risk of lung cancer (95% CI=2.00-10.9) as compared with those carrying *CYP1A1* wild type and *GSTM1* null genotype (Hung, Boffetta et al. 2003). The significant findings for *CYP1A1* Ile462Val reflect that the polymorphism Ile462Val maybe a potential risk factor for SHS-related lung cancer.

As described in the "Biomarkers of biologically effective does/early effect", genetic polymorphisms of *CYP1A1* MspI and A2455G, the combination of *CYP1A1* MspI/*GSTM1* null, *CYP1A1* MspI /*GSTP1* (Ile/Val), and *CYP1A1* MspI /*EPHX* slow phenotype were not significantly associated with the level of PAH-DNA adducts and aberrant chromosome after SHS exposure (Georgiadis, Demopoulos et al. 2004; Georgiadis, Topinka et al. 2005). SHS exposure and maternal genotypes of *CYP1A1 MspI* and Ile462Val and *CYP2E1 PstI* did not affect the level of neonatal oxidative damage MDA and 8-OHdG (Hong, Kim et al. 2001).

For childhood ALL, increased but not significant risk were found for children carrying the *CYP1A1**4 (C2453A) allele at high levels of maternal smoking in the last trimesters and at low level of paternal postnatal smoking (Infante-Rivard, Krajinovic et al. 2000). Decreased ALL risk was observed for the *CYP1A1**2B (A2455G) allele, which appeared to confer a protective advantage at low levels of maternal prenatal smoking and at high levels for paternal postnatal smoking (Infante-Rivard, Krajinovic et al. 2000). However, another study could not replicate these findings (Canalle, Burim et al. 2004).

CYP1B1

In an analyses of data from Surveillance, Epidemiology and End Results (SEER) database, Caucasian never-smokers carrying *CYP1B1* variant (Val) were found to have an increased risk of lung cancer (OR=2.87, 95% CI=1.63-5.07) (Wenzlaff, Cote et al. 2005). Gene-gene interactions have also been investigated. Never smokers carrying variant alleles of both *CYP1B1* Leu432Val and *NQO1* C609T had an elevated risk of lung cancer (OR=4.14, 95% CI=1.60-10.74), findings remained significant among those carrying *CYP1B1* Leu432Val and *GSTM1* null genotypes (OR=2.62, 95% CI=1.18-5.81), or *CYP1B1* Leu432Val and *GSTP1* Ile105Val (OR=3.21, 95% CI=1.34-7.74) (Wenzlaff, Cote et al. 2005). The consistent findings supported the contention that genetic polymorphisms of *CYP1B1* may play a role in lung carcinogenesis due to SHS exposure. As detailed in the "Biomarkers of biologically effective does/early effect", sequence variants of *CYP1B1* (Arg486Gly+Ala119Ser, Leu432Val, or Asn453Ser) were significantly associated with higher level of DNA adducts among SHS exposed individuals (Schoket, Papp et al. 2001; Georgiadis, Demopoulos et al. 2004).

GSTs (Glutathione-S-Transferase)

STT1

Though several studies have investigated the relationship between *GSTT1* and lung cancer risk among nonsmokers, most findings did not reach significance. Null findings were observed in a European Caucasian non-smoking population (Malats, Camus-Radon et al. 2000), a US Caucasian non-smoking female population (Bennett, Alavanja et al. 1999), two US Caucasian-predominant populations (Nazar-Stewart, Vaughan et al. 2003; Wenzlaff, Cote et al. 2005), nonsmokers in a pooled analysis of 14 Caucasian case-control studies (Hung, Boffetta et al. 2003), a Japanese non-smoking population (Sunaga, Kohno et al. 2002), and a Greek nonsmoking population (Georgiadis, Demopoulos et al. 2004). For joint effects, in a Chinese population of female nonsmokers, the combination of *GSTT1* null and *CYP1A1* MspI variant was significantly associated with increased risk of lung cancer (OR=2.7, 95% CI=1.1-6.9) (Ng, Tan et al. 2005), but not in a Greek nonsmoking population (Georgiadis, Demopoulos et al. 2004). However, the combination of *GSTT1* null and *CYP1A1* Ile462Val variants showed null association (Georgiadis, Demopoulos et al. 2004; Ng, Tan et al. 2005). In summary, *GSTT1* null genotype may not be a risk factor of lung cancer from SHS exposure.

As mentioned in the "Biomarkers of biologically effective does/early effect", *GSTT1* null genotype was not associated with significant change of urinary 1-OHP level among PAH exposed Italian police officers (Merlo, Andreassen et al. 1998). No significant association was observed for the maternal genotype, SHS exposure and the levels of neonatal oxidative damages (8-OHdG and MDA) (Hong, Kim et al. 2001).

GSTM1

GSTM1 null is a common polymorphism in Caucasians (Georgiadis, Demopoulos et al. 2004). Elevated risk of lung cancer was significantly linked to *GSTM1* null genotype in a US Caucasian non-smoking female population (OR=2.6, 95% CI=1.1-6.1) (Bennett, Alavanja et al. 1999), in Japanese nonsmokers (lung adenocarcinoma: OR=3.32, 95% CI=1.41-7.84) (Sunaga, Kohno et al. 2002), in another Japanese lifetime nonsmoking population (OR=2.27, 95% CI=1.13-4.57, high-dose SHS+*GSTM1* null vs. low-dose SHS +*GSTM1* present)

(Kiyohara, Wakai et al. 2003), in nonsmokers from the SEER database (OR=2.32, 95% CI= 1.05-5.13, □20 household SHS years +*GSTM1* null vs. no household SHS +*GSTM1* present) (Wenzlaff, Cote et al. 2005), and in a Chinese female population of never smokers (Ng, Tan et al. 2005). The magnitude of OR reported among nonsmokers was higher than those among smokers. For example, in a meta-analysis, *GSTM1* deficiency was associated with a 1.4-fold increased risk of lung cancer among smokers (95% CI=1.2-1.6) and accounted for 17% of all lung cancers because of its high prevalence (McWilliams, Sanderson et al. 1995). Insignificant association was observed in a Swedish nonsmoking population (Nyberg, Hou et al. 1998), a European Caucasian population (Malats, Camus-Radon et al. 2000), and two Caucasian-predominant populations (Tang, Rundle et al. 1998; Nazar-Stewart, Vaughan et al. 2003). Gene-gene interactions were observed in some studies. Among Swedish never-smokers, individual with *NAT2* slow acetylator and *GSTM1* present genotype had a 3.1-fold risk of lung cancer (95% CI=1.1-8.6), but no clear pattern was observed among smokers (Nyberg, Hou et al. 1998). In a pooled analysis of Caucasian nonsmokers, individuals carrying *GSTM1* null and *CYP1A1* Ile 462 Val variant were significantly associated with lung cancer risk (OR=4.67, 95% CI=1.00-10.9) (Hung, Boffetta et al. 2003). In a Caucasian-predominant population, significant association was detected among nonsmokers carrying *GSTM1* null and *GSTP1* Val (OR=4.67, 95% CI=1.00-10.9) (Wenzlaff, Cote et al. 2005). *GSTM1* null genotype is a sensitive marker for nonsmokers, it could be important for assessing the association between SHS exposure and lung cancer risk.

The *GSTM1* genotype may also play a role in asthma and wheezing because xenobiotic metabolism and antioxidant pathways are involved in asthma pathogenesis (Gilliland, McConnell et al. 1999; Hayes and Stange 2000; Ivashchenko, Sideleva et al. 2001; Piirila, Wikman et al. 2001). In a Caucasian-predominant population (61% Caucasian and 24.5% Hispanics), *in utero* tobacco smoke exposure was associated with increased risk of early onset of asthma (OR=1.6, 95% CI=1.0-2.5), asthma with current symptoms (OR=1.7, 95%CI=1.1-2.8), persistent asthma (OR=1.6, 95% CI=1.1-2.4), lifetime history of wheezing (OR=1.8, 95% CI=1.3-2.5), wheezing with exercise (OR=1.2, 95% CI=1.4-3.4), and emergency room visit in the past year (OR=3.7, 95% CI=1.4-3.4) among children carrying *GSTM1* null genotype (Gilliland, Li et al. 2002). The association between *GSTM1* and asthma has been limited and more studies are necessary to confirm these findings.

As mentioned in the "Biomarkers of biologically effective does/early effect", the *GSTM1* null genotype was not associated with elevated level of 1-OHP (Merlo, Andreassen et al. 1998) or DNA adducts (Butkiewicz, Grzybowska et al. 2000), but significantly associated with the neonatal oxidative damage (8-OHdG, but not MDA) when SHS-exposed mothers carrying the null genotype (P=0.007) (Hong, Kim et al. 2001). Genetic polymorphisms of the combination of *GSTM1* null and *CYP1A1* MspI were significantly associated with increased level of DNA adduct in one study (Georgiadis, Demopoulos et al. 2004) but not in the other (Butkiewicz, Grzybowska et al. 2000).

GSTP1

GST class p, encoded by *GSTP1* gene, is the most abundant isoform in the lung. It is highly expressed in many tissues (including the lung) and is one of the main detoxifiers of the activated form of BP (Awasthi, Sharma et al. 1994; Nakajima, Elovaara et al. 1995; Fields,

Morrow et al. 1998; Hecht 1999). A common nonsynonymous SNP in exon 5 of the *GSTP1* lead to amino acid exchange (Ile3Val) in codon 105 and reduced enzyme activity (Ali-Osman, Akande et al. 1997; Johansson, Stenberg et al. 1998). This SNP was in linkage disequilibrium with the other nonsynonymous SNP at codon 114 (Ala114Val) (Harris, Coggan et al. 1998). In a US Caucasian population, they found that SHS exposure among individuals carrying the *GSTP1* GG genotype was not significantly associated with lung cancer risk as compared with those without SHS exposure and carrying AA genotype (Miller, De Vivo et al. 2003). For joint effects, in the SEER database, individuals carrying the *GSTM1* null and *GSTP1* Val allele and exposed to SHS had a significantly elevated risk of lung cancer (OR=4.6, 95% CI=1.21-17.21) (Wenzlaff, Cote et al. 2005). Conflict results and limited studies make it difficult to reach any conclusion.

As detailed in the "Biomarkers of biologically effective does/early effect", DNA adducts levels were not affected by *GSTP1* variant genotype or the combination of genotypes of *GSTM1* and *GSTP1* genotypes among nonsmokers (Butkiewicz, Grzybowska et al. 2000; Georgiadis, Demopoulos et al. 2004).

NQO1 (NAD(P) H: Quinone Oxidoreductase 1)

The enzyme encoded by the gene *NAD(P)H:quinone oxidoreductase 1 (NQO1)* is a flavoprotein that catalyzes the reduction of quinones and activates compounds like antitumor quinones and some procarcinogens present in cigarette smoke (Bock, Wenzlaff et al. 2005). *NQO1* is highly expressed in normal lung tissue and overexpressed in non-small-cell lung cancer (Siegel, Franklin et al. 1998). In a Caucasian-predominant population, no significant protective effect was observed for the *NQO1* T allele among those either with or without SHS exposure (Bock, Wenzlaff et al. 2005). In a Japanese population, the same polymorphism was not associated with lung adenocarcinoma risk among non-smokers (Sunaga, Kohno et al. 2002). Among nonsmokers, individuals with the combined genotype of *NQO1* Pro/Pro and *GSTT1* null were not at significantly higher risk of lung adenocarcinoma compared with those who carried *NQO1* Ser/Ser and *GSTT1* positive (Sunaga, Kohno et al. 2002). Few studies have explored the association between sequence variants in *NQO1* and health effects related to SHS exposure; more studies are warranted.

EPHX (Microsomal Epoxide Hydrolase)

As detailed in the "Biomarkers of biologically effective does/early effect", *EPHX* "slow" phenotype (Arg139Arg) and its combination with *CYP1A1* MspI variant were significantly associated with higher DNA adduct levels among nonsmokers (Georgiadis, Demopoulos et al. 2004).

NAT2 (N-Acetyltransferase 2)

In a Chinese female population, nonsmokers carrying *NAT2* slow acetylator had a 2-fold higher risk of lung cancer than non-carriers (95% CI=1.1-3.7), but no effect was observed among smokers (Seow, Zhao et al. 1999). The association remained significant for adenocarcinoma (OR=2.1, 95% CI=1.1-4.0) (Seow, Zhao et al. 1999). In a Swedish population, there was a higher but insignificant increase of lung cancer risk when comparing *NAT2* slow to rapid acetylator genotypes among nonsmokers, but a lower risk was observed among smokers (Nyberg, Hou et al. 1998). In the same population, individuals carrying the combination of *NAT2* slow acetylator and *GSTM1* null genotype were significantly associated with lung cancer risk among nonsmokers (Nyberg, Hou et al. 1998). Results have been conflicting for studies without considering SHS exposure. Although there were few prior studies, these interesting findings indicate that variants of *NAT2* maybe a sensitive marker and is able to differentiate the metabolism profiles between smokers and nonsmokers. More studies are needed to assess this association.

DNA Repair

MGMT (O-6-Methylguanine-DNA Methyltransferase)/AGT (O6-Alkylguanine DNA Alkyltransferase)

Some nosynonymous SNPs (e.g. Gly160Arg, Ile143Val, and Lys178Arg) are located in exon 5 of *MGMT*. Among them, Ile143Val and Lys178Arg are in high linkage disequilibrium with each other (Deng, Xie et al. 1999). Other polymorphisms have been found in the promoter, exon 1, and exon 3 (Egyhazi, Ma et al. 2002). In a Caucasian population, *MGMT* 143Val and 178Arg variant carriers had a significantly higher risk of lung cancer (OR=2.05, 95% CI=1.03-4.07) (Cohet, Borel et al. 2004). The risk remained significant for adenocarcinoma (OR=2.67, 95% CI=1.21-5.87) but not for small cell carcinoma and squamous cell carcinoma (Cohet, Borel et al. 2004). However, SHS exposure did not modify this association (Cohet, Borel et al. 2004). This is the only association study explored the relationship between sequence variants of *MGMT* and the risk of lung cancer by SHS exposure. However, more studies are needed to replicate this association.

XPD (Xeroderma Pigmentosum Complementation Group D)

XPD is a DNA repair gene. Some nonsynonymous SNPs have been reported for the *XPD* gene, they are located at codons 312 (Asp>Asn, exon 10, G>A) and 751 (Lys>Gln, exon 23, A>C) (Shen, Jones et al. 1998). A Swedish study reported that *XPD* variant carriers were associated with an elevated risk of lung cancer among younger (<70 years) never smokers (exon 10: OR=2.6, 95% CI =1.1-6.5; exon 23: 3.2, 95% CI=1.3-8.0) (Hou, Falt et al. 2002). Sequence variants of *XPD* may affect its ability to repair DNA damage resulting from SHS exposure. However, only one study has assessed this association.

OGG1 (8-Oxoguanine DNA Glycosylase)

OGG1 is a DNA repair gene and encodes the enzyme responsible for the excision of a mutagenic base byproduct, 8-oxoguanine, after exposure to reactive oxygen (Hill, Hazra et al. 2001). There are two splice variants resulting from the alternative splicing of the C-terminal region. In a Japanese population, nonsmokers carrying the *OGG1* Cys was not associated with an increased risk of lung adenocarcinoma as compared to those carrying two Ser alleles (Sunaga, Kohno et al. 2002). However, no other studies have explored this association.

Immune Response

TNF (Tumor Necrosis Factor)

Tumor necrosis factor (TNF) is mainly secreted by macrophage and is involved in SHS-related inflammatory response and disease susceptibility (Vernooy, Kucukaycan et al. 2002; Churg, Wang et al. 2003). *TNF* G-308A is a common variant in the promoter region and has been associated with asthma (Noguchi, Yokouchi et al. 2002; Di Somma, Charron et al. 2003; Mitsuta, Matsuse et al. 2003).

In a population of US children (54% Caucasians, 32% Latino, 14% others), *TNF* G-308 variant carriers exposed to household SHS had an elevated risk of school absence due to respiratory illness (OR=2.13, 95% CI=1.34-3.40) or lower-respiratory illness-related school absence (OR=4.15, 95% CI=2.57-6.71) as compared to those without SHS exposure and carrying zero copies of variant (Wenten, Berhane et al. 2005). However, no other studies have explored this association.

IL-1 (Interleukin 1)

IL-1, produced by monocytes and macrophages, is involved in various immune responses, inflammatory processes, and hematopoiesis. About 30% of European adults are affected by periodontitis (Hugoson, Norderyd et al. 1998), of which smoking is a major environmental risk factor (Burgan 1997; Salvi, Lawrence et al. 1997; Gelskey 1999; Kinane and Chestnutt 2000). When compared with genotype-negative nonsmokers, increased risk of periodontitis was observed for genotype-negative smokers (OR=2.37, 95% CI=1.96-2.87) and genotype-positive smokers (OR=4.50, 95% CI=2.30-8.82) but not for genotype-positive non-smokers (Meisel, Schwahn et al. 2004). Therefore, little evidence showed that genetic polymorphisms of *IL-1* were associated with periodontitis among SHS-exposed nonsmokers.

CD14

In a Latino population, asthma patients who had *CD14* +1437 GG or GC genotypes and exposed to SHS had 8.6% lower mean baseline forced expiratory volume in the first second (FEV_1) than those without SHS exposure (p=0.03), significant changes of asthma severity and IgE level were observed for individuals carrying CD14 -159 variant genotype, and only IgE level significantly changed for those who carrying CD14 -810 variant genotype (Choudhry, Avila et al. 2005). As described in the "Biomarkers of biologically effective does/early effect", the *CD14* -159 TT genotype was significantly associated with lower level of IgE among SHS exposed individuals (Choudhry, Avila et al. 2005). This is the only study explored the interaction. Studies without stratification by smoking status and SHS exposure were conflicting (Baldini, Lohman et al. 1999; Koppelman, Reijmerink et al. 2001; Heinzmann, Dietrich et al. 2003; Leung, Tang et al. 2003; Sengler, Haider et al. 2003; Kabesch, Hasemann et al. 2004; O'Donnell, Toelle et al. 2004). Therefore, more studies will be needed to confirm these findings.

Nrf2-Dependent Antioxidant and Cytoprotective Genes

Nuclear factor, erythroidderived 2, like 2 (Nrf2) is a redox-sensitive basic leucine zipper protein transcription factor involving in the regulation of several many detoxification and antioxidant genes, which may counteract the oxidative stress and inflammation resulting from

SHS exposure. Mice study showed that disruption or deficiency of the *Nrf2* gene was related to SHS-induced emphysema, bronchoalveolar inflammation, and alveolar cell apoptosis (Rangasamy, Cho et al. 2004). No association studies have been reported before.

Others

α1-AT (Alpha1-Antitrypsin)

Alpha-1-antitrypsin is a plasma protease inhibitor (Gadek and Crystal 1982) and is encoded by the *PI* gene located on chromosome 14q. The pleomorphic protein inhibitor (Pi) α1-AT locus codes for several deficiency alleles with Z and S mutations, which are the most common in Northern Europeans (Gadek and Crystal 1982; Brantly, Nukiwa et al. 1988). Deficiency in *α1-AT* (homozygous PiZZ genotype) has been associated with emphysema, rapid decline in lung function among patients with COPD, and liver disease (Janus, Phillips et al. 1985; Burrows 1990). In a German population, children exposed to SHS who had low levels of α1-AT (□116 $mg*dL^{-1}$) showed small but significant decrements in baseline lung function (e.g., mid- to end-expiratory flow rates) as compared to SHS-exposed children with normal levels of α1-AT (von Ehrenstein, von Mutius et al. 2002). However, the genetic polymorphisms in *α1-AT* have not been linked to health effects related to SHS exposure.

ARG1 and ARG2 (Arginase)

Arginase catalyzes the hydrolysis of arginine to ornithine and urea. ARG1 and ARG2 are two isoforms of mammalian arginase, which differ in tissue distribution, subcellular localization, immunologic cross-reactivity, and physiologic function. Arginase is thought to play a role in nitric oxide and polyamine metabolism, which may contribute to asthma pathogenesis (Meurs, Maarsingh et al. 2003; Vercelli 2003). *ARG1* and *ARG2* are expressed in lung tissue; and *ARG1* was highly expressed in human asthmatic lung tissue (Zimmermann, King et al. 2003). The *ARG2* gene was shown in a linkage study to be close to chromosome 14q24.4, which has been linked to asthma (Hakonarson, Bjornsdottir et al. 2002).

In a Mexican case-parent triad population, *ARG1* SNPs and haplotypes were not associated with asthma risk, but *ARG1* SNPs were significantly associated with the number of positive skin tests ($P<0.05$)(Li, Romieu et al. 2006). For *ARG2*, childhood asthma was significantly increased among those who had smoking parents and were carrying two copies of variant arg2s2 (CC vs. TT: relative risk (RR) = 2.39, 95% CI = 1.48-3.86), but the result was insignificant for those with nonsmoking parents (P for gene*environment interaction =0.025 under recessive model). A similar result was observed for arg2s1 (CC vs.GG: RR = 2.1, 95% CI = 1.2-3.9) (Li, Romieu et al. 2006). However, we are unable to estimate the association between sequence variants in *ARG1* and *ARG2* and SHS-related health effects based on the single study.

Conclusion

In summary, for different health effects, significant associations have been observed in genetic markers, including risk modification by germline polymorphisms, gene expression changes, and somatic alterations. For lung cancer, genetic polymorphisms of *CYP1B1* MspI, *GSTM1* null, *NAT2* slow acetylator, *MGMT* variants (143Val and 178Arg) and its methylation level has been significantly related to SHS-related lung cancer. Lung adenocarcinoma is the most common histological type among nonsmoking females. G*STT1* null and the level of *MGMT* methylation have been significantly linked to this histological type among nonsmokers. In addition, *α1-AT* PiMS genotype was significantly associated with change of lung function. For asthma, *GSTM1* null, sequence variants *ARG2* (G→G, T→C) and *CD14* (+1437, -159) were related to SHS exposure. The levels of two neonatal oxidative damage markers (8-OHdG and MDA) and deletion in exon 2-3 of *HPRT* were significantly modified by *GSTM1* null genotype and SHS exposure. Childhood ALL was significantly related to *GSTP1* Ile/Val genotype and SHS exposure status. The association between DNA adducts and SHS exposure were modified by sequence variants of *CYP1A1* (MspI, MspI in combination of *GSTM1* null, *GSTP1* Ile/Val, or EPHX slow phenotype), *CYP1B1* (Arg48Gly + Ala119Ser, Leu432Val, and Asn453Ser), *EPHX* (His139Arg), and *NAT2* slower acetylator. Besides the markers identified above, it is important to find markers that can distinguish between exposure from SHS and active smoke. For example, *NAT2* slow acetylator was associated with "increased" risk of lung cancer, while there was "decreased" risk for fast acetylator carriers. In addition, levels of DNA adducts were significantly higher among those with *NAT2* slow acetylator and are high at low nicotine-cotinine levels.

Some gaps in our knowledge of SHS health effects remain. The associations between sequence variants of genes involved in phase I and II metabolism and cell cycle pathways and the risk of lung cancer have been widely explored for SHS exposure and conclusive findings are not yet available. Chronic inflammation (an innate immune response) has been associated with some cancers (e.g., cervix, breast, primary liver, bladder, and prostate cancers) (Kinlen 2004; Chen, Giovannucci et al. 2005). However, very few studies have assessed genes involved in angiogenesis and immune response and other pathways. Other than lung cancer and asthma, the association between genetic polymorphisms of genes discussed above and the risk of other health effects due to SHS exposure remains unclear.

The other point is that most association studies focused on the relationship between a few genotypes and SHS-related health effects or cytogenetic endpoints, and therefore failed to include other confounding factors (e.g., the level of personal exposure to genotoxic compounds, age, gender and nutritional habits) (Georgiadis, Demopoulos et al. 2004). In addition to SHS, ambient air pollution (e.g., traffic exhaust) is an important source of low-dose exposure to airborne carcinogens for large segments of the general population and may therefore influence cancer risk (1989; Woodward and McMichael 1991; Georgiadis, Topinka et al. 2005). In the occupational settings, exposure to components exist in SHS, e.g., PAHs, is common (Perera, Hemminki et al. 2002; Teixeira, Gaspar et al. 2002; Pavanello and Clonfero 2004). However, it is difficult to get individual exposure information. Other environmental or occupational factors may interact with SHS and lead to health effects (e.g., arsenic, asbestos, chromium, nickel, vinyl chloride, ionizing radiation, dietary aflatoxin, and infection).

Abundant evidence showed that environmental factors are major contributors to human carcinogenesis and that the risk of developing cancer is strongly influenced by genetically determined differences (Nebert, McKinnon et al. 1996; Perera and Weinstein 2000). Therefore, twin studies (Redline, Tishler et al. 1989; Schmitt, Prescott et al. 2005) provide another approach to explore environmental and genetic influences on health effects related to SHS.

The findings from previous association studies have been inconsistent due to (1) cancer risk differs between histological types, (2) small sample size, (3) population stratification, (4) small genetic effect of individual SNP, and (5) different approaches for outcome ascertainment. Lung adenocarcinoma incidence has increased and become the most frequent histological type of lung cancer (Wynder and Hoffmann 1994; Charloux, Quoix et al. 1997; Gazdar and Minna 1997; Thun, Lally et al. 1997), especially among non-smokers. However, few SHS-related studies have performed statistical analyses by histological subtypes. Past studies mainly assessed Caucasian populations, but results of association studies focused on genetic polymorphisms and the risk of health effects varied greatly according to ethnicity. For example, Puerto Ricans and Mexicans are both Latinos, but asthma morbidity and mortality were 4-fold higher among Puerto Ricans than among Mexicans (Carter-Pokras and Gergen 1993; Homa, Mannino et al. 2000). Therefore, it is important to consider the effect of population stratification in genetic epidemiologic studies.

Besides association and experimental studies, some other approaches are useful to resolve the mystery of pathogenesis of SHS-related health effects. Large regions in the human genome have not been investigated for SHS exposure. Linkage study is a nice tool to identify genomic regions related to SHS exposure. For example, chromosome 1p at 97 cM, 5q at 135 cM, and 9q at 106 cM were significant ly related to SHS exposure ($P<0.01$)(Colilla, Nicolae et al. 2003). From the region identified, we could explore genes harbor in these area. Currently, SNP and haplotype analyses are two popular ways to investigate the association between SHS exposure and the risk of an outcome. But haplotype analyses (Taioli, Crofts et al. 1995), which capture more genetic variations as compared to SNP analyses, have not been widely used. Because of the importance of gene-gene interaction, pathway analyses have recently become important. However, such analyses are very complicated. In addition, microarray analyses (Izzotti, Cartiglia et al. 2004; Landi, Gemignani et al. 2005) is a promising method to find susceptibility genes associated with SHS exposure. This approach can help us to find the genetic differences resulting from different histological types or ethnic groups. Once we find these susceptibility genes, they could be used to identify the populations susceptible to SHS exposure, develop drugs to treat related diseases or conditions, and produce gene chips for disease screening purposes. As a whole, more studies using various approaches are needed to access genetic susceptibility to SHS in order to better understand the pathogenesis of related health effects.

References

Abdel-Rahman, S. Z. and R. A. El-Zein (2000). "The 399Gln polymorphism in the DNA repair gene XRCC1 modulates the genotoxic response induced in human lymphocytes by the tobacco-specific nitrosamine NNK." *Cancer Lett. 159(1)*: 63-71.

Adgent, M. A. (2006). "Environmental tobacco smoke and sudden infant death syndrome: a review." *Birth Defects Res. B Dev. Reprod. Toxicol. 77(1)*: 69-85.

Ahijevych, K. L., R. F. Tyndale, et al. (2002). "Factors influencing cotinine half-life during smoking abstinence in African American and Caucasian women." *Nicotine Tob. Res.* 4(4): 423-31.

Al-Delaimy, W., T. Fraser, et al. (2001). "Nicotine in hair of bar and restaurant workers." *N Z Med. J. 114(1127)*: 80-3.

Alavanja, M. C. R., R. C. Brownson, et al. (1992). "Preexisting lung disease and lung cancer among nonsmoking women." *Am. J. Epidemiol. 136*: 623-632.

Ali-Osman, F., O. Akande, et al. (1997). "Molecular cloning, characterization, and expression in Escherichia coli of full-length cDNAs of three human glutathione S-transferase Pi gene variants. Evidence for differential catalytic activity of the encoded proteins." *J. Biol. Chem. 272(15)*: 10004-12.

Amos, C. I., W. Xu, et al. (1999). "Is there a genetic basis for lung cancer susceptibility?" *Recent Results Cancer Res. 151*: 3-12.

Arredondo, J., V. T. Nguyen, et al. (2001). "A receptor-mediated mechanism of nicotine toxicity in oral keratinocytes." *Lab. Invest 81(12)*: 1653-68.

Arshad, S. H., R. J. Kurukulaaratchy, et al. (2005). "Early life risk factors for current wheeze, asthma, and bronchial hyperresponsiveness at 10 years of age." *Chest 127(2)*: 502-8.

Attvall, S., J. Fowelin, et al. (1993). "Smoking induces insulin resistance--a potential link with the insulin resistance syndrome." *J. Intern. Med. 233(4)*: 327-32.

Awasthi, Y. C., R. Sharma, et al. (1994). "Human glutathione S-transferases." *Int. J. Biochem. 26(3)*: 295-308.

Bai, T. R., D. Zhou, et al. (1995). "Substance P (NK1)- and neurokinin A (NK2)-receptor gene expression in inflammatory airway diseases." *Am. J. Physiol. 269(3 Pt 1)*: L309-17.

Baker, J. A., O. O. Odunuga, et al. (2006). "Active and passive smoking and risk of ovarian cancer." *Int. J. Gynecol. Cancer 16 Suppl 1*: 211-8.

Baldini, M., I. C. Lohman, et al. (1999). "A Polymorphism* in the 5' flanking region of the CD14 gene is associated with circulating soluble CD14 levels and with total serum immunoglobulin E." *Am. J. Respir. Cell Mol. Biol. 20(5)*: 976-83.

Baldwin, R. T. and S. Preston-Martin (2004). "Epidemiology of brain tumors in childhood--a review." *Toxicol. Appl. Pharmacol. 199(2)*: 118-31.

Barnes, K. C. (1999). "Gene-environment and gene-gene interaction studies in the molecular genetic analysis of asthma and atopy." *Clin. Exp. Allergy 29 Suppl 4*: 47-51.

Bartsch, H., N. Caporaso, et al. (1990). "Carcinogen hemoglobin adducts, urinary mutagenicity, and metabolic phenotype in active and passive cigarette smokers.[comment]." *Journal of the National Cancer Institute. 82(23)*: 1826-31.

Bennett, W. P., M. C. Alavanja, et al. (1999). "Environmental tobacco smoke, genetic susceptibility, and risk of lung cancer in never-smoking women." *J. Natl. Cancer Inst. 91(23)*: 2009-14.

Besaratinia, A., L. M. Maas, et al. (2002). "A molecular dosimetry approach to assess human exposure to environmental tobacco smoke in pubs." *Carcinogenesis 23(7)*: 1171-6.

Bianchini, F., F. Donato, et al. (1998). "Urinary excretion of 5-(hydroxymethyl) uracil in healthy volunteers: effect of active and passive tobacco smoke." *Int. J. Cancer 77(1)*: 40-6.

Blum, M., A. Demierre, et al. (1991). "Molecular mechanism of slow acetylation of drugs and carcinogens in humans." *Proc. Natl. Acad. Sci. USA 88(12)*: 5237-41.

Bock, C. H., A. S. Wenzlaff, et al. (2005). "NQO1 T allele associated with decreased risk of later age at diagnosis lung cancer among never smokers: results from a population-based study." *Carcinogenesis 26(2)*: 381-6.

Boffetta, P. (1993). *Occupational factors of lun cancer. Prevention of respiratory disease*. A. Hirsh, M. Goldberg, J. P. Martin and R. Massw. New York, Marcek Dekker: 37-63.

Boffetta, P., A. Agudo, et al. (1998). "Multicenter case-control study of exposure to environmental tobacco smoke and lung cancer in Europe." *J. Natl. Cancer Inst. 90(19)*: 1440-50.

Bohr, V. A., C. A. Smith, et al. (1985). "DNA repair in an active gene: removal of pyrimidine dimers from the DHFR gene of CHO cells is much more efficient than in the genome overall." *Cell 40(2)*: 359-69.

Bonassi, S., L. Hagmar, et al. (2000). "Chromosomal aberrations in lymphocytes predict human cancer independently of exposure to carcinogens. European Study Group on Cytogenetic Biomarkers and Health." *Cancer Res. 60(6)*: 1619-25.

Borchers, M. T., M. P. Carty, et al. (1999). "Regulation of human airway mucins by acrolein and inflammatory mediators." *Am. J. Physiol. 276(4 Pt 1)*: L549-55.

Borchers, M. T., S. E. Wert, et al. (1998). "Acrolein-induced MUC5ac expression in rat airways." *Am. J. Physiol. 274(4 Pt 1)*: L573-81.

Borchers, M. T., S. Wesselkamper, et al. (1999). "Monocyte inflammation augments acrolein-induced Muc5ac expression in mouse lung." *Am. J. Physiol. 277(3 Pt 1)*: L489-97.

Brantly, M., T. Nukiwa, et al. (1988). "Molecular basis of alpha-1-antitrypsin deficiency." *Am. J. Med. 84(6A)*: 13-31.

Burgan, S. W. (1997). "The role of tobacco use in periodontal diseases: a literature review." *Gen. Dent. 45(5)*: 449-60; quiz 469-70.

Burns, D. M. (1994). *Tobacco smoking. Epidemiology of Lung Cancer*. J. M. Samet. New York, NT, Marcel Dekker Inc.: 15-50.

Burrows, B. (1990). "Airways obstructive diseases: pathogenetic mechanisms and natural histories of the disorders." *Med. Clin. North Am. 74(3)*: 547-59.

Butkiewicz, D., E. Grzybowska, et al. (2000). "Polymorphisms of the GSTP1 and GSTM1 genes and PAH-DNA adducts in human mononuclear white blood cells." *Environ. Mol. Mutagen. 35(2)*: 99-105.

Butler, M. A., N. P. Lang, et al. (1992). "Determination of CYP1A2 and NAT2 phenotypes in human populations by analysis of caffeine urinary metabolites." *Pharmacogenetics 2(3)*: 116-27.

Byrd, R. S. and C. R. Howard (1995). "Children's passive and prenatal exposure to cigarette smoke." *Pediatr Ann. 24(12)*: 640-2, 644-5.

Byun, D.-S., M.-G. Lee, et al. (2001). "Frequent Epigenetic Inactivation of RASSF1A by Aberrant Promoter Hypermethylation in Human Gastric Adenocarcinoma." *Cancer Res. 61(19)*: 7034-7038.

Canalle, R., R. V. Burim, et al. (2004). "Genetic polymorphisms and susceptibility to childhood acute lymphoblastic leukemia." *Environ. Mol. Mutagen. 43(2)*: 100-9.

Cardenas, V. M., M. J. Thun, et al. (1997). "Environmental tobacco smoke and lung cancer mortality in the American Cancer Society's Cancer Prevention Study. II." *Cancer Causes Control 8(1)*: 57-64.

Carrano, A. V. (1986). "Chromosomal alterations as markers of exposure and effect." *J. Occup. Med. 28(10)*: 1112-6.

Carter-Pokras, O. D. and P. J. Gergen (1993). "Reported asthma among Puerto Rican, Mexican-American, and Cuban children, 1982 through 1984." *Am. J. Public Health 83(4)*: 580-2.

Catusse, J., A. Liotard, et al. (2003). "Characterization of the molecular interactions of interleukin-8 (CXCL8), growth related oncogen alpha (CXCL1) and a non-peptide antagonist (SB 225002) with the human CXCR2." *Biochem. Pharmacol. 65(5)*: 813-21.

Charloux, A., E. Quoix, et al. (1997). "The increasing incidence of lung adenocarcinoma: reality or artifact? A review of the epidemiology of lung adenocarcinoma." International *Journal of Epidemiology 26*: 14-23.

Chen, Y., D. C. Rennie, et al. (1998). "Evidence for major genetic control of wheeze in relation to history of respiratory allergy: Humboldt family study." *Am. J. Med. Genet. 75(5)*: 485-91.

Chen, Y. C., J. H. Chen, et al. (2004). "Lung adenocarcinoma and human papillomavirus infection." *Cancer 101(6)*: 1428-36.

Chen, Y. C., E. Giovannucci, et al. (2005). "Sequence Variants of Toll-Like Receptor 4 (TLR4) and Susceptibility to Prostate Cancer." *Cancer Research 65(24)*: 11771-11778.

Chen, Y. C., H. J. Su, et al. (2005). "Interaction between environmental tobacco smoke and arsenic methylation ability on the risk of bladder cancer." *Cancer Causes Control 16(2)*: 75-81.

Cherpillod, P. and P. A. Amstad (1995). "Benzo[a]pyrene-induced mutagenesis of p53 hot-spot codons 248 and 249 in human hepatocytes." *Mol. Carcinog 13(1)*: 15-20.

Choudhry, S., P. C. Avila, et al. (2005). "CD14 tobacco gene-environment interaction modifies asthma severity and immunoglobulin E levels in Latinos with asthma." *Am. J. Respir. Crit. Care Med. 172(2)*: 173-82.

Churg, A., R. D. Wang, et al. (2003). "Macrophage metalloelastase mediates acute cigarette smoke-induced inflammation via tumor necrosis factor-alpha release." *Am. J. Respir. Crit. Care Med. 167(8)*: 1083-9.

Clearing the air: asthma and indoor exposure. Washington, DC, Committee on the assessment of Asthma and Indoor Air, National Academy of Sciences (2000).

Cohet, C., S. Borel, et al. (2004). "Exon 5 polymorphisms in the O6-alkylguanine DNA alkyltransferase gene and lung cancer risk in non-smokers exposed to second-hand smoke." *Cancer Epidemiol. Biomarkers Prev. 13(2)*: 320-3.

Colilla, S., D. Nicolae, et al. (2003). "Evidence for gene-environment interactions in a linkage study of asthma and smoking exposure." *J. Allergy Clin. Immunol. 111(4)*: 840-6.

Collier, A. C. and C. A. Pritsos (2003). "Environmental tobacco smoke in the workplace: markers of exposure, polymorphic enzymes and implications for disease state." *Chem. Biol. Interact. 146(3)*: 211-24.

Cook, D. G. and D. P. Strachan (1997). "Health effects of passive smoking. 3. Parental smoking and prevalence of respiratory symptoms and asthma in school age children." *Thorax 52(12)*: 1081-94.

Crawford, F. G., J. Mayer, et al. (1994). "Biomarkers of environmental tobacco smoke in preschool children and their mothers." *J. Natl. Cancer Inst. 86(18)*: 1398-402.

Cribb, A. E., R. Isbrucker, et al. (1994). "Acetylator phenotyping: the urinary caffeine metabolite ratio in slow acetylators correlates with a marker of systemic NAT1 activity." *Pharmacogenetics 4(3)*: 166-70.

Dammann, R., U. Schagdarsurengin, et al. (2003). "Epigenetic inactivation of the Ras-association domain family 1 (RASSF1A) gene and its function in human carcinogenesis." *Histol. Histopathol. 18(2)*: 665-77.

Daniel, V. (1993). "Glutathione S-transferases: gene structure and regulation of expression." *Crit. Rev. Biochem. Mol. Biol. 28(3)*: 173-207.

Daube, H., G. Scherer, et al. (1997). "DNA adducts in human placenta in relation to tobacco smoke exposure and plasma antioxidant status." *J. Cancer Res. Clin. Oncol. 123(3)*: 141-51.

Dautzenberg, B. (2004). "[Tobacco-related diseases]." *Rev. Prat. 54(17)*: 1877-82.

de Boer, J. and J. H. Hoeijmakers (2000). "Nucleotide excision repair and human syndromes." *Carcinogenesis 21(3)*: 453-60.

De Flora, S., R. M. Balansky, et al. (2003). "Molecular alterations and lung tumors in p53 mutant mice exposed to cigarette smoke." *Cancer Res. 63(4)*: 793-800.

De Flora, S., A. Izzotti, et al. (2005). "Induction and modulation of lung tumors: genomic and transcriptional alterations in cigarette smoke-exposed mice." *Exp. Lung Res. 31(1)*: 19-35.

Dejin-Karlsson, E., B. S. Hanson, et al. (1998). "Does passive smoking in early pregnancy increase the risk of small-for-gestational-age infants?" *Am. J. Public Health 88(10)*: 1523-7.

Deng, C., D. Xie, et al. (1999). "Genetic polymorphism of human O6-alkylguanine-DNA alkyltransferase: identification of a missense variation in the active site region." *Pharmacogenetics 9(1)*: 81-7.

Denissenko, M. F., A. Pao, et al. (1996). "Preferential formation of benzo[a]pyrene adducts at lung cancer mutational hotspots in P53." *Science 274(5286)*: 430-2.

Di Somma, C., D. Charron, et al. (2003). "Atopic asthma and TNF-308 alleles: linkage disequilibrium and association analyses." *Hum. Immunol. 64(3)*: 359-65.

Divine, K. K., L. C. Pulling, et al. (2005). "Multiplicity of abnormal promoter methylation in lung adenocarcinomas from smokers and never smokers." *Int. J. Cancer 114(3)*: 400-5.

Dockery, D. W. and D. Trichopoulos (1997). "Risk of lung cancer from environmental exposures to tobacco smoke." *Cancer Causes Control 8(3)*: 333-45.

Dogliotti, E., P. Hainaut, et al. (1998). "Mutation spectra resulting from carcinogenic exposure: from model systems to cancer-related genes." *Recent Results Cancer Res. 154*: 97-124.

Egyhazi, S., S. Ma, et al. (2002). "Novel O6-methylguanine-DNA methyltransferase SNPs: a frequency comparison of patients with familial melanoma and healthy individuals in Sweden." *Hum. Mutat. 20(5)*: 408-9.

Ehrlich, R., E. Jordaan, et al. (2001). "Household smoking and bronchial hyperresponsiveness in children with asthma." *J. Asthma 38(3)*: 239-51.

Environmental Tobacco Smoke. *Measuring Exposures and Assessing Health Effects.* National Research Council. Board on Environmental Studies and Toxicology. Committee on Passive Smoking. Washington, DC, National Academy Press (1986).

Esteller, M., S. R. Hamilton, et al. (1999). "Inactivation of the DNA repair gene O6-methylguanine-DNA methyltransferase by promoter hypermethylation is a common event in primary human neoplasia." *Cancer Res. 59(4)*: 793-7.

Esteller, M., M. Toyota, et al. (2000). "Inactivation of the DNA repair gene O6-methylguanine-DNA methyltransferase by promoter hypermethylation is associated with G to A mutations in K-ras in colorectal tumorigenesis." *Cancer Res. 60(9)*: 2368-71.

Exposure to Environmental Tobacco Smoke and Cotinine Levels ? Fact Sheet. National Center for Chronic Disease Prevention and Health Promotion, Centers for Disease Control and Prevention, US Department of Health and Human Services (2006).

Faraglia, B., S. Y. Chen, et al. (2003). "Evaluation of 4-aminobiphenyl-DNA adducts in human breast cancer: the influence of tobacco smoke." *Carcinogenesis 24(4)*: 719-25.

Fields, W. R., C. S. Morrow, et al. (1998). "Overexpression of stably transfected human glutathione S-transferase P1-1 protects against DNA damage by benzo[a]pyrene diol-epoxide in human T47D cells." *Mol. Pharmacol. 54(2)*: 298-304.

Finette, B. A., J. P. O'Neill, et al. (1998). "Gene mutations with characteristic deletions in cord blood T lymphocytes associated with passive maternal exposure to tobacco smoke." *Nat. Med. 4(10)*: 1144-51.

Fontham, E. T. (1990). "Protective dietary factors and lung cancer." *Int. J. Epidemiol. 19 Suppl 1*: S32-42.

Fontham, E. T., P. Correa, et al. (1994). "Environmental tobacco smoke and lung cancer in nonsmoking women. A multicenter study." *Jama 271(22)*: 1752-9.

Frederickson, S. M., E. M. Messing, et al. (1994). "Relationship between in vivo acetylator phenotypes and cytosolic N-acetyltransferase and O-acetyltransferase activities in human uroepithelial cells." *Cancer Epidemiol. Biomarkers Prev. 3(1)*: 25-32.

Gadek, J. E. and R. G. Crystal (1982). *Alpha1Antitrypsin deficiency. The metabolic basis of inherited disease.* J. B. Stanbury, J. B. Wyngaarden, D. S. Fredrickson, J. L. Goldstein and M. S. Brown. New York, McGraw Hill Book Company: 1450-1467.

Gao, Y. T. (1996). "Risk factors for lung cancer among nonsmokers with emphasis on lifestyle factors." *Lung Cancer 14 Suppl 1*: S39-45.

Gazdar, A. F. and J. D. Minna (1997). "Cigarettes, sex, and lung adenocarcinoma." *J. Natl. Cancer Inst. 89(21)*: 1563-5.

Gealy, R., L. Zhang, et al. (1999). "Comparison of mutations in the p53 and K-ras genes in lung carcinomas from smoking and nonsmoking women." *Cancer Epidemiol. Biomarkers Prev. 8(4 Pt 1)*: 297-302.

Gebremichael, A., K. Tullis, et al. (1996). "Ah-receptor-dependent modulation of gene expression by aged and diluted sidestream cigarette smoke." *Toxicol. Appl. Pharmacol. 141(1)*: 76-83.

Gelskey, S. C. (1999). "Cigarette smoking and periodontitis: methodology to assess the strength of evidence in support of a causal association." *Community Dent Oral Epidemiol. 27(1)*: 16-24.

General, U. S. S. (1986). The health consequences of involuntary smoking. A report of the surgeon general Rockville, Maryland, Office of Smoking and Health.

Georgiadis, P., N. A. Demopoulos, et al. (2004). "Impact of phase I or phase II enzyme polymorphisms on lymphocyte DNA adducts in subjects exposed to urban air pollution and environmental tobacco smoke." *Toxicol Lett. 149(1-3)*: 269-80.

Georgiadis, P., J. Topinka, et al. (2001). "Biomarkers of genotoxicity of air pollution (the AULIS project): bulky DNA adducts in subjects with moderate to low exposures to airborne polycyclic aromatic hydrocarbons and their relationship to environmental tobacco smoke and other parameters." *Carcinogenesis 22(9)*: 1447-57.

Georgiadis, P., J. Topinka, et al. (2005). "Interactions between CYP1A1 polymorphisms and exposure to environmental tobacco smoke in the modulation of lymphocyte bulky DNA adducts and chromosomal aberrations." *Carcinogenesis 26(1)*: 93-101.

Gerde, P., B. A. Muggenburg, et al. (1998). "A relevant dose of 4-(methylnitrosamino)-1-(3-pyridyl)-1-butanone is extensively metabolized and rapidly absorbed in the canine tracheal mucosa." *Cancer Res. 58(7)*: 1417-22.

Gerde, P., B. A. Muggenburg, et al. (1997). "Benzo[a]pyrene at an environmentally relevant dose is slowly absorbed by, and extensively metabolized in, tracheal epithelium." *Carcinogenesis 18(9)*: 1825-32.

Gergen, P. J., J. A. Fowler, et al. (1998). "The burden of environmental tobacco smoke exposure on the respiratory health of children 2 months through 5 years of age in the United States: Third National Health and Nutrition Examination Survey, 1988 to 1994." *Pediatrics 101(2)*: E8.

Gilliland, F. D., Y. F. Li, et al. (2002). "Effects of glutathione S-transferase M1, maternal smoking during pregnancy, and environmental tobacco smoke on asthma and wheezing in children." *Am. J. Respir. Crit. Care Med. 166(4)*: 457-63.

Gilliland, F. D., Y. F. Li, et al. (2001). "Effects of maternal smoking during pregnancy and environmental tobacco smoke on asthma and wheezing in children." *Am. J. Respir. Crit. Care Med. 163(2)*: 429-36.

Gilliland, F. D., R. McConnell, et al. (1999). "A theoretical basis for investigating ambient air pollution and children's respiratory health." *Environ Health Perspect 107 Suppl 3*: 403-7.

Girod, C. E. and T. E. King, Jr. (2005). "COPD: a dust-induced disease?" *Chest 128(4)*: 3055-64.

Gold, D. R. (2000). "Environmental tobacco smoke, indoor allergens, and childhood asthma." *Environ. Health Perspect. 108 Suppl 4*: 643-51.

Hackshaw, A. K., M. R. Law, et al. (1997). "The accumulated evidence on lung cancer and environmental tobacco smoke." *Bmj 315(7114)*: 980-8.

Hainaut, P. and G. P. Pfeifer (2001). "Patterns of p53 G-->T transversions in lung cancers reflect the primary mutagenic signature of DNA-damage by tobacco smoke." *Carcinogenesis 22(3)*: 367-74.

Hakonarson, H., U. S. Bjornsdottir, et al. (2002). "A major susceptibility gene for asthma maps to chromosome 14q24." *Am. J. Hum. Genet. 71(3)*: 483-91.

Hammond, E. C. and H. Seidman (1980). "Smoking and cancer in the United States." *Prev. Med. 9(2)*: 169-74.

Hammond, S. K., J. Coghlin, et al. (1993). "Relationship between environmental tobacco smoke exposure and carcinogen-hemoglobin adduct levels in nonsmokers." *J. Natl. Cancer Inst. 85(6)*: 474-8.

Hanke, W., J. Kalinka, et al. (1999). "Passive smoking and pregnancy outcome in central Poland." *Hum. Exp. Toxicol. 18(4)*: 265-71.

Harris, M. J., M. Coggan, et al. (1998). "Polymorphism of the Pi class glutathione S-transferase in normal populations and cancer patients." *Pharmacogenetics 8(1)*: 27-31.

Harris, R. E., E. A. Zang, et al. (1993). "Race and sex differences in lung cancer risk associated with cigarette smoking." *Int. J. Epidemiol. 22(4)*: 592-9.

Hasday, J. D., R. Bascom, et al. (1999). "Bacterial endotoxin is an active component of cigarette smoke." *Chest 115(3)*: 829-35.

Hassett, C., L. Aicher, et al. (1994). "Human microsomal epoxide hydrolase: genetic polymorphism and functional expression in vitro of amino acid variants." *Hum. Mol. Genet. 3(3)*: 421-8.

Hayashi, S., J. Watanabe, et al. (1991). "Genetic linkage of lung cancer-associated MspI polymorphisms with amino acid replacement in the heme binding region of the human cytochrome P450IA1 gene." *J. Biochem. (Tokyo) 110(3)*: 407-11.

Hayes, J. D. and R. C. Stange (2000). "Glutathione S-transferase polymorphisms and their biological consequences." *Pharmacology 61*: 154-166.

Hayes, R. B., W. Bi, et al. (1993). "N-acetylation phenotype and genotype and risk of bladder cancer in benzidine-exposed workers." *Carcinogenesis 14(4)*: 675-8.

Health effects of exposure to environmental tobacco smoke. Sacramento, CA, California Environmental Protection Agency (1997).

Hecht, S. S. (1998). "Biochemistry, biology, and carcinogenicity of tobacco-specific N-nitrosamines." *Chem. Res. Toxicol. 11(6)*: 559-603.

Hecht, S. S. (1999). "Tobacco smoke carcinogens and lung cancer." *J. Natl. Cancer Inst. 91(14)*: 1194-210.

Hecht, S. S. (2002). "Human urinary carcinogen metabolites: biomarkers for investigating tobacco and cancer." *Carcinogenesis 23(6)*: 907-22.

Hecht, S. S., S. G. Carmella, et al. (2006). "4-(methylnitrosamino)-1-(3-pyridyl)-1-butanol and its glucuronides in the urine of infants exposed to environmental tobacco smoke." *Cancer Epidemiol. Biomarkers Prev. 15(5)*: 988-92.

Hecht, S. S., S. G. Carmella, et al. (1993). "A tobacco-specific lung carcinogen in the urine of men exposed to cigarette smoke." *N Engl. J. Med. 329(21)*: 1543-6.

Heeschen, C., J. J. Jang, et al. (2001). "Nicotine stimulates angiogenesis and promotes tumor growth and atherosclerosis." *Nat. Med. 7(7)*: 833-9.

Hein, D. W. (1988). "Acetylator genotype and arylamine-induced carcinogenesis." *Biochim. Biophys. Acta 948(1)*: 37-66.

Hein, D. W., M. A. Doll, et al. (1993). "Metabolic activation and deactivation of arylamine carcinogens by recombinant human NAT1 and polymorphic NAT2 acetyltransferases." *Carcinogenesis 14(8)*: 1633-8.

Heinzmann, A., H. Dietrich, et al. (2003). "Promoter polymorphisms of the CD14 gene are not associated with bronchial asthma in Caucasian children." *Eur. J. Immunogenet. 30(5)*: 345-8.

Hernandez-Boussard, T. M. and P. Hainaut (1998). "A specific spectrum of p53 mutations in lung cancer from smokers: review of mutations compiled in the IARC p53 database." *Environ. Health Perspect. 106(7)*: 385-91.

Hill, J. W., T. K. Hazra, et al. (2001). "Stimulation of human 8-oxoguanine-DNA glycosylase by AP-endonuclease: potential coordination of the initial steps in base excision repair." *Nucl. Acids Res. 29(2)*: 430-438.

Hoffjan, S., D. Nicolae, et al. (2003). "Association studies for asthma and atopic diseases: a comprehensive review of the literature." *Respir. Res. 4*: 14.

Hoffjan, S. and C. Ober (2002). "Present status on the genetic studies of asthma." *Curr. Opin. Immunol. 14(6)*: 709-17.

Hoffmann, D. and I. Hoffmann (2001). The changing cigarette: chemical studies and bioassays. Risks associated with smoking cigarettes with low machine-measured yields of tar and nicotine. D. R. Shopland, D. M. Burns and N. L. Benowitz, National Cancer Institute.

Holt, P. G., P. D. Sly, et al. (1997). "Atopic versus infectious diseases in childhood: a question of balance?" *Pediatr Allergy Immunol. 8(2)*: 53-8.

Holz, O., R. Meissner, et al. (1993). "Detection of DNA single-strand breaks in lymphocytes of smokers." *Int. Arch Occup. Environ. Health 65(2)*: 83-8.

Homa, D. M., D. M. Mannino, et al. (2000). "Asthma mortality in U.S. Hispanics of Mexican, Puerto Rican, and Cuban heritage, 1990-1995." *Am. J. Respir. Crit. Care Med. 161(2 Pt 1)*: 504-9.

Hong, Y. C., H. Kim, et al. (2001). "Maternal genetic effects on neonatal susceptibility to oxidative damage from environmental tobacco smoke." *J. Natl. Cancer Inst. 93(8)*: 645-7.

Hong, Y. C., K. H. Lee, et al. (2003). "Effects of the GSTM1 and GSTT1 polymorphisms on the relationship between maternal exposure to environmental tobacco smoke and neonatal birth weight." *J. Occup. Environ. Med. 45(5)*: 492-8.

Hou, S. M., S. Falt, et al. (2002). "The XPD variant alleles are associated with increased aromatic DNA adduct level and lung cancer risk." *Carcinogenesis 23(4)*: 599-603.

Houston, T. K., T. K. Houston, et al. (2006). "Active and passive smoking and development of glucose intolerance among young adults in a prospective cohort: CARDIA study." *BMJ*: *bmj*.38779.584028.55.

Hu, W., Z. Feng, et al. (2004). "Chromium(VI) enhances (+/-)-anti-7beta,8alpha-dihydroxy-9alpha,10alpha-epoxy-7,8,9,10-tetrahydro benzo[a]pyrene-induced cytotoxicity and mutagenicity in mammalian cells through its inhibitory effect on nucleotide excision repair." *Biochemistry 43(44)*: 14282-9.

Hugoson, A., O. Norderyd, et al. (1998). "Distribution of periodontal disease in a Swedish adult population 1973, 1983 and 1993." *J. Clin. Periodontol. 25(7)*: 542-8.

Humble, C., J. Croft, et al. (1990). "Passive smoking and 20-year cardiovascular disease mortality among nonsmoking wives, Evans County, Georgia." *Am. J. Public Health 80(5)*: 599-601.

Hung, R. J., P. Boffetta, et al. (2003). "CYP1A1 and GSTM1 genetic polymorphisms and lung cancer risk in Caucasian non-smokers: a pooled analysis." *Carcinogenesis 24(5)*: 875-82.

Husgafvel-Pursiainen, K., P. Boffetta, et al. (2000). "p53 mutations and exposure to environmental tobacco smoke in a multicenter study on lung cancer." *Cancer Res. 60(11)*: 2906-11.

IARC *Monographs on The Evaluation of Carcinogenic Risk to Human.* Lyon, IARC. 46 (1989).

IARC, Ed. (2004). Tobacco smoke and involuntary smoking. *IARC Monographs on the Evaluation of Carocinogenic Risks to Humans.* Lyon, France, IARC.

Infante-Rivard, C., M. Krajinovic, et al. (2000). "Parental smoking, CYP1A1 genetic polymorphisms and childhood leukemia (Quebec, Canada)." *Cancer Causes Control 11(6)*: 547-53.

Ivashchenko, T. E., O. G. Sideleva, et al. (2001). "[Genetic factors in predisposition to bronchial asthma]." *Genetika 37(1)*: 107-11.

Izzotti, A., C. Cartiglia, et al. (2004). "Gene expression in the lung of p53 mutant mice exposed to cigarette smoke." *Cancer Res. 64(23)*: 8566-72.

Jaakkola, J. J., P. Nafstad, et al. (2001). "Environmental tobacco smoke, parental atopy, and childhood asthma." *Environ. Health Perspect 109(6)*: 579-82.

Janerich, D. T., W. D. Thompson, et al. (1990). "Lung cancer and exposure to tobacco smoke in the household." *N Engl. J. Med. 323(10)*: 632-6.

Janus, E. D., N. T. Phillips, et al. (1985). "Smoking, lung function, and alpha 1-antitrypsin deficiency." *Lancet 1(8421)*: 152-4.

Janzon, L., K. Berntorp, et al. (1983). "Glucose tolerance and smoking: a population study of oral and intravenous glucose tolerance tests in middle-aged men." *Diabetologia 25(2)*: 86-8.

Jarmalaite, S., A. Kannio, et al. (2003). "Aberrant p16 promoter methylation in smokers and former smokers with nonsmall cell lung cancer." *Int. J. Cancer 106(6)*: 913-8.

Jemal, A., R. Siegel, et al. (2006). "Cancer statistics, 2006." *CA Cancer J. Clin. 56(2)*: 106-30.

Ji, B. T., X. O. Shu, et al. (1997). "Paternal cigarette smoking and the risk of childhood cancer among offspring of nonsmoking mothers." *J. Natl. Cancer Inst. 89(3)*: 238-44.

Jindal, S. K., A. N. Aggarwal, et al. (2006). "A multicentric study on epidemiology of chronic obstructive pulmonary disease and its relationship with tobacco smoking and environmental tobacco smoke exposure." *Indian J. Chest Dis. Allied Sci. 48(1)*: 23-9.

Johansson, A. S., G. Stenberg, et al. (1998). "Structure-activity relationships and thermal stability of human glutathione transferase P1-1 governed by the H-site residue 105." *J. Mol. Biol. 278(3)*: 687-98.

Jordaan, E. R., R. I. Ehrlich, et al. (1999). "Environmental tobacco smoke exposure in children: household and community determinants." *Arch Environ. Health 54(5)*: 319-27.

Kabat, G. C. (1996). "Aspects of the epidemiology of lung cancer in smokers and nonsmokers in the United States." *Lung Cancer 15(1)*: 1-20.

Kabesch, M., K. Hasemann, et al. (2004). "A promoter polymorphism in the CD14 gene is associated with elevated levels of soluble CD14 but not with IgE or atopic diseases." *Allergy 59(5)*: 520-5.

Kawakami, N., N. Takatsuka, et al. (1997). "Effects of smoking on the incidence of non-insulin-dependent diabetes mellitus. Replication and extension in a Japanese cohort of male employees." *Am. J. Epidemiol. 145(2)*: 103-9.

Kharrazi, M., G. N. DeLorenze, et al. (2004). "Environmental tobacco smoke and pregnancy outcome." *Epidemiology 15(6)*: 660-70.

Kinane, D. F. and I. G. Chestnutt (2000). "Smoking and periodontal disease." *Crit. Rev. Oral. Biol. Med. 11(3)*: 356-65.

Kinlen, L. (2004). "Infections and immune factors in cancer: the role of epidemiology." *Oncogene 23(38)*: 6341-8.

Kiyohara, C. (2000). "Genetic polymorphism of enzymes involved in xenobiotic metabolism and the risk of colorectal cancer." *J. Epidemiol. 10(5)*: 349-60.

Kiyohara, C., K. Wakai, et al. (2003). "Risk modification by CYP1A1 and GSTM1 polymorphisms in the association of environmental tobacco smoke and lung cancer: a case-control study in Japanese nonsmoking women." *Int. J. Cancer 107(1)*: 139-44.

Klebanoff, M. A., J. D. Clemens, et al. (1996). "Maternal smoking during pregnancy and childhood cancer." *Am. J. Epidemiol. 144(11)*: 1028-33.

Ko, Y. C., C. H. Lee, et al. (1997). "Risk factors for primary lung cancer among non-smoking women in Taiwan." *International Journal of Epidemiology 26(1)*: 24-31.

Koo, L. C. and J. H. C. Ho (1990). "Worldwide epidemiological patterns of lung cancer in nonsmokers." *Int. J. Epidemiol. 19(Suppl 1)*: S14-23.

Koppelman, G. H., N. E. Reijmerink, et al. (2001). "Association of a promoter polymorphism of the CD14 gene and atopy." *Am. J. Respir. Crit. Care Med. 163(4)*: 965-9.

Krajinovic, M., H. Sinnett, et al. (2002). "Role of NQO1, MPO and CYP2E1 genetic polymorphisms in the susceptibility to childhood acute lymphoblastic leukemia." *Int. J. Cancer 97(2)*: 230-6.

Kramer, U., C. H. Lemmen, et al. (2004). "The effect of environmental tobacco smoke on eczema and allergic sensitization in children." *Br. J. Dermatol. 150(1)*: 111-8.

Kukla, L., D. Hruba, et al. (2001). "Smoking and damages of reproduction: evidence of ELSPAC." *Cent. Eur. J. Public Health 9(2)*: 59-63.

Kurie, J. M. and R. N. Dubois (2001). "Prostaglandin E Synthase: Another Enzyme in the Cyclooxygenase Pathway Driving Epithelial Cancer?" *Clin. Cancer Res. 7(9)*: 2608-2610.

Kurz, T. and C. Ober (2004). "The role of environmental tobacco smoke in genetic susceptibility to asthma." *Curr. Opin. Allergy Clin. Immunol. 4(5)*: 335-9.

Landi, S., F. Gemignani, et al. (2005). "A database of single-nucleotide polymorphisms and a genotyping microarray for genetic epidemiology of lung cancer." *Exp. Lung Res. 31(2)*: 223-58.

Larsson, L., B. Szponar, et al. (2004). "Tobacco smoking increases dramatically air concentrations of endotoxin." *Indoor Air 14(6)*: 421-4.

Larsson, M. L., M. Frisk, et al. (2001). "Environmental tobacco smoke exposure during childhood is associated with increased prevalence of asthma in adults." *Chest 120(3)*: 711-7.

Lee, C. Z., F. H. Royce, et al. (2000). "Effect of in utero and postnatal exposure to environmental tobacco smoke on the developmental expression of pulmonary cytochrome P450 monooxygenases." *J. Biochem. Mol. Toxicol. 14(3)*: 121-30.

Lee, J. H., S. B. Rho, et al. (2005). "Programmed Cell Death 6 (PDCD6) Protein Interacts with Death-Associated Protein Kinase 1 (DAPk1): Additive Effect on Apoptosis via Caspase-3 Dependent Pathway." *Biotechnology Letters 27(14)*: 1011-1015.

Leung, T. F., N. L. Tang, et al. (2003). "The C-159T polymorphism in the CD14 promoter is associated with serum total IgE concentration in atopic Chinese children." *Pediatr Allergy Immunol. 14(4)*: 255-60.

Li, H., I. Romieu, et al. (2006). "Genetic polymorphisms in arginase I and II and childhood asthma and atopy." *J. Allergy Clin. Immunol. 117(1)*: 119-26.

Li, Q. J., S. Lu, et al. (2000). "Isolation and characterization of a new chemokine receptor gene, the putative chicken CXCR1." *Gene 257(2)*: 307-17.

Liggett, W. H., Jr. and D. Sidransky (1998). "Role of the p16 tumor suppressor gene in cancer." *J. Clin. Oncol. 16(3)*: 1197-1206.

Little, J., A. Cardy, et al. (2004). "Smoking and orofacial clefts: a United Kingdom-based case-control study." *Cleft Palate Craniofac J. 41(4)*: 381-6.

Liu, L., J. H. Yoon, et al. (2002). "Frequent hypermethylation of the RASSF1A gene in prostate cancer." *Oncogene 21(44)*: 6835-40.

Liu, Z. (1992). "Smoking and lung cancer in China: combined analysis of eight case-control studies." *Int. J. Epidemiol. 21(2)*: 197-201.

London, S. J., J. Smart, et al. (2000). "Lung cancer risk in relation to genetic polymorphisms of microsomal epoxide hydrolase among African-Americans and Caucasians in Los Angeles County." *Lung Cancer 28(2)*: 147-55.

Lu, K. P., N. F. Alejandro, et al. (2002). "Differential expression of ribosomal L31, Zis, gas-5 and mitochondrial mRNAs following oxidant induction of proliferative vascular smooth muscle cell phenotypes." *Atherosclerosis 160(2)*: 273-80.

MacLennan, R., J. Da Costa, et al. (1977). "Risk factors for lung cancer in Singapore Chinese, a population with high female incidence rates." *Int. J. Cancer 20(6)*: 854-60.

Maclure, M., R. B. Katz, et al. (1989). "Elevated blood levels of carcinogens in passive smokers." *Am. J. Public Health 79(10)*: 1381-4.

Mainous, A. G., 3rd and W. J. Hueston (1994). "Passive smoke and low birth weight. Evidence of a threshold effect." *Arch Fam. Med. 3(10)*: 875-8.

Malats, N., A. M. Camus-Radon, et al. (2000). "Lung cancer risk in nonsmokers and GSTM1 and GSTT1 genetic polymorphism." *Cancer Epidemiol. Biomarkers Prev. 9(8)*: 827-33.

Manna, S. K., T. Rangasamy, et al. (2006). "Long term environmental tobacco smoke activates nuclear transcription factor-kappa B, activator protein-1, and stress responsive kinases in mouse brain." *Biochem. Pharmacol. 71(11)*: 1602-9.

Martin, T. R. and M. B. Bracken (1986). "Association of low birth weight with passive smoke exposure in pregnancy." *Am. J. Epidemiol. 124(4)*: 633-42.

Martinez, F. D., M. Cline, et al. (1992). "Increased incidence of asthma in children of smoking mothers." *Pediatrics 89(1)*: 21-6.

Matikainen, T., G. I. Perez, et al. (2001). "Aromatic hydrocarbon receptor-driven Bax gene expression is required for premature ovarian failure caused by biohazardous environmental chemicals." *Nat. Genet. 28(4)*: 355-60.

Matsuda, T., M. Kawanishi, et al. (1998). "Specific tandem GG to TT base substitutions induced by acetaldehyde are due to intra-strand crosslinks between adjacent guanine bases." *Nucleic Acids Res. 26(7)*: 1769-74.

Mayer, A. S. and L. S. Newman (2001). "Genetic and environmental modulation of chronic obstructive pulmonary disease." *Respir. Physiol. 128(1)*: 3-11.

McWilliams, J. E., B. J. Sanderson, et al. (1995). "Glutathione S-transferase M1 (GSTM1) deficiency and lung cancer risk." *Cancer Epidemiol. Biomarkers Prev. 4(6)*: 589-94.

Meisel, P., C. Schwahn, et al. (2004). "Dose-effect relation of smoking and the interleukin-1 gene polymorphism in periodontal disease." *J. Periodontol. 75(2)*: 236-42.

Merlo, F., A. Andreassen, et al. (1998). "Urinary excretion of 1-hydroxypyrene as a marker for exposure to urban air levels of polycyclic aromatic hydrocarbons." *Cancer Epidemiol. Biomarkers Prev. 7(2)*: 147-55.

Meurs, H., H. Maarsingh, et al. (2003). "Arginase and asthma: novel insights into nitric oxide homeostasis and airway hyperresponsiveness." *Trends Pharmacol. Sci. 24(9)*: 450-5.

Meyers, D. A., D. S. Postma, et al. (2005). "Genome screen for asthma and bronchial hyperresponsiveness: interactions with passive smoke exposure." *J. Allergy Clin. Immunol. 115(6)*: 1169-75.

Miller, D. P., I. De Vivo, et al. (2003). "Association between self-reported environmental tobacco smoke exposure and lung cancer: modification by GSTP1 polymorphism." *International Journal of Cancer. 104(6)*: 758-63.

Mitchell, K. R. and D. Warshawsky (1999). "Frequent Ha-ras mutations in murine skin and liver tumors induced by 7H-dibenzo[c,g]carbazole." *Mol. Carcinog. 25(2)*: 107-12.

Mitsuta, K., H. Matsuse, et al. (2003). "Production of TNF-alpha by peripheral blood mononuclear cells through activation of nuclear factor kappa B by specific allergen stimulation in patients with atopic asthma." *Allergy Asthma Proc. 24(1)*: 19-26.

Mooney, L. A., R. M. Santella, et al. (1995). "Decline of DNA damage and other biomarkers in peripheral blood following smoking cessation." *Cancer Epidemiol. Biomarkers Prev. 4(6)*: 627-34.

Morimoto, K., K. Miura, et al. (1984). "Human health situation and chromosome alterations: sister chromatid exchange frequency in lymphocytes from passive smokers and patients with hereditary diseases." *Basic Life Sci. 29 Pt B*: 801-11.

Murphy, V. E., T. Zakar, et al. (2002). "Reduced 11beta-hydroxysteroid dehydrogenase type 2 activity is associated with decreased birth weight centile in pregnancies complicated by asthma." *J. Clin. Endocrinol. Metab. 87(4)*: 1660-8.

Nakajima, T., E. Elovaara, et al. (1995). "Expression and polymorphism of glutathione S-transferase in human lungs: risk factors in smoking-related lung cancer." *Carcinogenesis 16(4)*: 707-11.

National Health Survey 1002 Highlights of Main Survey Findings (Report), Research and Evaluation Department, Ministry of Health, Singapore (1993).

National Research Council (U.S.). Committee on Passive Smoking. (1986). *Environmental tobacco smoke: measuring exposures and assessing health effects*. Washington, D.C., National Academy Press.

National Research Council, C. o. P. S. (1986). *Environmental tobacco smoke: measuring exposures and assessing health effects.* Washington, D.C., National Academy Press.

National Research Council, N. A. o. S. (1993). *Pesticides in the diets of infants and children.* Washington, DC, National Academy Press.

Nazar-Stewart, V., T. L. Vaughan, et al. (2003). "A population-based study of glutathione S-transferase M1, T1 and P1 genotypes and risk for lung cancer." *Lung Cancer 40(3)*: 247-58.

Nebert, D. W., R. A. McKinnon, et al. (1996). "Human drug-metabolizing enzyme polymorphisms: effects on risk of toxicity and cancer." *DNA Cell Biol. 15(4)*: 273-80.

Nelson, H. H., D. C. Christiani, et al. (1999). "k-ras mutation and occupational asbestos exposure in lung adenocarcinoma: asbestos-related cancer without asbestosis." *Cancer Research. 59(18)*: 4570-3.

Ng, D. P., K. W. Tan, et al. (2005). "CYP1A1 polymorphisms and risk of lung cancer in non-smoking Chinese women: influence of environmental tobacco smoke exposure and GSTM1/T1 genetic variation." *Cancer Causes Control 16(4)*: 399-405.

Noguchi, E., Y. Yokouchi, et al. (2002). "Association between TNFA polymorphism and the development of asthma in the Japanese population." *Am. J. Respir. Crit. Care Med. 166(1)*: 43-6.

Norppa, H. (2004). "Cytogenetic biomarkers and genetic polymorphisms." *Toxicol. Lett. 149(1-3)*: 309-34.

Nyberg, F., S. M. Hou, et al. (1998). "Glutathione S-transferase mu1 and N-acetyltransferase 2 genetic polymorphisms and exposure to tobacco smoke in nonsmoking and smoking lung cancer patients and population controls." *Cancer Epidemiol. Biomarkers Prev. 7(10)*: 875-83.

O'Donnell, A. R., B. G. Toelle, et al. (2004). "Age-specific relationship between CD14 and atopy in a cohort assessed from age 8 to 25 years." *Am. J. Respir. Crit. Care Med. 169(5)*: 615-22.

Olds, D. L., C. R. Henderson, Jr., et al. (1994). "Intellectual impairment in children of women who smoke cigarettes during pregnancy." *Pediatrics 93(2)*: 221-7.

Parain, K., C. Hapdey, et al. (2003). "Cigarette smoke and nicotine protect dopaminergic neurons against the 1-methyl-4-phenyl-1,2,3,6-tetrahydropyridine Parkinsonian toxin." *Brain Res. 984(1-2)*: 224-32.

Parkin, D. M., C. S. Muir, et al. (1992). Cancer incidence in five continetns Vol VI. IARC Scientific Publication No. 120. Lyon, France, International Agency of Research on Cancer.

Parkin, D. M., P. Pisani, et al. (1999). "Global cancer statistics." *CA Cancer J. Clin. 49(1)*: 33-64, 1.

Parsons, W. D., S. G. Carmella, et al. (1998). "A metabolite of the tobacco-specific lung carcinogen 4-(methylnitrosamino)-1-(3-pyridyl)-1-butanone in the urine of hospital workers exposed to environmental tobacco smoke." *Cancer Epidemiol. Biomarkers Prev. 7(3)*: 257-60.

Pavanello, S. and E. Clonfero (2004). "[Individual susceptibility to occupational carcinogens: the evidence from biomonitoring and molecular epidemiology studies]." *G Ital. Med. Lav. Ergon. 26(4)*: 311-21.

Perera, F., K. Hemminki, et al. (2002). "In utero DNA damage from environmental pollution is associated with somatic gene mutation in newborns." *Cancer Epidemiol Biomarkers Prev. 11(10 Pt 1)*: 1134-7.

Perera, F. P. (1997). "Environment and cancer: who are susceptible?" *Science 278(5340)*: 1068-73.

Perera, F. P. and I. B. Weinstein (2000). "Molecular epidemiology: recent advances and future directions." *Carcinogenesis 21(3)*: 517-24.

Pershagen, G., A. Ericson, et al. (1992). "Maternal smoking in pregnancy: does it increase the risk of childhood cancer?" *Int. J. Epidemiol. 21(1)*: 1-5.

Petruzzelli, S., A. Celi, et al. (1998). "Serum antibodies to benzo(a)pyrene diol epoxide-DNA adducts in the general population: effects of air pollution, tobacco smoking, and family history of lung diseases." *Cancer Res. 58(18)*: 4122-6.

Phillips, D. H. (2002). "Smoking-related DNA and protein adducts in human tissues." *Carcinogenesis 23(12)*: 1979-2004.

Piirila, P., H. Wikman, et al. (2001). "Glutathione S-transferase genotypes and allergic responses to diisocyanate exposure." *Pharmacogenetics 11(5)*: 437-45.

Pirkle, J. L., K. M. Flegal, et al. (1996). "Exposure of the US population to environmental tobacco smoke: the Third National Health and Nutrition Examination Survey, 1988 to 1991." *Jama 275(16)*: 1233-40.

Pluth, J. M., M. J. Ramsey, et al. (2000). "Role of maternal exposures and newborn genotypes on newborn chromosome aberration frequencies." *Mutat. Res. 465(1-2)*: 101-11.

Pulling, L. C., K. K. Divine, et al. (2003). "Promoter hypermethylation of the O6-methylguanine-DNA methyltransferase gene: more common in lung adenocarcinomas from never-smokers than smokers and associated with tumor progression." *Cancer Res. 63(16)*: 4842-8.

Raherison, C., A. Taytard, et al. (2003). "[Smoking, asthma and associated phenotypes. An epidemiological approach]." *Rev. Mal. Respir. 20(2 Pt 1)*: 233-47.

Rangasamy, T., C. Y. Cho, et al. (2004). "Genetic ablation of Nrf2 enhances susceptibility to cigarette smoke-induced emphysema in mice." *J. Clin. Invest. 114(9)*: 1248-59.

Redline, S., P. V. Tishler, et al. (1989). "Genotypic and phenotypic similarities in pulmonary function among family members of adult monozygotic and dizygotic twins." *Am. J. Epidemiol. 129(4)*: 827-36.

Repace, J. L., J. Jinot, et al. (1998). "Air nicotine and saliva cotinine as indicators of workplace passive smoking exposure and risk." *Risk Anal. 18(1)*: 71-83.

Report of the scientific committee on tobacco and health. UK: Her Majesty's Stationery Office, Scientific Committee on Tobacco and Health (SCPTH) (1998).

Report on carcinogens. 11th Edition. P. H. S. U.S. Department of Health and Human Services, National Toxicology Program (2005).

Respiratory health effects of passive smoking: lung cancer and other disorders. US Environmental Protection Agency. Washington, DC (1992).

Reynolds, P., S. Hurley, et al. (2004). "Active smoking, household passive smoking, and breast cancer: evidence from the California Teachers Study." *J. Natl. Cancer Inst. 96(1)*: 29-37.

Rimm, E. B., J. Chan, et al. (1995). "Prospective study of cigarette smoking, alcohol use, and the risk of diabetes in men." *Bmj 310(6979)*: 555-9.

Rimm, E. B., J. E. Manson, et al. (1993). "Cigarette smoking and the risk of diabetes in women." *Am. J. Public Health 83(2)*: 211-4.

Ronmark, E., E. Jonsson, et al. (1999). "Different pattern of risk factors for atopic and nonatopic asthma among children--report from the Obstructive Lung Disease in Northern Sweden Study." *Allergy 54(9)*: 926-35.

Rushton, L., C. Courage, et al. (2003). "Estimation of the impact on children's health of environmental tobacco smoke in England and Wales." *J. R Soc. Health 123(3)*: 175-80.

Salvi, G. E., H. P. Lawrence, et al. (1997). "Influence of risk factors on the pathogenesis of periodontitis." *Periodontol. 2000 14*: 173-201.

Samet, J. M., D. Brenner, et al. (1998). *Health effects of exposure to radon: BEIR VI.* Washington DC, National Academy Press.

Sardas, S., B. Karahalil, et al. (1995). "The effect of smoking on sister chromatid exchange rate of newborn infants born to smoking mothers." *Mutat. Res. 341(4)*: 249-53.

Schmitt, J. E., C. A. Prescott, et al. (2005). "The differential heritability of regular tobacco use based on method of administration." *Twin Res. Hum. Genet. 8(1)*: 60-2.

Schoket, B., G. Papp, et al. (2001). "Impact of metabolic genotypes on levels of biomarkers of genotoxic exposure." *Mutat. Res. 482(1-2)*: 57-69.

Schonberger, H. J. and C. P. Van Schayck (1998). "Prevention of asthma in genetically predisposed children in primary care--from clinical efficacy to a feasible intervention programme." *Clin. Exp. Allergy 28(11)*: 1325-31.

Sellers, T. A., J. D. Potter, et al. (1992). "Lung cancer detection and prevention: evidence for an interaction between smoking and genetic predisposition." *Cancer Res. 52(9 Suppl)*: 2694s-2697s.

Sengler, C., A. Haider, et al. (2003). "Evaluation of the CD14 C-159 T polymorphism in the German Multicenter Allergy Study cohort." *Clin. Exp. Allergy 33(2)*: 166-9.

Seow, A., B. Zhao, et al. (1999). "NAT2 slow acetylator genotype is associated with increased risk of lung cancer among non-smoking Chinese women in Singapore." *Carcinogenesis 20(9)*: 1877-81.

Sepkovic, D. W., N. J. Haley, et al. (1986). "Elimination from the body of tobacco products by smokers and passive smokers." *Jama 256(7)*: 863.

Shen, M. R., I. M. Jones, et al. (1998). "Nonconservative amino acid substitution variants exist at polymorphic frequency in DNA repair genes in healthy humans." *Cancer Res. 58(4)*: 604-8.

Shu, X. O., J. A. Ross, et al. (1996). "Parental alcohol consumption, cigarette smoking, and risk of infant leukemia: a Childrens Cancer Group study." *J. Natl. Cancer Inst. 88(1)*: 24-31.

Siegel, D., W. A. Franklin, et al. (1998). "Immunohistochemical detection of NAD(P)H:quinone oxidoreductase in human lung and lung tumors." *Clin. Cancer Res. 4(9)*: 2065-70.

Silverman, E. K. and F. E. Speizer (1996). "Risk factors for the development of chronic obstructive pulmonary disease." *Med. Clin. North Am. 80(3)*: 501-22.

Slezak, R. and M. Sasiadek (2000). "[Poland's syndrome]." Pol Merkuriusz Lek 9(50): 568-71.

Smoking and tobacco control monograph 10: Health effects of exposure to environmental tobacco smoke. Bethesda, MD: National Cancer Institute (1999).

Song, N., W. Tan, et al. (2001). "CYP 1A1 polymorphism and risk of lung cancer in relation to tobacco smoking: a case-control study in China." *Carcinogenesis 22(1)*: 11-6.

Song, S., S. M. Lippman, et al. (2005). "Induction of cyclooxygenase-2 by benzo[a]pyrene diol epoxide through inhibition of retinoic acid receptor-beta 2 expression." *Oncogene 24(56)*: 8268-76.

Sorahan, T., P. Prior, et al. (1997). "Childhood cancer and parental use of tobacco: deaths from 1971 to 1976." *Br. J. Cancer 76(11)*: 1525-31.

Sorsa, M., K. Husgafvel-Pursiainen, et al. (1989). "Cytogenetic effects of tobacco smoke exposure among involuntary smokers." *Mutat. Res. 222(2)*: 111-6.

"State-specific prevalence of cigarette smoking among adults, and children's and adolescents' exposure to environmental tobacco smoke -- United States, 1996." *MMWR Morb. Mortal. Wkly Rep. 46(44)*: 1038-43 (1997).

Stewart, P. M., F. M. Rogerson, et al. (1995). "Type 2 11 beta-hydroxysteroid dehydrogenase messenger ribonucleic acid and activity in human placenta and fetal membranes: its relationship to birth weight and putative role in fetal adrenal steroidogenesis." *J. Clin. Endocrinol. Metab. 80(3)*: 885-90.

Stierum, R. H., G. J. Hageman, et al. (1997). "Age-related negative associations between parameters of cytogenetic damage and ex vivo (+/-)-anti-benzo(a)pyrene diolepoxide-induced unscheduled DNA synthesis in smoking humans." *Cancer Epidemiol. Biomarkers Prev. 6(11)*: 943-8.

Stoney, C. M., L. M. Lentino, et al. (1998). "Environmental tobacco smoke: association with cardiovascular function at rest and during stress." *Int. J. Behav. Med. 5(3)*: 230-44.

Strachan, D. P. and D. G. Cook (1998). "Health effects of passive smoking. 6. Parental smoking and childhood asthma: longitudinal and case-control studies." *Thorax. 53(3)*: 204-12.

Streissguth, A. P., P. D. Sampson, et al. (1994). *The effects of prenatal exposure to alcohol and tobacco: contributions from the Seattle Longitudinal Prospective Study and implications for public policy.* H. L. Needleman and D. Bellinger. Beltimore, The Johns Hopkins University Press: 148-183.

Sunaga, N., T. Kohno, et al. (2002). "Contribution of the NQO1 and GSTT1 polymorphisms to lung adenocarcinoma susceptibility." *Cancer Epidemiol. Biomarkers Prev. 11(8)*: 730-8.

Taioli, E., F. Crofts, et al. (1995). "Radical differences in CYP1A1 genotype and function." *Toxicol. Lett. 77(1-3)*: 357-62.

Talamini, G., C. Bassi, et al. (1999). "Alcohol and smoking as risk factors in chronic pancreatitis and pancreatic cancer." *Dig. Dis. Sci. 44(7)*: 1303-11.

Tang, D., D. Warburton, et al. (1999). "Molecular and genetic damage from environmental tobacco smoke in young children." *Cancer Epidemiol. Biomarkers Prev. 8(5)*: 427-31.

Tang, D. L., A. Rundle, et al. (1998). "Associations between both genetic and environmental biomarkers and lung cancer: evidence of a greater risk of lung cancer in women smokers." *Carcinogenesis 19(11)*: 1949-53.

Tang, X., F. R. Khuri, et al. (2000). "Hypermethylation of the death-associated protein (DAP) kinase promoter and aggressiveness in stage I non-small-cell lung cancer." *J. Natl. Cancer Inst. 92(18)*: 1511-6.

Teixeira, J. P., J. Gaspar, et al. (2002). "Aromatic DNA adduct levels in coke oven workers: correlation with polymorphisms in genes GSTP1, GSTM1, GSTT1 and CYP1A1." *Mutat. Res. 517(1-2)*: 147-55.

The Health Consequences of Involuntary Exposure to Tobacco Smoke: A Report of the Surgeon General. US Department of Health and Human Services (2006).

The health consequences of involuntary smoking. A report of the Surgeon General. Public Health Service. U.S. Department of Health and Human Services, Centers for Disease Control, Center for Health Promotion and Education, Office on Smoking and Health. Rockville, MD (1986).

Thorn, J., J. Brisman, et al. (2001). "Adult-onset asthma is associated with self-reported mold or environmental tobacco smoke exposures in the home." *Allergy 56(4)*: 287-92.

Thun, M. J., C. A. Lally, et al. (1997). "Cigarette smoking and changes in the histopathology of lung cancer." *J. Natl. Cancer Inst. 89(21)*: 1580-1586.

Tobacco free initiative: consultative report. International Consultation on Environmental Tobacco Smoke and Child Health proceedings. Geneva, Switzerland, WHO (1999).

Tucker, J. D., D. A. Eastmond, et al. (1997). *Application of Biomarkers in Cancer Epidemiology. Cytogenetic end-points as biological dosimeters and predictors of risk in epidemiological studies.* P. Toniolo, P. Boffetta, D. E. G. Shukeret al. Lyon, France, IARC: 185–200.

Ueta, E., Y. Tadokoro, et al. (2003). "The effect of cigarette smoke exposure and ascorbic acid intake on gene expression of antioxidant enzymes and other related enzymes in the livers and lungs of Shionogi rats with osteogenic disorders." *Toxicol Sci. 73(2)*: 339-47.

Vahakangas, K. H., W. P. Bennett, et al. (2001). "p53 and K-ras mutations in lung cancers from former and never-smoking women." *Cancer Res. 61(11)*: 4350-6.

Vatsis, K. P., W. W. Weber, et al. (1995). "Nomenclature for N-acetyltransferases." *Pharmacogenetics 5(1)*: 1-17.

Vercelli, D. (2003). "Arginase: marker, effector, or candidate gene for asthma?" *J. Clin. Invest 111(12)*: 1815-7.

Vercelli, D. (2004). "Genetics, epigenetics, and the environment: switching, buffering, releasing." *J. Allergy Clin. Immunol. 113(3)*: 381-6; quiz 387.

Vernooy, J. H., M. Kucukaycan, et al. (2002). "Local and systemic inflammation in patients with chronic obstructive pulmonary disease: soluble tumor necrosis factor receptors are increased in sputum." *Am. J. Respir. Crit. Care Med. 166(9)*: 1218-24.

Vineis, P., H. Bartsch, et al. (1994). "Genetically based N-acetyltransferase metabolic polymorphism and low-level environmental exposure to carcinogens." *Nature 369(6476)*: 154-6.

Vineis, P., F. Veglia, et al. (2003). "CYP1A1 T3801 C polymorphism and lung cancer: a pooled analysis of 2451 cases and 3358 controls." *Int. J. Cancer 104(5)*: 650-7.

Vinke, J. G., A. KleinJan, et al. (1999). "Passive smoking causes an 'allergic' cell infiltrate in the nasal mucosa of non-atopic children." *Int. J. Pediatr. Otorhinolaryngol. 51(2)*: 73-81.

von Ehrenstein, O. S., E. von Mutius, et al. (2002). "Lung function of school children with low levels of alpha1-antitrypsin and tobacco smoke exposure." *Eur. Respir. J. 19(6)*: 1099-106.

von Mutius, E. (2002). "Environmental factors influencing the development and progression of pediatric asthma." *J. Allergy Clin. Immunol. 109(6 Suppl)*: S525-32.

Walter, R., D. J. Gottlieb, et al. (2000). "Environmental and genetic risk factors and gene-environment interactions in the pathogenesis of chronic obstructive lung disease." *Environ. Health Perspect 108 Suppl 4*: 733-42.

Wang, T. J., B. S. Zhou, et al. (1996). "Lung cancer in nonsmoking Chinese women: a case-control study." *Lung Cancer 14 Suppl 1*: S93-8.

Wang, Y., Z. Zhang, et al. (2005). "Tobacco smoke-induced lung tumorigenesis in mutant A/J mice with alterations in K-ras, p53, or Ink4a/Arf." *Oncogene 24(18)*: 3042-9.

Wannamethee, S. G., A. G. Shaper, et al. (2001). "Smoking as a modifiable risk factor for type 2 diabetes in middle-aged men." *Diabetes Care 24(9)*: 1590-5.

Weiss, W. (1997). "Cigarette smoking and lung cancer trends. A light at the end of the tunnel?" *Chest 111(5)*: 1414-6.

Wenten, M., K. Berhane, et al. (2005). "TNF-308 modifies the effect of second-hand smoke on respiratory illness-related school absences." *Am. J. Respir. Crit. Care Med. 172(12)*: 1563-8.

Wenzlaff, A. S., M. L. Cote, et al. (2005). "CYP1A1 and CYP1B1 polymorphisms and risk of lung cancer among never smokers: a population-based study." *Carcinogenesis 26(12)*: 2207-12.

Wenzlaff, A. S., M. L. Cote, et al. (2005). "GSTM1, GSTT1 and GSTP1 polymorphisms, environmental tobacco smoke exposure and risk of lung cancer among never smokers: a population-based study." *Carcinogenesis 26(2)*: 395-401.

Whyatt, R. M., S. J. Garte, et al. (1995). "CYP1A1 messenger RNA levels in placental tissue as a biomarker of environmental exposure." *Cancer Epidemiol. Biomarkers Prev. 4(2)*: 147-53.

Whyatt, R. M., R. M. Santella, et al. (1998). "Relationship between ambient air pollution and DNA damage in Polish mothers and newborns." *Environ. Health Perspect 106 Suppl 3*: 821-6.

Wilce, M. C. and M. W. Parker (1994). "Structure and function of glutathione S-transferases." *Biochim. Biophys. Acta 1205(1)*: 1-18.

Will, J. C., D. A. Galuska, et al. (2001). "Cigarette smoking and diabetes mellitus: evidence of a positive association from a large prospective cohort study." *Int. J. Epidemiol. 30(3)*: 540-6.

Williams, M. D. and A. B. Sandler (2001). "The epidemiology of lung cancer." *Cancer Treatment & Research 105*: 31-52.

Witschi, H., V. I. Oreffo, et al. (1995). "Six-month exposure of strain A/J mice to cigarette sidestream smoke: cell kinetics and lung tumor data." *Fundam. Appl. Toxicol. 26(1)*: 32-40.

Wolf, A., A. Kutz, et al. (2005). "The effect of benzo(a)pyrene on porcine urinary bladder epithelial cells analyzed for the expression of selected genes and cellular toxicological endpoints." *Toxicology 207(2)*: 255-69.

Wong, S. S., N. N. Sun, et al. (2002). "Tissue-specific patterns of neurokinin-1 receptor (NK-1R) gene expression in mice exposed to sidestream cigarette smoke." *Toxicol Ind. Health 18(9-10)*: 435-44.

Woodward, A. and A. J. McMichael (1991). "Passive smoking and cancer risk: the nature and uses of epidemiological evidence." *Eur. J. Cancer 27(11)*: 1472-9.

World cancer report. B. W. Stewart and P. Kleihues. Lyon, IARC Press: 182 (2003).

Wu, D., X. Q. Zhang, et al. (2001). "[Analysis of association between gene polymorphisms of microsomal epoxide hydrolase (EPHX1) and infant birthweight]." *Yi Chuan Xue Bao 28(7)*: 595-600.

Wu, M. F., W. J. Wu, et al. (2004). "Increased expression of cytochrome P4501B1 in peripheral leukocytes from lung cancer patients." *Toxicol. Lett. 150(2)*: 211-9.

Wynder, E. L. and D. Hoffmann (1994). "Smoking and lung cancer: scientific challenges and opportunities." *Cancer Res. 54(20)*: 5284-95.

Yang, K., L. Julan, et al. (2006). "Cadmium reduces 11 beta-hydroxysteroid dehydrogenase type 2 activity and expression in human placental trophoblast cells." *Am. J. Physiol. Endocrino.l Metab 290(1)*: E135-E142.

Yang, M. and M. Y. Pyo (2005). "Molecular epidemiology of lung cancer in female passive smokers." *J. Environ. Sci. Health C Environ. Carcinog. Ecotoxicol. Rev. 23(1)*: 75-97.

Yao, R., Y. Wang, et al. (2005). "K-ras mutations in lung tumors from p53 mutant mice exposed to cigarette smoke." *Exp. Lung Res. 31(2)*: 271-81.

Zenzes, M. T., L. A. Puy, et al. (1998). "Immunodetection of benzo[a]pyrene adducts in ovarian cells of women exposed to cigarette smoke." *Mol. Hum. Reprod. 4(2)*: 159-65.

Zhu, B. Q., C. Heeschen, et al. (2003). "Second hand smoke stimulates tumor angiogenesis and growth." *Cancer Cell 4(3)*: 191-6.

Zimmermann, N., N. E. King, et al. (2003). "Dissection of experimental asthma with DNA microarray analysis identifies arginase in asthma pathogenesis." *J. Clin. Invest 111(12)*: 1863-74.

In: Smoking and Lung Cancer
Editors: E. N. Powers and J. B. Cabbot
ISBN 978-1-60692-367-2

Chapter VIII

Passive Smoking as a Conditioner of Food Habits and Nutritional Status: Repercussions on Health

Rosa M. Ortega, Ana M. López-Sobaler, Aranzazu Aparicio, Laura M. Bermejo, Elena Rodríguez-Rodríguez and M. Carmen Mena
Departamento de Nutrición. Facultad de Farmacia.
Universidad Complutense. Ciudad Universitaria s/n. 28040- Madrid, Spain

Abstract

Many studies have associated passive smoking with an increased risk of developing certain diseases. Smoking during pregnancy increases the risk of the newborn having a low birth weight (at term or pre-term), and of suffering impaired respiratory function and ischaemic heart disease etc. In children and adolescents, environmental exposure to tobacco smoke has been associated with abnormal lipid profiles and an increased risk of atherosclerosis. Passive smoking can also be the cause of reduced female fertility in the general population. The food habits of both active and passive smokers may also be negatively affected.

The diets of smokers tend to be less adequate than those of non-smokers. Exposure to tobacco smoke modifies the sense of taste and smell, leading to changes in food preferences and food intake, and eventually to a more imbalanced diet. Matters are made worse in that smokers may have greater needs of certain nutrients such as antioxidants. Thus, even with a normal intake of these nutrients, the nutritional status of smokers can be inadequate.

As with active smokers, passive smokers may show slightly unhealthy food habits and more imbalanced diets than non-smokers – either as a consequence of living with smokers (and therefore sharing their food habits) or via the direct modification of their food choices. Passive smokers consume fewer fruits and vegetables and have lower intakes of a number of nutrients, which might be reflected at the serum level. For example, exposure to tobacco smoke is associated with reduced folate levels, via which some of the effects of active and passive smoking on health may be made manifest. Like active smokers, passive smokers may have a greater need of certain nutrients. For example, they show lower plasma concentrations of antioxidants than do non-smokers not exposed to smoke, independent of the differences in dietary antioxidant intake.

The diet of passive smokers may be an important factor in the relationship between tobacco smoke exposure and health problems. Although the cessation of smoking and the avoidance of passive smoking is the ideal goal, it cannot always be attained. Dietary intervention may therefore be a useful and indeed necessary strategy to prevent or delay smoking-related pathologies.

Introduction

Tobacco smoke is composed of mainstream smoke, which is directly inhaled by the smoker, and sidestream smoke, generated by the spontaneous combustion of the cigarette. Environmental tobacco smoke (ETS) consists of sidestream smoke and the smoke exhaled by the smoker, also known as second-hand smoke. "Passive smoking" is the involuntary inhalation by a non-smoker of smoke generated in his neighbourhood by one or more smokers (Romero-Palacios, 2004).

Tobacco smoke contains over 4000 chemicals in the form of particles and gases. The particulate phase includes tar (itself composed of many compounds), nicotine, benzene and benzo(a)pyrene. The gas phase includes carbon monoxide, ammonia, dimethylnitrosamine, formaldehyde, hydrogen cyanide and acrolein (Bermúdez et al., 1994; Eiserich et al., 1995). Some of these have markedly irritant properties and some 60 are known or suspected carcinogens (Romero-Palacios, 2004). Thus, tobacco smoke is an important source of oxidative stress, whether exposure is active of passive (Cross et al., 1999).

Currently, exposure to ETS, or passive smoking, affects between 20% and 80% of the population depending on the country, and is associated with long- and short-term health risks, especially ischaemic heart disease and lung cancer (Romero-Palacios, 2004). Smoking and exposure to ETS are the main causes of preventable morbidity and premature disease and death in developed countries (US Department of Health Education and Welfare, 1971).

Exposure to ETS may occur in the home, at the workplace, or in public places. The degree of exposure depends on several factors, e.g., the number of smokers in the vicinity, how much they smoke, the duration of exposure, and the characteristics of the exposure location (Romero-Palacios, 2004).

The exposure of children to ETS is a worldwide problem. In 1996, a national survey carried out in China found that 53.6% of non-smoker children and adults were exposed to ETS, with exposure defined as being in the presence of tobacco smoke for at least 15 minutes per day for more than 1 day per week (Yang et al., 1999). In 1998, nearly half of all US children under 5 years of age were reported to be exposed to ETS (Samet and Yang, 2001). In the UK, 42% of English children and 60% of Scottish children were reported exposed to ETS by parental smoking (Samet and Yang, 2001). According to a number of studies from Spain, between 48% and 69% of children and teenagers are exposed to smoke in their homes (Fuertes et al., 2001). A recent study in Granada on a sample of 504 children between the ages of 3 and 6 found that 57.6% lived in houses polluted with tobacco smoke by their parents and other relatives (Muñoz et al., 2003) Such data, however, is not available in most countries. According to the World Health Organization, some 1000 million adult smokers, and at least 700 million children, breath household ETS (WHO, 1999).

The determination of cotinine in serum, urine, and saliva is commonly used as a measure of exposure (active or passive) to tobacco smoke (Pirkle et al., 1996). Cotinine is the major metabolite of nicotine and has a half-life of about 16 - 20 hours (Jarvis et al., 1988; Benowitz et al., 1983). The serum cotinine level reflects exposure to nicotine largely from the previous 1 - 2 days. Both the children of smokers (Pirkle et al., 1996) and other adults who live with smokers (Kim et al., 2004) have higher concentrations of cotinine in their blood and saliva.

Relationship between Passive Smoking and Health Problems

For many years it was thought that passive smoking was ofohittle or no importance, causing only mild irritation of the conjunctiva and upper respiratory tract. However, the sanitary and social importance of passive smoking is becoming ever more evident, and its many repercussions affect all population groups.

The evidence regarding the health risks of passive smoking comes from epidemiological studies that have assessed the association between exposure to ETS and its negative effects on health, and from our growing knowledge regarding the components of ETS and their toxicities.

Health Problems in Expectant Mothers and their in Utero-Exposed Children

Some of the studies published over the last 15 years show that smoking, both active and passive, is related to reduced female fertility (Nizard, 2005). Others suggest that exposure during pregnancy can have negative effects on the child such as delayed intauterine development, low birth weight, and an increased risk of sudden death (Kalinka et al., 2005; Ortega et al., 2004; Tong et al., 2005). The children of mothers who are passively exposed to ETS during pregnancy are more likely to suffer asthma and are at greater risk of negative developmental outcomes (Barber et al., 1996). Such exposure also seems to be related to the cognitive capacity of child, who might experience difficulties in the comprehension of written texts and show learning difficulties (Rauh et al., 2004; Ortega et al., 2004; Yolton et al., 2005).

Health Problems in Child Passive Smokers

Passive smoking in children has been the subject of many studies. Exposure occurs basically at home and in play environments. As children grow up, exposure to maternal smoking decreases and the influence of smoke from other sources, such as ETS in public places, increases. Such exposure, particularly maternal smoking, undoubtedly influences the development of asthma in children (Heraud and Herbelin-Wagne, 2002; Gilliland et al., 2002).

ETS clearly has an effect on the respiratory system. In newborns and young infants, this may lead to an increased risk of suffering infections, including pneumonia and bronchitis (which can more be more severe than normal). Chronic respiratory problems such as childhood asthma may develop, and lung development may be slowed down (Mannino et al., 2001; Klerman, 2004).

Exposure to ETS has also been related to acute otitis in the first four years of life (the most common cause of deafness in children) (Klerman, 2004), and bacterial meningitis, the prevalence of which is greater among children exposed for longer periods (Iles et al., 2001).

Some authors report exposure to ETS to be associated with a greater risk of sudden death in babies (Tong et al., 2005), and with a greater probability of complications developing during surgery requiring general anaesthesia (Drongowski et al., 2003).

The results of other studies indicate ETS to have neurotoxic activity. Thus, constant exposure to ETS could have a negative influence on certain cognitive abilities in children and adolescents, e.g., greater difficulty in learning to read, greater difficulty in correctly solving mathematical problems, and perhaps even defects in the development of spatial vision (Yolton et al., 2005).

In adolescents, exposure is associated with an increased prevalence of headaches and eye irritation (Borzecki et al., 2005), and with the appearance of metabolic syndrome, perhaps including increased resistance to insulin (Weitzman et al., 2005).

Currently there is no clear scientific evidence of a direct relationship between exposure to ETS and an increased risk of childhood cancer (World Health Organization International Agency for Research on Cancer, 2002).

Health Problems in Adult Passive Smokers

Exposure to ETS has been causally related to lung cancer; this has been reported in many large epidemiological studies and by numerous groups of experts (National Research Council, 1986; US Environmental Protection Agency, 1992; Scientific Committee on Tobacco and Health, 1998; World Health Organisation, International Agency for Research on Cancer, 2002). Some studies also suggest that constant, prolonged exposure to ETS leads to other types of cancer such as leukaemia (Kasim et al., 2005).

Numerous observational and experimental studies have also causally related ETS exposure to coronary heart disease (California Environmental Protection Agency, 1997; Scientific Committee on Tobacco and Health, 1998; Samet., 2002); some studies also indicate that the risk of myocardial infarction is increased (Qureshi et al., 2005). Passive smokers (both children and adults) show increased total cholesterol, LDL-C and VLDL-C levels. Their total/HDL-C ratio is also increased and their HDL-C levels are lower (Holay et al., 2004; Azizi et al., 2002; Zhang, 1992; Neufeld et al., 1997; Whig et al., 1992; Feldman et al., 1991) – all of which increases the risk of developing atherosclerosis (Ambrose and Barua, 2004; Feldman et al., 1991).

Evidence also exists linking ETS to the worsening of asthma, reduced lung function, and other respiratory problems. However, these associations have not yet been declared causal (California Environmental Protection Agency, 1997; Scientific Committee on Tobacco and Health, 1998). Other studies show that people exposed to ETS are also at greater risk of periodontal problems (Arbes et al., 2001), and that they more commonly suffer allergies such as allergic rhinitis. This suggests ETS to be linked to a weakening of the immune system (Topp et al., 2005).

Recent studies associate ETS exposure to a reduction in bone mineral density, which may have a negative effect on development and the appearance of osteoporosis. Serum cotinine levels have been shown to be inversely correlated with bone mineral content in both males and females (Benson and Shulman, 2005).

Health Problems in Elderly Passive Smokers

In elderly people, exposure to tobacco smoke may have the same negative effects as in adults, but also appears to be directly related to the appearance and development of macular degeneration and even blindness (Khan et al., 2006). It has also been related to an increased incidence of cataracts (Ortega et al., 1994a).

Some studies have related prolonged and constant exposure to ETS to hearing losses, both in adults and the elderly (Nomura et al., 2005), although long-term longitudinal studies are need to confirm this.

It should be borne in mind that elderly people tend to remain indoors more often than younger people. If these places were smoke-polluted they would be in contact with ETS for longer, which might have a negative effect on their health (Simoni et al., 2003)

In summary, the disease load caused by smoking is huge, and its impact on public health around the world enormous – reason enough for programmes aimed at controlling smoking to be given high priority.

Changes in the Food Habits and Nutritional Status of Passive Smokers That May Increase Risks to Health

Reasons for Changes in Food Habits in Passive Smokers

Smokers' diets tend to be less adequate than those of non-smokers (Ortega et al., 1994b; Ortega, 2003; Ortega et al., 2004). Chronic cigarette smokers consume a smaller amount of phytonutrient-rich foods; this has been reported for smokers in the UK (Pollard et al., 2001), Canada (Palaniappan et al., 2001), the United States (Subar et al., 1990), and the Netherlands (Zondervan et al., 1996). The available evidence also indicates that the heaviest smokers invariably consume fewer fruits and vegetables than those who smoke fewer cigarettes per day (Ma et al., 2000; Birkett, 1999; Ortega et al., 1994b; Ortega et al., 2004). While the evidence is more limited, some epidemiological data suggest that male smokers are more likely than female smokers to consume fewer fruits and vegetables (Ma et al., 2000). Cigarette smokers appear to make up for the energy deficit created by consuming more dietary fats, especially saturated fats (Palaniappan et al., 2001; Ma et al., 2000; Birkett, 1999).

Non-smokers who live with smokers also have poorer dietary habits than those who live in non-smoking households. This relationship may be due to shared family lifestyle patterns. Some studies show that women married to smokers are significantly less likely to eat cooked or fresh vegetables more than once a day than women not exposed to ETS (Forastiere et al., 2000). In the study by Emmons et al., (1995), which involved 10,833 non-smokers, those exposed to ETS at home had significantly lower intakes of all the micronutrients studied compared to those free of household exposure. Exposure to ETS at the workplace was associated with lower intakes of vitamin C (but not the other micronutrients examined), fruits and vegetables. These authors indicate that home exposure to ETS was a stronger predictor of intake than workplace exposure (Table 1).

It should be remembered that parents have a decisive influence on the food habits and physical activity patterns of their children (Nicklas et al., 2004). Early childhood and the social environment in which the child takes his/her meals are widely assumed to be critical in the establishment of lifelong healthy eating habits. In their family life, the children of smokers are exposed to more imbalanced diets (Table 1).

Exposure to tobacco smoke modifies the sense of taste and smell, leading to changes in food preferences and food intake; the diets of passive smokers could therefore be more imbalanced. Active smokers certainly have a reduced sense of taste and smell (Reibel, 2003). Some studies indicate that smokers have a reduced capacity to recognise sweet, salty and sour tastes, and that the sensitivity of their tongue receptors to electric stimuli is slightly lower than that of non-smokers (Suliburska et al., 2004; Sato et al., 2002). The same can occur in passive smokers, and has been recorded in children. The children of smokers were found to be less able to identify certain smells than those who lived in generally smoke-free environments (Nageris et al., 2001).

It may also be the case that the lifestyles of passive smokers are more inadequate, perhaps because of the influence of the smokers with whom they live. In the U.K a study of 5036 non-smokers showed that those living with smokers ate more fried food, chips and butter, and less fruit and margarine than those living with other non-smokers (Thompson and Warburton, 1992). Koo et al., (1997), investigated the characteristics of non-smoking women from different countries (530 from Hong Kong, 13,047 from Japan, 87 from Sweden, and 144 from the U.S) who were married to either smokers or non-smokers. Independent of the country of residence, wives with smoking husbands generally ate less healthy diets, with a tendency to eat more fried food and less fruit than wives of non-smoking husbands. In addition, the women married to smokers scored worse in terms of behaviour regarded as healthy, e.g., avoiding obesity, controlling dietary cholesterol and alcohol, or taking vitamins and participating in preventive screening. These patterns suggest that wives who have never smoked but who have smoker husbands tend to share their less healthy dietary traits, and therefore to have dietary habits associated with an increased risk for lung cancer and heart disease.

Non-smoker women married to smokers also tend to be less well educated, to take fewer supplements, to drink alcohol more frequently, and to have lower vitamin A, C and calcium intakes, which may increase the risk of developing cancer (Matanoski et al., 1995). Passive smokers also have a lower consumption of vegetables and a lower folic acid intake than non-smoking women not exposed to EST (Ortega et al., 2004) (Tables 1 and 2).

Reasons for the Poorer Nutritional Status of Passive Smokers Even when their Intakes are Similar to those of Non-Smokers

Passive smokers may have higher requirements for some nutrients, such as antioxidants; thus, even with the same intake as non-smokers, they may have a poorer nutritional status.

Tobacco smoke contains a great variety of reactive oxygen species, reactive nitrogen species, free radicals, and many toxic compounds that together act as an important source of oxidative stress. Therefore, the antioxidant defences of both active and passive smokers can be placed under strain (Aycicek et al., 2005; Jacob, 2000). As seen in active smokers, passive smokers have lower levels of certain micronutrients, especially antioxidants. Exposure to even small quantities of tobacco smoke can affect the concentrations of antioxidant nutrients (Alberg, 2000), and thus lead to adverse effects. It should be remembered that the association between exposure and lower blood levels of nutrients might be underestimated if passive smokers classify themselves as non-smokers (Alberg, 2002) – something often seen.

Second hand smoke contains numerous oxidants and pro-oxidants that can produce free radicals and perhaps initiate lipid peroxidation (Church and Pryor, 1985). Free radicals are sequestered by antioxidants in the serum, thus providing greater protection against oxidation reactions. However, if this protection fails, peroxidation of LDL cholesterol may occur. This, plus the accumulation of cholesterol in macrophages, signals the start of atherosclerosis (Brown and Goldstein, 1983), and may be one of the reasons why cardiovascular diseases are more common among active smokers (Schectman et al., 1991). The circulating concentration of antioxidants in passive smokers is also lower than in non-smokers not exposed to EST (Valkonen and Kuusi, 1998).

Ascorbic acid levels can become reduced by two thirds within 90 minutes of being exposed to EST – something not seen with other antioxidants such as vitamin E, retinol, beta-carotene and uric acid (Valkonen and Kuusi, 1998). Acute exposure in non-smokers may therefore lead to deteriorated antioxidant defences in the serum, accelerate lipid peroxidation, and the accumulation of LDL cholesterol in the macrophages. It has even been suggested that the oxidative stress induced by second hand smoke may be worse in non-smokers than in active smokers, who are more accustomed to dealing with tobacco smoke (Glantz and Parmley, 1995)

Nutrient Intake and Nutritional Status: Changes in Passive Smokers

Differences in Energy Intake

Exposure to tobacco smoke leads to a reduction in appetite, which in turn leads to a reduction in the intake of food, and therefore of energy (Curtin et al., 1999) (Table 2). This loss of appetite has been associated with a reduction in neuropeptide Y in the hypothalamus in animals (Chen et al., 2005; Chen et al., 2006). In addition, nicotine can increase energy expenditure by 10 fold, leading to a reduction in body fat and body weight in active and passive smokers (Powledge, 2004; Pfeffer and Kaufer-Horwitz, 2001). One of the most representative examples of this is the often low birth weight of children borne to mothers who smoke (Ortega et al., 1998a; Steyn et al., 2006) - although it is also true that expectant mothers who smoke have a lower energy intake compared to their non-smoking counterparts (Ortega et al., 1998a).

Differences in the Intake of Macronutrients

Numerous studies have shown that the food habits of smokers are very different – and generally less healthy – than those of non-smokers (Dyer et al., 2003). Smokers consume fewer fruits, vegetables and wholemeal cereals than non-smokers (Ortega, 2003; Osler, 1998; Palaniappan et al., 2001), and thus their intake of carbohydrates, fibre, antioxidant vitamins and polyunsaturated fats is also lower (Reynolds et al., 2004; Schroder et al., 2002; Palaniappan et al., 2001; Dallongeville et al., 1998). In addition, they consume more meat, alcoholic drinks and coffee than non-smokers (Osler, 1998), which favours a higher intake of saturated fat and cholesterol (Palaniappan et al., 2001; Dallongeville et al., 1998) (Table 2). These habits are also taken up by those who live with smokers (Osler, 1998), and even though they are non-smokers their diets are also less healthy than those of other non-smokers (see Reynolds et al., 2004; Curtin et al., 1999; Crawley and While, 1996). It has been shown that people exposed to tobacco smoke have food habits similar to those of smokers, with a lower intake of water, fruits and vegetables (Alberg et al., 2000; Koo et al., 1997; Matanoski et al., 1995). This translates into a lower intake in fibre and vitamins than that seen in non-smokers (Hampl et al., 2001). They also have a higher consumption of alcohol and fried foods (Koo et al., 1997; Matanoski et al., 1995), and therefore greater intakes of ethanol and saturated fats and cholesterol than do non-smokers (Table 2).

Differences in Vitamin Intake and Vitamin Status

As mentioned above, passive smokers have less healthy food habits and tend to consume smaller quantities of fruits and vegetables. Therefore, their intake of vitamins and minerals also tends to be inferior. This, along with the direct effect of tobacco on antioxidant levels could lead to lower concentrations of these vitamins in the blood (Alberg et al., 2000; Lewis et al., 2005) (Table 3).

Plasma concentrations of antioxidant vitamins are significantly lower in passive smoker infants and their mothers than in non-passive smoker infants and their mothers. In addition, lipid peroxidation and the oxidative stress index is remarkably higher in passive smoker infants and their mothers than in their non-passive counterparts. Significant correlations also exist between the oxidative and antioxidative parameters of passive smoker infants and their mothers (Aycicek et al., 2005).

As mentioned above, the compounds present in tobacco smoke are an important source of oxidative stress, and therefore the antioxidant capacity of active and smokers can be strongly challenged. Several studies report that active and passive smokers have lower levels of vitamin C, tocopherol, and carotenes (Alberg et al., 2000; Lykkesfeldt et al., 2000; Valkonen and Kuusi, 1998). This could be due to their greater use in the protection of cells from free radicals induced by tobacco smoke (Marangon et al., 1998), to a reduced intake of vitamin-rich foods (Ma et al., 2000), or both (Dallongeville et al., 1998).

Vitamin C is an effective free radical scavenger and is among the strongest determinants of plasma total antioxidant defence capability (Lykkesfeldt et al., 2000). The intake of vitamin C is lower in passive smokers than in non-smokers (Trobs et al., 2002). In addition, several studies that have quantified exposure to EST in passive smokers in terms of urine cotinine levels have shown that individuals with high cotinine levels take in smaller quantities of vitamin C (Wei et al., 2001). As with folates, the greater the duration of exposure to EST, the less vitamin C is consumed (Farchi et al., 2001) (Table 2). Numerous studies have shown that smoking, or being exposed to tobacco smoke, reduces the plasma concentration of this vitamin (Ayaori et al., 2000), even when exposure is minimal (Preston et al., 2003). In one study involving active, passive and non-smokers it was found that passive smokers had a plasma concentration of ascorbic acid intermediate between those of the others two groups, even when the intake of the vitamin was similar in all three groups (Tribble et al., 1993). In another study, a reduction in ascorbic acid levels was seen after exposure to EST (Valkonen and Kuusi, 1998). Even a short exposure led to a significant reduction, and therefore to an impairment of the antioxidant defence system (Valkonen and Kuusi, 1998) (Table 3).

During their intrauterine development, the children of smokers are effectively passive smokers, and thus suffer similar problems of low vitamin C levels. In addition, even though maternal blood levels of vitamin C may be similar to those of non-smokers, the milk of mothers who smoke contains less vitamin C than that of non-smokers. Thus, the breast-fed newborns of smoker mothers continue to have lower vitamin C levels after birth (Ortega et al., 1998b).

The length of time spent exposed to EST has an important effect on plasma vitamin C levels. One study involving passive smokers showed that women who spent 2 hours per day or less in the presence of EST had a higher plasma ascorbic acid level than those who were exposed for 2-8 hours per day (Mena, 2003).

Vitamin E is also a powerful antioxidant, and is the main lipophilic antioxidant in cell membranes. Protection against lipid peroxidation is achieved by its acting directly on a wide range of oxygen radicals (Jialal and Gruñid, 1993). However, the data coming from studies performed on vitamin E levels in smokers have been the centre of controversy.

The intake of vitamin E would appear to be lower in passive smokers than in non-smokers (Bruno and Traber, 2005). In addition, the concentration of this vitamin in the maternal milk of smokers is lower than that of non-smokers, even though dietary intake of the vitamin during pregnancy and maternal serum levels are similar to those of non-smoker mothers. Thus, children born to mothers who smoke (already intrauterine passive smokers) receive less vitamin E via their mothers' milk than do those born to non-smokers (Ortega et al., 1998a).

In vitro investigations have consistently demonstrated that cigarette smoke depletes plasma vitamin E as well as other antioxidants (Handelman et al., 1996). However, the plasma alpha- and gamma-tocopherol concentrations of smokers either do not differ (Leonard et al., 2003) or are lower (Bolton-Smith et al., 1991) than those that, compared to non-smokers, smokers and passive smokers have higher plasma concentrations of gamma-tocopherol, but not alpha-tocopherol (Dietrich et al., 2003b). Marangon et al., (1998) observed a plasma alpha-tocopherol level increase of 5% in smokers in comparison with non-smokers. Sobczak et al., (2004), however, indicate a statistically significant reduction in plasma alpha-tocopherol level in passive and active smokers compared to non-smokers, whereas smoking had virtually no influence on the gamma-tocopherol level.

It should be remembered that one of the reasons why lower tocopherol levels are not always seen in smokers is that, even though this vitamin suffers the oxidising effects of tobacco smoke it can be regenerated to its active form via the action of other antioxidants. This helps to maintain total tocopherol levels in plasma (Halliwell, 1996a).

The intake of beta-carotene is also lower in passive smokers compared to non-smokers, and is inversely related to the magnitude of exposure to ETS (Curtin et al., 1999; Dallongeville et al., 1998). In addition, people exposed to a greater degree show significantly lower serum beta-carotene levels (Farchi et al., 2001) (Table 3). This may be a reflection of the lower fruit and vegetable consumption of passive smokers since beta-carotene is the best biomarker of their recent intake (Ziegler et al., 1996).

In passive smokers, the duration of exposure to tobacco smoke seems to have an important influence on nutritional status. Mena (2003) found that women exposed to ETS for eight or more hours per day were more likely to show deficient serum beta-carotene levels (80%) than those exposed for 2-8 hours (20%) or those exposed for two hours or less (36.4%).

The fact that passive smokers have lower serum retinol concentrations than non-smokers may be due to the greater use of this antioxidant vitamin in the neutralisation of the free radicals in tobacco smoke, although they could also be a reflection of the effect of tobacco smoke on diet (Chelchowska et al., 2001) (Tables 2 and 3).

Both active and passive smoking are associated with a lower intake of folates (which is often low in the general population anyway) (Ortega et al., 2004), and with lower levels of serum and erythrocyte folic acid (Mannino et al., 2003). In addition, folate intake decreases with the duration of exposure (Ortega et al., 2004).

Exposure to tobacco smoke remains associated with lower serum and erythrocyte folate levels even after adjustment for folic acid intake (Mannino et al., 2003; Voutilainen et al.,

2001) (Table 3). These reduced folate levels may be one of the ways via which some of the health effects of active and passive smoking are eventually made manifest.

Differences in Mineral Intake and Status

Serum iron concentration can be higher in people most exposed to tobacco smoke since the carbon monoxide it contains provokes tissue hypoxia, to which the body reacts by increasing the synthesis of haemoglobin. This, of course, requires iron (Smith and Fischer, 2001) (Table 3). However, higher serum iron levels can be harmful since this mineral can contribute to increased oxidative stress (Whitfield et al., 2001).

The newborns of mothers who smoke (and who were therefore intra-uterine passive smokers) have lower levels of zinc, although an adequate maternal dietary intake of this mineral can resolve this problem (King, 2000). However, it is quite normal for such mothers – and indeed non-smoker mothers – not to take in sufficient zinc (Ortega et al., 1998a).

The dietary intake of calcium by passive smokers is often lower than that of non-smokers. The effects on health can be serious since tobacco also reduces the absorption of this mineral (Morabia et al., 2000) (Table 2).

Table 1. Differences in food intake in active, passive and non-smokers

Food	Non smokers	Active smokers	Passive smokers	Reference
Animal Fat (servings/week)	8.2	9.4	8.3	Osler, 1998
Coffee (servings/week)	4.1	6.2	4.5	Osler, 1998
Cereals (g/day)	169		131	Curtin et al., 1999
(servings/week)	22.2	21.7	21.7	Osler, 1998
Eggs (servings/week)	1.8	1.8	1.7	Osler, 1998
Fish (servings/week)	1	0.7	0.8	Osler, 1998
Fruits (g/day)	235.5±142.4	203.5±187.5	197.0±160.0	Ortega et al., 2004
(servings/day)	1.3	0.7	1.2	Dietrich et al., 2003b
(servings/day)	0.96±0.03	0.52±0.04	0.86±0.06	Strauss, 2001
(servings/week)	5.8	4.2	5.6	Osler, 1998
Meat (g)	40.9		31.3	Curtin et al., 1999
(servings/week)	4.7	5.4	5.1	Osler, 1998
Vegetables (g/day)	272.1±124.1	235.8±122.0	231.1±108.4	Ortega et al., 2004
(g/day)	230		186	Curtin et al., 1999
(servings/day)	2.5	2.2	2.5	Dietrich et al., 2003b
(servings/week)	6.1	3.7	5.8	Osler, 1998
Alcoholic drinks (g/day)	34.8±82.0	71.6±111.3	31.7±66.8	Ortega et al., 2004

Table 2. Differences in nutrient intake in active, passive and non-smokers

Nutrien	Non smokers	Active smokers	Passive smokers	Reference
Carbohydrates (%)	22.3		21.0	Curtin et al., 1999
Energy (Kcal)	1822		1636	Curtin et al., 1999
(MJ/day)	8.5±2.2	8.0±2.1	8.5±1.8	Ortega et al., 2004
Fiber (g/day)	15.0		13.0	Curtin et al., 1999
(g/day)	20.1±6.4	15.3±4.5	18.0±5.9	Tröbs et al., 2002
Alcohol (g/day)	2.5±5.4	5.2±8.4	2.6±5.1	Ortega et al., 2004
Linoleic Acid (g/day)	12.4±4.6	10.5±3.1	10.9±4.5	Tröbs et al., 2002
Beta-carotene (mg/day)	3.2±2.7	2.0±1.4	2.7±1.7	Trobs et al., 2002
(mg/day)	2,5	1,8	2,0	Dietrich et al., 2003b
(mg/day)	3,3		2,4	Curtin et al., 1999
(μg/day)	3429± 2044		-22.4±206.0 *	Farchi et al., 2001
Lycopene (μg/day)	4629	3197	3328	Dietrich et al., 2003b
Retinol (μg/day)	392	351	358	Dietrich et al., 2003b
(μg/day)	611.9±606.4		-37.1±63.4 *	Farchi et al., 2001
Vitamin E (alpha TE/day)	8.8	8.0	9.5	Dietrich et al., 2003b
(mg/day)	11.4±4.1	9.3±3.0	10.0±3.9	Tröbs et al., 2002
(mg/day)	9.0±3.8		0.01±0.38*	Farchi et al., 2001
Vitamin C (mg/day)	96.7±49.5	73.9±37.0	92.4±42.8	Tröbs et al., 2002
(mg/day)	86.5	66.4	89.1	Dietrich et al., 2003b
(mg/day)	94.2		83.8	Preston et al., 2003
(mg/day)	111.3±3.3	95.8±7.2	104.8±5.0	Strauss, 2001
(mg/day)	113	142	104	Tribble et al., 1993
(mg/day)	151.0±90.2		-5.2±7.7 *	Farchi et al., 2001
Cobalamin (μg/día)	5.4±3.5	5.3±2.5	4.9±2.8	Tröbs et al., 2002
Folate (μg/day)	181.7±72.4	159.1±65.7	165.2±66.6	Ortega et al., 2004
(μg/day)	318±173	252±110	276±173	Trobs et al., 2002
Iron (mg/day)	9.7		8.4	Curtin et al., 1999

* Difference with Non Smoker

In conclusion, passive smokers have less adequate food habits rendering them more susceptible to the serious health problems that can be provoked by tobacco. Active and passive smoking both lead to lower circulating concentrations of micronutrients, and consequently to a poorer nutritional status and increased health risks. The diet of passive smokers may be an important factor in the relationship between tobacco smoke exposure and health problems. Although the cessation of smoking and the avoidance of passive smoking is the ideal goal, it cannot always be attained. Dietary intervention may therefore be a useful and indeed necessary strategy to prevent or delay smoking-related pathologies.

Table 3. Differences in serum concentration/biochemical data in active, passive and non-smokers

Parameter	Non smokers	Active smokers	Passive smokers	Reference
Ascorbic acid (µmol/L)	42.6±12.9	41.8±14.7	43.4±12.4	Tröbs et al., 2002
(µmol/L)	60.8	40.3	59.1	Dietrich et al., 2003b
(µmol/L)	59±3.8		44±4.4	Valkonen y Kuusi, 1998
(µmol/L)	54.5	43.6	54.6	Dietrich et al., 2003b*
(µmol/L)	52.1		48.9	Preston et al., 2003
(µmol/L)	70	40	53	Tribble et al., 1993
(ng/mL)	0.94±0.30		-0.06±0.04 *	Farchi et al., 2001
(mg/dL)	0.94±0.36		-0.04±0.02*	Forastiere et al., 2000
Alpha tocopherol (µmol/L)	30.0	30.0	29.3	Dietrich et al., 2003b
(µmol/L)	22±1.4		21±1.4	Valkonen y Kuusi, 1998
(ng/mL)	10972±5023		-636.9±512.3 *	Farchi et al., 2001
(ng/mL)	10934±4902		-78.4±292*	Forastiere et al., 2000
(µmol/ mg cholesterol/L)	01.5±0.3	1.4±0.2	1.5±0.2	Tröbs et al., 2002
Gamma-tocopherol (µmol/L)	6.0	7.9	7.8	Dietrich et al., 2003b
Alpha carotene (µmol/L)	0.064	0.036	0.039	Dietrich et al., 2003b
(ng/mL)	57.1± 70.0		-7.8±7.6 *	Farchi et al., 2001
(ng/mL)	57.0±69.4		-1.24±4.34*	Forastiere et al., 2000
Beta Carotene (µmol/L)	0.25	0.16	0.15	Dietrich et al., 2003b
(µmol/L)	1.06±0.75	0.73±0.43	0.97±0.56	Trobs et al., 2002
(ng/mL)	345.6±351.3		-32.0±32.9 *	Farchi et al., 2001
(ng/mL)	346.9±350.5		-21.9±19.1*	Forastiere et al., 2000
Total corotenoids (µmol/L)	1.84	1.51	1.52	Dietrich et al., 2003b
Plasma retinol (µmol/L)	2.21		1.86	Hozyasz and Chelchowska, 2004
(µmol/L)	2.17	2.33	2.06	Dietrich et al., 2003b
(ng/mL)	523.0±292.7		-13.4±29.5 *	Farchi et al., 2001
(ng/mL)	520.5±291.5		-10.6±17.0*	Forastiere et al., 2000
Cobalamin (pmol/L)	238±111	241±83	239±127	Tröbs et al., 2002
Folate (serum) (nmol/L)	18.7±6.1	17.1±6.6	18.8±6.3	Tröbs et al., 2002
(nmol/L)	18.4±6.7	16.5±5.5	16.7±6.5	Ortega et al., 2004
(log nmol/L)		-0.29*	-0.16 *	Mannino et al., 2003
Folate (Erythrocyte) (nmol/L)	889.3±421.5	879.6±393.1	828.9±385.0	Ortega et al., 2004
(nmol/L)		-86 *	-50 *	Mannino et al., 2003
Total Cholesterol (mg/dL)	227.3±49.7		-1.34±2.86*	Forastiere et al., 2000
HDL-Cholesterol (mg/dL)	43±11	38±10	42±11	Azizi et al., 2002
(mg/dL)	59±15	53±13	60±15	Tröbs et al., 2002
(mg/dL)	50.7±13.5		-0.80±0.79*	Forastiere et al., 2000
Tryglicerides (mg/dL)	89.8±52.7		-0.12±3.0*	Forastiere et al., 2000
(mg/dL)	92±64	101±61	90±46	Tröbs et al., 2002
Homocystein (µmol/L)	11.9±4.9	12.4±4.0	11.1±3.4	Tröbs et al., 2002
(µmol/L)	8.8±2.4	9.4±2.9	8.27±1.99	Ortega et al., 2004
Lycopene (µmol/L)	0.73	0.71	0.67	Dietrich et al., 2003b
(ng/mL)	357.4±221.9		-32.7±30.0 *	Farchi et al., 2001
(ng/mL)	358.9±224.2		18.8±17.6*	Forastiere et al., 2000
(µmol/mmol cholesterol)	0.48		0.33	Hozyasz y Chelchowska, 2004

* Difference with Non Smoker

Proposed Dietary Modifications for Passive Smokers

Dietary intervention could be helpful in preventing or delaying smoking-related disease.

With the aim of reducing the oxidative effects of tobacco smoke, several national and international bodies have indicated that the requirements of vitamin C in smokers (and by extension passive smokers) are greater than those of non-smokers (see Ortega, 2003; Cross et al., 1999). Taking a daily supplement of vitNªin C for two months reduces the level of F2-isoprostanes (an indicator of lipid peroxidation) in passive smokers (Dietrich et al., 2003a).

The Institute of Medicine (2000) estimates that smokers require 35 mg/day of vitamin C more than non-smokers since the metabolic turnover of this vitamin is double in these people (70 mg/day compared to 35.7 mg/day in non-smokers). Thus, the recommended vitamin C intake for smokers has been raised from 60 to 100 mg/day. However, it is not clear whether this is the most appropriate intake. Ortega et al., (2003) have calculated the intake of vitamin C necessary to bring the percentage of serum deficiencies in smokers down to that of non-smokers would require an intake of 150-200 mg/day. The same may be true for passive smokers.

Data available on vitamin E levels in smokers are controversial. Sobczak et al., (2004) indicate the plasma levels of alpha-tocopherol in passive and active smokers to be lower than those of non-smokers, whereas smoking had virtually no influence on the gamma-tocopherol level. Mena (2003) reports similar serum vitamin E levels in active and/or passive smokers, while Dietrich et al., (2003b) report smokers and passive smokers to have higher plasma concentrations of gamma-tocopherol but not alpha-tocopherol. Some studies have shown that certain indicators of oxidative stress can be improved with vitamin supplementation. For example, Jendryczko et al., (1993) found that despite their having similar plasma vitamin E concentrations, the erythrocytes of 25 children of smoker parents had an increased tendency ($p<0.01$) to peroxidise *in vitro* compared to those of 28 children of non-smoker parents. However, after supplementing both sets of children with 100 mg alpha-tocopherol acetate for 14 days, the susceptibility to erythrocyte peroxidation in the children of the smoker parents was partially improved.

One of the reasons why lower serum vitamin E levels in active and/or passive smokers have not been generally found is the regeneration of the vitamin by other antioxidants (Halliwell, 1996b; Packer, 1992). Given this type of controversy it is currently questioned whether recommending smokers to increase their vitamin E intake via their diet or by supplements is a sound idea (Ortega, 2003).

Beta-carotene only has an antioxidant effect at certain doses and at certain concentrations of oxygen: at high concentrations and high partial pressures of oxygen it can, in fact, have pro-oxidant effects (Zhang and Omaye, 2000). More peroxidised radicals of beta-carotene are formed under such conditions, and there is a higher incidence of beta-carotene auto-oxidation (Palozza, 1998). There are some reports in the literature that supplementation with high doses of beta-carotene may be dangerous for smokers (Modnicki and Matlawska, 2005), even conditioning an increase in the incidence of lung cancer (Arora et al., 2001). It would therefore seem more appropriate to recommend smokers increase their intake of fruits and vegetables rather than take supplements (Modnicki and Matlawska, 2005; Ortega, 2003). In a study on ferrets administered a supplement with a physiological (low) or pharmacological (high) dose of beta-carotene (0.43 mg compared to 2.4 mg/kg body wt/day; equivalent to 6 and 30 mg/day respectively in humans) that were exposed to cigarette smoke for 6 months, it was seen that, in contrast with the pharmacological dose, the physiological dose had no potentially detrimental effects and may have afforded weak protection against the lung damage induced by cigarette smoke.

However, the use of antioxidant supplements by passive smokers may provide some protection against the increased oxidative stress they suffer. Taking a supplement of 3000 □g of beta-carotene, 60 mg of vitamin C, 30 I.U. of alpha-tocopherol, 40 mg of zinc, 40 □g of selenium, and 2 mg of copper for 60 days reduced the level of 8-hydroxy-2-deoxyguanosine, a marker of oxidative DNA damage (Howard et al., 1998). In addition, Moller et al., (2004) observed that long-term vitamin C supplementation at high doses (500 mg) together with vitamin E in moderate dose (182 mg) for four weeks reduced the steady-state level of oxidative DNA damage in the mononuclear blood cells of smokers.

Active and passive exposure to tobacco smoke has been associated with a lower intake of folate (Ortega et al., 2004) and lower serum and erythrocyte folate levels (Mannino et al., 2003). However, by tripling the recommended intake of folic acid (400 µg/day) serum levels similar to those of non-smokers can be attained (Ortega, 2003). Cafolla et al., (2002) indicate that following supplementation with 5 mg/day of folic acid, the serum and erythrocyte folate levels of smokers became similar to those of non-smokers. Therefore, active and passive smokers may be able to improve their health by increasing their intake of folates via fruits and vegetables or folate-fortified foods, or by taking folate supplements.

In summary, the question remains as to whether the recommended intakes of certain vitamins should be increased for smokers and passive smokers. More research is needed to determine the most appropriate levels of nutrients for these groups.

References

Alberg AJ, Chen JC, Zhao H, Hoffman SC, Comstock GW, Helzlsouer KJ. Household exposure to passive cigarette smoking and serum micronutrient concentrations. *Am. J. Clin. Nutr.* 2000; 72(6):1576-82.

Ambrose JA, Barua RS. The pathophysiology of cigarette smoking and cardiovascular disease: an update. *J. Am. Coll. Cardiol.* 2004;43(10):1731-7.

Arbes SJ Jr, Agustsdottir H, Slade GD. Environmental tobacco smoke and periodontal disease in the United Status. *Am. J. Public Health.* 2001;91(2):253-7.

Arora A, Willhite CA, Liebler DC. Interactions of beta-carotene and cigarette smoke in human bronchial epithelial cells. *Carcinogenesis.* 2001;22(8):1173-8.

Ayaori M, Hisada T, Suzukawa M, Yoshida H, Nishiwaki M, Ito T, Nakajima K,Higashi K, Yonemura A, Ohsuzu F, Ishikawa T, Nakamura H. Plasma levels and redox status of ascorbic acid and levels of lipid peroxidation products in active and passive smokers. *Environ Health Perspect.* 2000;108(2):105-8.

Aycicek A, Erel O, Kocyigit A. Decreased total antioxidant capacity and increased oxidative stress in passive smoker infants and their mothers. *Pediatr. Int.* 2005;47(6):635-9.

Azizi F, Raiszadeh F, Salehi P, Rahmani M, Emami H, Ghanbarian A, Hajipour R. Determinants of serum HDL-C level in a Tehran urban population: the Tehran Lipid and Glucose Study. *Nutr. Metab. Cardiovasc. Dis.* 2002;12(2):80-9.

Barber K, Mussin E, Taylor DK. Fetal exposure to involuntary maternal smoking and childhood respiratory disease. *Ann. Allergy Asthma Immunol.* 1996;76(5):427-30.

Benowitz NL, Kuyt F, Jacob P, Jones RT, Osman AL. Cotinine disposition and effects. *Clin. Pharmacol. Ther.* 1983;34:604-611

Benson BW, Shulman JD. Inclusion of tobacco exposure as a predictive factor for decreased bone mineral content. *Nicotine Tob. Res.* 2005;7(5):719-24.

Bermudez E, Stone K, Carter KM, Pryor WA. Environmental tobacco smoke is just as damaging to DNA as mainstream smoke. *Environ. Health Perspect.* 1994;102(10):870-4.

Birkett NJ. Intake of fruits and vegetables in smokers. *Public Health Nutr.* 1999;2:217-222.

Bolton-Smith, C., Casey, C. E., Gey, K. F., Smith, W. C. and Tunstall-Pedoe, H. Antioxidant vitamin intakes assessed using a food-frequency questionnaire: correlation with biochemical status in smokers and non-smokers. *Br. J. Nutr.* 1991; 65:337-346.

Borzecki A, Brzeski Z, Sodolski W, Wojcik A, Krakowska A, Pajak A. Tobacco smoking among adolescents-self-reported psycho-somatic health. *Przegl. Lek.* 2005;62(10):1099-101.

Brown MS, Goldstein JL. Lipoprotein metabolism in the macrophage: implications for cholesterol deposition in atherosclerosis. *Annu. Rev. Biochem.* 1983;52:223–261.

Bruno RS, Traber MG. Cigarette smoke alters human vitamin E requirements. *J. Nutr.* 2005;135(4):671-4.

Cafolla A, Dragoni F, Girelli G, Tosti ME, Costante A, De Luca AM, Funaro D, Scott CS. Effect of folic acid and vitamin C supplementation on folate status and homocysteine level: a randomised controlled trial in Italian smoker-blood donors. *Atherosclerosis.* 2002;163(1):105-11.

California Environmental Protection Agency. Health effects of exposureto environmental tobacco smoke. Sacramento, CA: Office of Environmental Health Hazard Assessment; 1997. Available at: *www.oehha.org/pdf/exec.pdf.*

Chelchowska M, Laskowska-Klita T, Szymborski J. Level of retinol and beta-carotene in plasma of smoking and non-smoking women. *Wiad. Lek.* 2001;54(5-6):248-54.

Chen H, Hansen MJ, Jones JE, Vlahos R, Bozinovski S, Anderson GP, Morris MJ. Cigarette Smoke Exposure Reprograms the Hypothalamic Neuropeptide Y Axis to Promote Weight Loss. *Am. J. Respir. Crit. Care Med.* 2006; [Epub ahead of print]

Chen H, Vlahos R, Bozinovski S, Jones J, Anderson GP, Morris MJ. Effect of short-term cigarette smoke exposure on body weight, appetite and brain neuropeptide Y in mice. *Neuropsychopharmacology.* 2005;30(4):713-9.

Church DF, Pryor WA. Free-radical chemistry of cigarette smoke and its toxicological implications. *Environ. Health Perspect.* 1985;64:111–126.

Crawley HF, While D. Parental smoking and the nutrient intake and food choice of British teenagers aged 16-17 years. *J. Epidemiol. Community Health.* 1996;50(3):306-12.

Cross CE, Traber M, Eiserich J, van der Vliet A. Micronutrient antioxidants and smoking. *Br. Med. Bull.* 1999;55(3):691-704.

Curtin F, Morabia A, Bernstein MS. Relation of environmental tobacco smoke to diet and health habits: variations according to the site of exposure. *J. Clin. Epidemiol.* 1999;52(11):1055-62.

Dallongeville J, Marecaux N, Fruchart JC, Amouyel P. Cigarette smoking is associated with unhealthy patterns of nutrient intake: a meta-analysis. *J. Nutr.* 1998;128(9):1450-7.

Dietrich M, Block G, Benowitz NL, Morrow JD, Hudes M, Jacob P 3rd, Norkus EP, Packer L. Vitamin C supplementation decreases oxidative stress biomarker f2-isoprostanes in plasma of nonsmokers exposed to environmental tobacco smoke. *Nutr. Cancer* 2003a;45(2):176-84.

Dietrich M, Block G, Norkus EP, Hudes M, Traber MG, Cross CE, Packer L. Smoking and exposure to environmental tobacco smoke decrease some plasma antioxidants and increase gamma-tocopherol in vivo after adjustment for dietary antioxidant intakes. *Am. J. Clin. Nutr.* 2003b;77(1):160-6.

Drongowski RA, Lee D, Reynolds PI, Malviya S, Harmon CM, Geiger J, Lelli JL, Coran AG. Increased respiratory symptoms following surgery in children exposed to environmental tobacco smoke. *Paediatr. Anaesth.* 2003;13(4):304-10.

Dyer AR, Elliott P, Stamler J, Chan Q, Ueshima H, Zhou BF. Dietary intake in male and female smokers, ex-smokers, and never smokers: the INTERMAP study. *J. Hum. Hypertens.* 2003;17(9):641-54.

Eiserich JP, van der Vliet A, Handelman GJ, Halliwell B, Cross CE. Dietary antioxidants and cigarette smoke-induced biomolecular damage: a complex interaction. *Am. J. Clin. Nutr.* 1995;62(6 Suppl):1490S-1500S.

Emmons KM, Thompson B, Feng Z, Hebert JR, Heimendinger J, Linnan L. Dietary intake and exposure to environmental tobacco smoke in a worksite population. *Eur. J. Clin. Nutr.* 1995;49(5):336-45.

Farchi S, Forastiere F, Pistelli R, Baldacci S, Simoni M, Perucci CA, Viegi G; On behalf of the SEASD Group. Exposure to environmental tobacco smoke is associated with lower plasma beta-carotene levels among nonsmoking women married to a smoker. *Cancer Epidemiol. Biomarkers Prev.* 2001;10(8):907-9.

Feldman J, Shenker IR, Etzel RA, Spierto FW, Lilienfield DE, Nussbaum M, Jacobson MS. Passive smoking alters lipid profiles in adolescents. *Pediatrics.* 1991;88(2):259-64.

Forastiere F, Mallone S, Lo Presti E, Baldacci S, Pistelli F, Simoni M, Scalera A, Pedreschi M, Pistelli R, Corbo G, Rapiti E, Agabiti N, Farchi S, Basso S, Chiaffi L, Matteelli G, Di Pede F, Carrozzi L, Viegi G. Characteristics of nonsmoking women exposed to spouses who smoke: epidemiologic study on environment and health in women from four Italian areas. *Environ. Health Perspect.* 2000;108(12):1171-7.

Fuertes Fernández-Espinar J, Meriz Rubio J, Pardos Martínez C, López Cortés V, Ricarte Díez JI, González Pérez-Yarza E.. Prevalencia actual del asma, alergia e hiperrespuesta bronquial en niños de 6-8 años. *An. Esp. Pediatr.* 2001;54:18-26.

Gilliland FD, Li YF, Dubeau L, Berhane K, Avol E, McConnell R, et al.. Effects of glutation S-transferase M1, maternal smoking during pregnancy, and environmental tobacco smoke on asthma and wheezing in children. *Am. J. Respir. Crit. Care Med.* 2002; 166:457-63.

Glantz SA, Parmley WW. Passive smoking and heart disease: mechanisms and risk. *JAMA.* 1995;273:1047–1053.

Halliwell B. Antioxidants in human health and disease. *Annu. Rev. Nutr.* 1996b;16:33-50.

Halliwell B. Oxidative stress, nutrition and health. Experimental strategies for optimization of nutritional antioxidant intake in humans. *Free Radic. Res.* 1996a;25(1):57-74.

Hampl JS, Taylor CA, Booth CL, Differences in dietary patterns of nonsmoking adults married to smokers vs. nonsmokers. *Am. J. Health Promot.* 2001; 16(1):1-6.

Handelman GJ, Packer L, Cross CE. Destruction of tocopherols, carotenoids, and retinol in human plasma by cigarette smoke. *Am. J. Clin. Nutr.* 1996;63(4):559-65.

Heraud MC, Herbelin-Wagner ML, Risk factors: environment, tobacco smoke. *Arch. Pediatr.* 2002;9(Suppl 3):377-83.

Holay MP, Paunikar NP, Joshi PP, Sahasrabhojney VS, Tankhiwale SR. Effect of passive smoking on endothelial function in: healthy adults. *J. Assoc. Physicians India.* 2004;52:114-7.

Howard DJ, Ota RB, Briggs LA, Hampton M, Pritsos CA. Oxidative stress induced by environmental tobacco smoke in the workplace is mitigated by antioxidant supplementation. *Cancer Epidemiol. Biomarkers Prev.* 1998;7(11):981-8.

Hozyasz KK, Chelchowska M. [Vitamin A levels among nonsmoking mothers of children with orofacial clefts married to a smoker]. *Przegl. Lek.* 2004;61(10):1083-5.

Iles K, Poplawski NK, Couper RT. Passive exposure to tobacco smoke and bacterial meningitis in children. *J. Paediatr. Child Health.* 2001;37(4):388-91.

Institute of Medicine, Food and Nutrition Borrad. Dietary references intakes for vitamin C, vitamin E, selenium and carotenoids, chapter 5: vitamin C. Washington DC: *National Academy Press*, 2000; 95:185.

Jacob RA. Passive smoking induces oxidant damage preventable by vitamin C. *Nutr. Rev.* 2000;58(8):239-41.

Jarvis MJ, Russell MAH, Benowitz NL, Feyerabend C. Elimination of cotinine from body fluids: implications for noninvasive measurement of tobacco smoke exposure. *Am. J. Public Health.* 1988; 78:696-698.

Jendryczko A, Szpyrka G, Gruszczynski J, Kozowicz M. Cigarette smoke exposure of school children: effect of passive smoking and vitamin E supplementation on blood antioxidant status. *Neoplasma.* 1993;40(3):199-203.

Jialal I, Grundy SM. Effect of combined supplementation with alpha-tocopherol, ascorbate, and beta carotene on low-density lipoprotein oxidation. *Circulation.* 1993;88(6):2780-6.

Kalinka J, Hanke W, Sobala W. Impact of prenatal tobacco smoke exposure, as measured by midgestation serum cotinine levels, on fetal biometry and umbilical flow velocity waveforms. *Am. J. Perinatol.* 2005;22(1):41-7.

Kasim K, Levallois P, Abdous B, Auger P, Johnson KC; Canadian Cancer Registries Epidemiology Research Group. Environmental tobacco smoke and risk of adult leukemia. *Epidemiology.* 2005;16(5):672-80.

Khan JC, Thurlby DA, Shahid H, Clayton DG, Yates JR, Bradley M, Moore AT, Bird AC; Genetic Factors in AMD Study. Smoking and age related macular degeneration: the number of pack years of cigarette smoking is a major determinant of risk for both geographic atrophy and choroidal neovascularisation. *Br. J. Ophthalmol.* 2006;90(1):75-80.

Kim H, Lim Y, Lee S, Park S, Kim C, Hong C, Shin D.Relationship between environmental tobacco smoke and urinary cotinine levels in passive smokers at their residence. *J. Expo. Anal. Environ. Epidemiol.* 2004;14 Suppl 1:S65-70.

King JC. Determinants of maternal zinc status during pregnancy. *Am. J. Clin. Nutr.* 2000;71(5 Suppl):1334S-43S.

Klerman L. Protecting children: reducing their environmental tobacco smoke exposure. *Nicotine Tob. Res.* 2004;6 Suppl 2:S239-53.

Koo LC, Kabat GC, Rylander R, Tominaga S, Kato I, Ho j H-C. Dietary and lifestyles correlates of passive smoking in Hong-Kong, Japan, Sweeden and the USA. *Soc. Sci. Med.* 1997; 45:159-69.

Leonard, S. W., Bruno, R. S., Paterson, E., Schock, B. C., Atkinson, J., Bray, T. M., Cross, C. E. and Traber, M. G. 5-Nitro--tocopherol increases in human plasma exposed to cigarette smoke in vitro and in vivo. *Free Radic. Biol. Med.* 2003;35:1560-1567.

Lewis SA, Antoniak M, Venn AJ, Davies L, Goodwin A, Salfield N, Britton J, Fogarty AW. Secondhand smoke, dietary fruit intake, road traffic exposures, and the prevalence of asthma: a cross-sectional study in young children. *Am. J. Epidemiol.* 2005;161(5):406-11.

Lykkesfeldt J, Christen S, Wallock LM, Chang HH, Jacob RA, Ames BN. Ascorbate is depleted by smoking and repleted by moderate supplementation: a study in male smokers and nonsmokers with matched dietary antioxidant intakes. *Am. J. Clin. Nutr.* 2000;71(2):530-6.

Ma A, Hampl JS, Betts NM. Antioxidants intakes and smoking status: data from the Continuing survey of Food Intakes by Individuals 1994-1996. *Am. J. Clin. Nutr.* 2000;71:774-80.

Mannino DM, Moorman JE, Kingsley B, Rose D, Repace J. Health effects related to environmental tobacco smoke exposure in children in the United States: data from the Third National Health and Nutrition Examination Survey. *Arch. Pediatr. Adolesc. Med.* 2001;155(1):36-41.

Mannino DM, Mulinare J, Ford ES, Schwartz J. Tobacco smoke exposure and decreased serum and red blood cell folate levels: data from the Third National Health and Nutrition Examination Survey. *Nicotine Tob. Res.* 2003;5(3):357-62.

Marangon K, Herbeth B, Lecomte E, Paul-Dauphin A, Grolier P, Chancerelle Y, Artur Y, Siest G. Diet, antioxidant status, and smoking habits in French men. *Am. J. Clin. Nutr.* 1998;67(2):231-9.

Matanoski G, Kanchanaraska S, Lantry D, Chang Y. Characteristics of nonsmoking women in NHANES I and NHANES I Epidemiologic Follow-up Study with exposure to spouses who smoke. *Am. J. Epidemiol.* 1995; 142:149-57.

Mena MC. El hábito de fumar como condicionante del estado nutricional en población femenina. *Tesis Doctoral Madrid.* 2003.

Modnicki D, Matlawska I. Carotenoids as components of dietary supplements recommended for smokers and persons passively exposed to cigarette smoke. *Przegl. Lek.* 2005;62(10):1188-9.

Moller P, Viscovich M, Lykkesfeldt J, Loft S, Jensen A, Poulsen HE.Vitamin C supplementation decreases oxidative DNA damage in mononuclear blood cells of smokers. *Eur. J. Nutr.* 2004;43(5):267-74

Morabia A, Bernstein MS, Antonini S. Smoking, dietary calcium and vitamin D deficiency in women: a population-based study. *Eur. J. Clin. Nutr.* 2000;54(9):684-9.

Muñoz C, Jurado D, Luna JD.. Exposición al humo de tabaco ambiental en niños en el medio familiar: creencias, actitudes y prácticas de los padres. *Prev. Tab.* 2003;5:11-8.

Nageris B, Braverman I, Hadar T, Hansen MC, Frenkiel S. Effects of passive smoking on odour identification in children. *J. Otolaryngol.* 2001;30(5):263-5.

National Research Council. *Environmental Tobacco Smoke: Measuring Exposures and Assessing Health Effects.* Washington, DC: Committee on Passive Smoking, Board on Environmental Studies and Toxicology, National Research Council; 1986.

Neufeld EJ, Mietus-Snyder M, Beiser AS, Baker AL, Newburger JW. Passive cigarette smoking and reduced HDL cholesterol levels in children with high-risk lipid profiles. Passive cigarette smoking and reduced HDL cholesterol levels in children with high-risk lipid profiles. *Circulation.* 1997;96(5):1403-7.

Nicklas T, Johnson R; American Dietetic Association. Position of the American Dietetic Association: Dietary guidance for healthy children ages 2 to 11 years. *J. Am. Diet. Assoc.* 2004;104(4):660-77.

Nizard J. What are the epidemiological data on maternal and paternal smoking?. *J. Gynecol. Obstet. Biol. Reprod* (Paris). 2005;34 Spec No 1:3S347-52.

Nomura K, Nakao M, Morimoto T. Effect of smoking on hearing loss: quality assessment and meta-analysis. *Prev. Med.* 2005;40(2):138-44.

Ortega RM, Andres P, Zamora MJ, Ortega A. The nutritional problems of the smoker. The role of diet in the appearance and progress of cataracts. *Rev. Clin. Esp.* 1994a;194(11):982-4.

Ortega RM, Lopez-Sobaler AM, Gonzalez-Gross MM, Redondo RM, Marzana I, Zamora MJ, Andres P. Influence of smoking on folate intake and blood folate concentrations in a group of elderly Spanish men. *J. Am. Coll. Nutr.* 1994b;13(1):68-72.

Ortega RM, Lopez-Sobaler AM, Martinez RM, Andres P, Quintas ME. Influence of smoking on vitamin E status during the third trimester of pregnancy and on breast-milk tocopherol concentrations in Spanish women. *Am. J. Clin. Nutr.* 1998a;68(3):662-7.

Ortega RM, Lopez-Sobaler AM, Quintas ME, Martinez RM, Andres P. The influence of smoking on vitamin C status during the third trimester of pregnancy and on vitamin C levels in maternal milk. *J. Am. Coll. Nutr.* 1998;17(4):379-84.

Ortega RM, Requejo AM, Lopez-Sobaler AM, Navia B, Mena MC, Basabe B, Andres P. Smoking and passive smoking as conditioners of folate status in young women. *J. Am. Coll. Nutr.* 2004;23(4):365-71.

Ortega RM. Nutrición del fumador. En: Requejo AM y Ortega RM, eds. Nutriguía. Manual de nutrición clínica en atención primaria. Ed. Complutense. *Madrid.* 2003. p. 324-331.

Osler M. The food intake of smokers and nonsmokers: the role of partner's smoking behavior. *Prev. Med.* 1998;27(3):438-43.

Packer L. Interactions among antioxidants in health and disease: vitamin E and its redox cycle. *Proc. Soc. Exp. Biol. Med.* 1992;200(2):271-6.

Palaniappan U, Jacobs Starkey L, O'Loughlin J, Gray-Donald K. Fruit and vegetable consumption is lower and saturated fat intake is higher among Canadians reporting smoking. *J. Nutr.* 2001;131:1952-1958.

Palozza P. Prooxidant actions of carotenoids in biologic systems. *Nutr. Rev.* 1998;56(9):257-65.

Pfeffer F, Kaufer-Horwitz M. *Nutrición en el adulto.* En: Casanueva E, Kaufer-Horwitz M, Pérez-Lizaur AB, Arroyo P. Nutriología Médica 2ª ed. 2001. Editorial Médica Panamericana. México. 104-119.

Pirkle JL, Flegal KM, Bernert JT, Brody DJ, Etzel RA, Maurer KR.. Exposure of the US population to environmental tobacco smoke: the Third National Health and Nutrition Examination Survey, 1988-91. *JAMA* 1996;275:1233-40.

Pollard J, Greenwood D, Kirk S, Cade J. Lifestyle factors affecting fruit and vegetable consumption in the UK Women's Cohort Study. *Appetite* 2001;37:71-79.

Powledge TM. Nicotine as therapy. PLoS. Biol. 2004;2(11):e404. *Epub* 2004 Nov 16.

Preston AM, Rodriguez C, Rivera CE, Sahai H. Influence of environmental tobacco smoke on vitamin C status in children. *Am. J. Clin. Nutr.* 2003;77(1):167-72.

Qureshi AI, Suri MF, Kirmani JF, Divani AA. Cigarette smoking among spouses: another risk factor for stroke in women. *Stroke.* 2005;36(9):e74-6. *Epub* 2005 Aug 4.

Rauh VA, Whyatt RM, Garfinkel R, Andrews H, Hoepner L, Reyes A, Diaz D, Camann D, Perera FP. Developmental effects of exposure to environmental tobacco smoke and material hardship among inner-city children. Neurotoxicol. *Teratol.* 2004;26(3):373-85.

Reibel J. Tobacco and oral diseases. Update on the evidence, with recommendations. *Med. Princ. Pract.* 2003;12 Suppl 1:22-32.

Reynolds P, Hurley SE, Hoggatt K, Anton-Culver H, Bernstein L, Deapen D, Peel D, Pinder R, Ross RK, West D, Wright W, Ziogas A, Horn-Ross PL. Correlates of active and passive smoking in the California Teachers Study cohort. *J. Womens Health* (Larchmt). 2004;13(7):778-90.

Romero-Palacios PJ. Asthma and tobacco smoke. *Arch. Bronconeumol.* 2004;40(9):414-8.

Samet JM, Yang G.. Passive smoking women and children. In: Samet JM, Yoon SY, editors. Women and the tobacco epidemic. Challenges for the 21st Century. The World Health Organization in collaboration with the Institute for Global Tobacco Control and the Johns Hopkins School of Public Health. *Geneva: World Health Organization*, 2001.

Samet JM. Risks of active and passive smoking. *Salud. Publica. Mex.* 2002;44 Suppl. 1:S144-60.

Sato K, Endo S, Tomita H. Sensitivity of three loci on the tongue and soft palate to four basic tastes in smokers and non-smokers. *Acta Otolaryngol. Suppl.* 2002;(546):74-82.

Schectman G, Byrd JC, Hoffman R. Ascorbic acid requirements for smokers: analysis of a population survey. *Am. J. Clin. Nutr.* 1991;53: 1466–1470

Schroder H, Marrugat J, Elosua R, Covas MI. Tobacco and alcohol consumption: impact on other cardiovascular and cancer risk factors in a southern European Mediterranean population. *Br. J. Nutr.* 2002; 88(3):273-81.

Scientific Committee on Tobacco and Health, HSMO. *Report of the Scientific Committee on Tobacco and Health.* The Stationari Office.1998. 011322124x.

Simoni M, Jaakkola MS, Carrozzi L, Baldacci S, Di Pede F, Viegi G. Indoor air pollution and respiratory health in the elderly. *Eur. Respir. J. Suppl.* 2003;40:15s-20s.

Smith CJ, Fischer TH. Particulate and vapor phase constituents of cigarette mainstream smoke and risk of myocardial infarction. *Atherosclerosis.* 2001;158(2):257-67.

Sobczak A, Golka D, Szoltysek-Boldys I. The effects of tobacco smoke on plasma alpha- and gamma-tocopherol levels in passive and active cigarette smokers. *Toxicol. Lett.* 2004;151(3):429-37.

Steyn K, de Wet T, Saloojee Y, Nel H, Yach D. The influence of maternal cigarette smoking, snuff use and passive smoking on pregnancy outcomes: the Birth To Ten Study. *Paediatr. Perinat. Epidemiol.* 2006;20(2):90-9.

Strauss RS. Environmental tobacco smoke and serum vitamin C levels in children. *Pediatrics.* 2001;107(3):540-2.

Subar AF, Harlan LC, Mattson ME. Food and nutrient intake differences between smokers and non-smokers in the US. *Am. J. Public Health.* 1990;80:1323-1329.

Suliburska J, Duda G, Pupek-Musialik D. Effect of tobacco smoking on taste sensitivity in adults. *Przegl. Lek.* 2004;61(10):1174-6.

Thompson, D. H. and Warburton, D. M. (1992) Lifestyle differences between smokers, ex-smokers and non-smokers, and their implications for their health. *Psychology and Health* 1992;7: 311-321.

Tong EK, England L, Glantz SA. Changing conclusions on secondhand smoke in a sudden infant death syndrome review funded by the tobacco industry. *Pediatrics.* 2005;115(3):e356-66.

Topp R, Thefeld W, Wichmann HE, Heinrich J. The effect of environmental tobacco smoke exposure on allergic sensitization and allergic rhinitis in adults. *Indoor Air.* 2005;15(4):222-7.

Tribble DL, Giuliano LJ, Fortmann SP. Reduced plasma ascorbic acid concentrations in nonsmokers regularly exposed to environmental tobacco smoke. *Am. J. Clin. Nutr.* 1993;58(6):886-90.

Trobs M, Renner T, Scherer G, Heller WD, Geiss HC, Wolfram G, Haas GM, Schwandt P. Nutrition, antioxidants, and risk factor profile of nonsmokers, passive smokers and smokers of the Prevention Education Program (PEP) in Nuremberg, Germany. *Prev. Med.* 2002;34(6):600-7.

US Department of Health Education and Welfare. *The health consequences of smoking.* A report of the Surgeon General (DHEW Publication No. HSM 73-8704). Washington, DC: US Government Printing Office, 1971.

US Environmental Protection Agency. *Respiratory health effects of passive smoking: lung cancers and other disorders.* Washington, DC: Office of Research and Development, Office of Health and Environmental Assessment; 1992. US EPA Publication No. EPA/600/6-90/006F. Available at: *http://cfpub.epa.gov/ncea/cfm/recordisplay.cfm?deid_2835*

Valkonen M, Kuusi T. Passive smoking induces atherogenic changes in low-density lipoprotein. *Circulation.* 1998;97(20):2012-6.

Voutilainen S, Rissanen TH, Virtanen J, Lakka TA, Salonen JT; Kuopio Ischemic Heart Disease Risk Factor Study. Low dietary folate intake is associated with an excess incidence of acute coronary events: The Kuopio Ischemic Heart Disease Risk Factor Study. *Circulation.* 2001;103(22):2674-80.

Wei W, Kim Y, Boudreau N. Association of smoking with serum and dietary levels of antioxidants in adults: NHANES III, 1988-1994. *Am. J. Public Health.* 2001;91(2):258-64.

Weitzman M, Cook S, Auinger P, Florin TA, Daniels S, Nguyen M, Winickoff JP. Tobacco smoke exposure is associated with the metabolic syndrome in adolescents. *Circulation.* 2005;112(6):862-9

Whig J, Singh CB, Soni GL, Bansal AK. Serum lipids and lipoprotein profiles of cigarette smokers and passive smokers. *Indian J. Med. Res.* 1992;96:282-7.

Whitfield JB, Zhu G, Heath AC, Powell And LW, Martin NG. Effects of alcohol consumption on indices of iron stores and of iron stores on alcohol intake markers. Alcohol. *Clin. Exp. Res.* 2001;25(7):1037-45.

World Health Organization Division of Noncommunicable Disease Tobacco Free Initiative.. International consultation on environmental tobacco smoke (ETS) and child health consultation report. *Geneva: WHO*, 1999. Available from *http://www.who.int./toh*

World Health Organization International Agency for Research on Cancer IARC. Monographs on the Evaluation of Carcinogenic Risks to Humans. Volume 83 Tobacco Smoke and Involuntary Smoking Summary of Data Reported and Evaluation Tobacco smoking and tobacco smoke Involuntary smoking. 2002. Available at: *http://monographs.iarc.fr/ENG/Monographs/vol83/volume83.pdf*

Yang G, Fant L, Tan J, et al.. Smoking in China. Findings of the 1996 National Prevalence Survey. *JAMA* 1999;2892:1247-53.

Yolton K, Dietrich K, Auinger P, Lanphear BP, Hornung R. Exposure to environmental tobacco smoke and cognitive abilities among U.S. children and adolescents. *Environ. Health Perspect.* 2005;113(1):98-103.

Zhang P, Omaye ST. Beta-carotene and protein oxidation: effects of ascorbic acid and alpha-tocopherol. *Toxicology.* 2000;146(1):37-47.

Zhang Y. Influence of smoking on cholesterol concentrations in serum lipo-protein of healthy subjects. *Zhonghua Liu Xing Bing Xue Za Zhi.* 1992 Apr;13(2):97-100.

Ziegler RG, Mayne ST, Swanson CA. Nutrition and lung cancer. *Cancer Causes Control.* 1996;7(1):157-77. Review.

Zondervan KT, Ocke MC, Smit HA, Seidell JC. Do dietary and supplementary intakes of antioxidants differ with smoking status? *Int. J. Epidemiol.* 1996;25:70-79.

In: Smoking and Lung Cancer
Editors: E. N. Powers and J. B. Cabbot
ISBN 978-1-60692-367-2

Chapter IX

Women and Lung Cancer: A Neglected Epidemic

***C. Ho*[1], *P. N. Lara*[2,3], *D. R. Gandara*[2,3] *and A. M. Davies*[2,3,*]**
[1]British Columbia Cancer Agency, Vancouver, British Columbia, Canada
[2]UC Davis Cancer Center, Sacramento, California, USA;
[3]University of California, Davis School of Medicine, USA

Abstract

Lung cancer has reached nearly epidemic proportions in women; the incidence has quadrupled over the past 40 years. Multiple studies have been conducted to identify reasons for the dramatic increase in lung cancer over the past decades. Smoking behaviors, pathways of carcinogenesis and the impact of the hormonal milieu have all been examined as possible explanations. Although many studies have attempted to address these questions, they have been retrospective or case-control studies and results have been inconsistent. With the recognition that lung cancer may behave differently in men versus women, current studies are prospectively examining this question.

Introduction

Lung cancer is the leading cause of cancer-related death in both men and women. While lung cancer deaths in men have declined, they have risen for women [1]. Women will account for almost half (47%) of the projected new diagnoses of lung cancer (174,470) in the United States this year[1]. Mortality closely parallels incidence with an anticipated 162,460 deaths and an estimated 72,130 women's lives lost. In comparison, breast cancer accounts for

* Correspondence concerning this article should be addressed to Angela Davies, M.D. Assistant Professor of Medicine, UC Davis Cancer Center 4501 X Street, Suite 3016, Sacramento, California 95817. Phone: (916) 734-3771; Fax: (916) 734-7946; Email: Angela.davies@ucdmc.ucdavis.edu.

41,430 deaths per year, making lung cancer the leading cause of cancer death for women by a wide margin.

A significant increase in tobacco usage by women during and after World War II has been identified as the major contributor to this dramatic rise in incidence and mortality in lung cancer [2]. While changes in smoking behavior have been implicated, there has been much speculation about whether women have an increased susceptibility to develop lung cancer. Researchers have evaluated the role of sex, carcinogen metabolism, and the hormonal milieu as factors influencing lung cancer development and progression. This chapter will review the data currently available addressing these areas of interest in an effort to gain a better understanding of this disease in women.

Smoking Behavior

Smoking and Lung Cancer

Although exposures to asbestos, arsenic, benzene, radon and radiation have been connected to lung cancer development, the agent with the most significant causal association is tobacco smoke. While only 20% of smokers develop this disease, the majority of lung cancer patients have a history of past or current tobacco use with a clear dose response curve for amount smoked and the development of lung cancer [3]. Although more difficult to quantify, secondhand or passive smoke exposure has also been linked to lung cancer. A meta-analysis of 37 published epidemiologic studies of lung cancer in non-smokers indicates that a woman who has never smoked has a 24% greater risk of developing lung cancer if she lives with a smoker [4]. Workplace smoke exposure is also associated with a 16-19% increase in risk to develop lung cancer [5]. With the delayed recognition of the perils of environmental smoke exposure, it is not surprising that non-smoking individuals represent approximately 15% of the lung cancer population [1].

Smoking and Lung Cancer Trends over Time

Smoking became a popular habit in the early 20th century due to mass production of cigarettes, increased marketing and subsequent social acceptability [2]. The epidemic began when smoking rates increased in men in higher socioeconomic groups in the 1940s-50s, with smoking in women lagging 10-20 years behind [6]. The impact of this negative behavior has manifested several years later due to a process of malignant transformation that occurs over decades. By 1987, lung cancer deaths began to exceed breast cancer mortality in women in the USA.

While overall rates have decreased, smoking is now paradoxically a habit of lower socioeconomic groups with less formal education [2]. The prevalence of smoking in 1965 in American women 18 years and older was 34% and over the years has declined; in 1970 the rate was 32%; 1980, 30%; 1990, 23% and in 2000, 22% [7]. Paralleling the prevalence of smoking, lung cancer incidence and mortality rates in women increased drastically in the 1970s through the mid-1990s and is only now finally beginning to stabilize [1].

Smoking and Youths

The National Survey on Drug Use and Health for 2004 [8] showed that while trends in smoking have declined overall, there was a significant and concerning rate of usage in younger populations. In youths aged 12 to 17, the rate of current smokers was 12.5% for females and 11.3% for males with young adults aged 18-25 having the highest rate of current tobacco use (44.6%). This trend of early smoking behavior was more prominently observed in young women. It was hypothesized that young women seek to emulate social images associated with glamour, independence and equality. A desire to bond with peers, improve self-image and maintain low body weight has also been suggested as factors.

Adolescents are clearly influenced by exposure through the media; a study noted that adolescents in the highest quartile of exposure to movie smoking were more likely to initiate smoking compared to those in the lowest quartile [9]. Recognizing the impact of media images, tobacco companies have spent over $200 million per year between 1995-2000 in marketing, with 50-60% of the funds directed towards youth-oriented magazines [10].

Risk of Lung Cancer

Smoke Exposure

The increase in the incidence of lung cancer observed in women has prompted epidemiological studies examining the relationship between sex, toxin exposure and disease development. While a number of large case-control and cohort studies have examined this relationship, it remains unclear whether women are more susceptible to the carcinogenic effects of cigarette smoke than men and even more difficult to determine susceptibility to second hand smoke exposure.

Harris et al, used the American Health Foundation data to perform a case-control study of over 8,000 patients examining race and sex differences in lung cancer risk for smokers (Table 1) [11]. Women were at increased risk (RR 1.7) compared to men for a given level of smoke exposure. Zang et al updated this in 1996, adding more than 600 cases, equivalent controls and with more precise information regarding histological classification, smoking exposure and body size [12]. Similar to the initial study, women had a 1.5 fold higher relative risk of developing lung cancer compared to men given the same level of cigarette smoke exposure. Case control analysis of data collected by the Cancer Surveillance Program in Orange County California found an age and ethnicity adjusted odds ratio for ever smokers compared to never smokers of 19.7 for women and 15 for men [13]. Risch et al performed a case control study in Canada; the risk of lung cancer for both sexes was associated with cigarette consumption and increased with the number of pack years [14]. The odds ratio for 40 pack year smokers compared to lifelong non-smokers was 27.9 for women and 9.6 for men, indicating a substantially higher risk for women than men. A CT lung cancer screening study also found an increased risk of lung cancer for women; after controlling for age and smoking history, the odds ratio was 2.7 for females compared to males [15]. All of these studies, the majority of which are case-control in design, suggest that women are more susceptible than men to the negative effects of cigarette smoking, resulting in higher lung cancer rates.

In contrast, in the Cancer Prevention Study II (CPS II) the relative risk of a smoker developing lung cancer compared to a never smoker was 22.3 for men and 11.9 for women [16]. Kreuzer et al, using pooled data from 6 European case-control studies from 1988-94, found that the risk of lung cancer in ever smokers compared to never smokers was higher in men than women [17]. However, when controlled for duration of smoking, average daily consumption and time since quitting, the risk was the same for both genders. Two other large cohort studies have demonstrated similar results; the Carotene and Retinol Efficacy trial (n=18,172) had a hazard ratio of 0.9 (female compared to male smokers) when adjusted for age, asbestos exposure, smoking duration, dose and time since quitting [18]. In the data extracted from the Nurse Health Study of women and the Health Professionals Follow-up study of men (total n=85,693), the hazard ratio in women ever-smokers compared to men was 1.08, adjusted for pack years and time since quitting [19]. These latter studies have demonstrated no increased risk of lung cancer in women compared to men when variables like dose and duration are taken into account.

Sex difference in susceptibility to lung cancer with smoke exposure continues to be a topic of controversy. These differences were initially observed in case-control studies but are not supported by subsequent cohort observations. All of these studies are confounded by the retrospective nature of reporting smoking history. In addition, they were unable to account for environmental smoke exposure. While this debate will likely never be settled, it has prompted investigations into biological variations in lung cancer between sexes.

Table 1. Summary of studies evaluating the risk of lung cancer in women versus men

Year	Author	Source Data	Study design	n	Women increased risk
1973-1993	Harris	American Health Foundation	Case-control		Yes
1981-1985	Risch	Canada	Case-control	1617	Yes
1981-1994	Zang	American Health Foundation	Case-control	3959	Yes
1982-1988	Halpern	American Cancer Society's Cancer Prevention Study II	Cohort	1.2 million	No
1984-1986	Osann	Cancer Surveillance Program Orange County	Case-control	5493	Yes
1985-1994	Bach	Carotene and Retinol Efficacy Trial	Cohort	18,172	No
1986-2000	Bain	Nurses Health Study and Health Professionals Follow up study	Cohort	85,693	No
1988-1994	Kreuzer	European	Case-control	9792	No
1993-2001	Henschke	CT screening study	Screening	2490	Yes

Carcinogen metabolism

A model of carcinogenesis proposes that activation of pro-carcinogens in smoke leads to the formation of DNA adducts which, if unrepaired, leads to critical mutations resulting in cancer. Sex differences in carcinogen metabolism have been proposed at multiple levels in this model including pro-carcinogen activation, carcinogen neutralization, DNA repair and mutagenesis of key cell signaling proteins (Figure 1).

Cytochrome P450

The first step of the carcinogenesis process involves the metabolism of polycyclic aromatic hydrocarbons (PAH) in cigarette smoke by the cytochrome P450 pathway. The CYP1A1 isoform activates aryl hydrocarbon hydroxylase, an enzyme that metabolizes PAH into highly reactive diol-epoxides. Cigarette smoking induces gene expression of CYP1A1 leading to pro-carcinogen activation [20,21]. Mollerup et al observed that female smokers had a higher expression of CYP1A1 and aromatic DNA adducts than their male counterparts in their non-tumor lung tissue [22]. Consistent with this observation, women had higher levels of DNA adducts per pack years as compared to men indicating a higher degree of DNA damage for the amount of exposure.

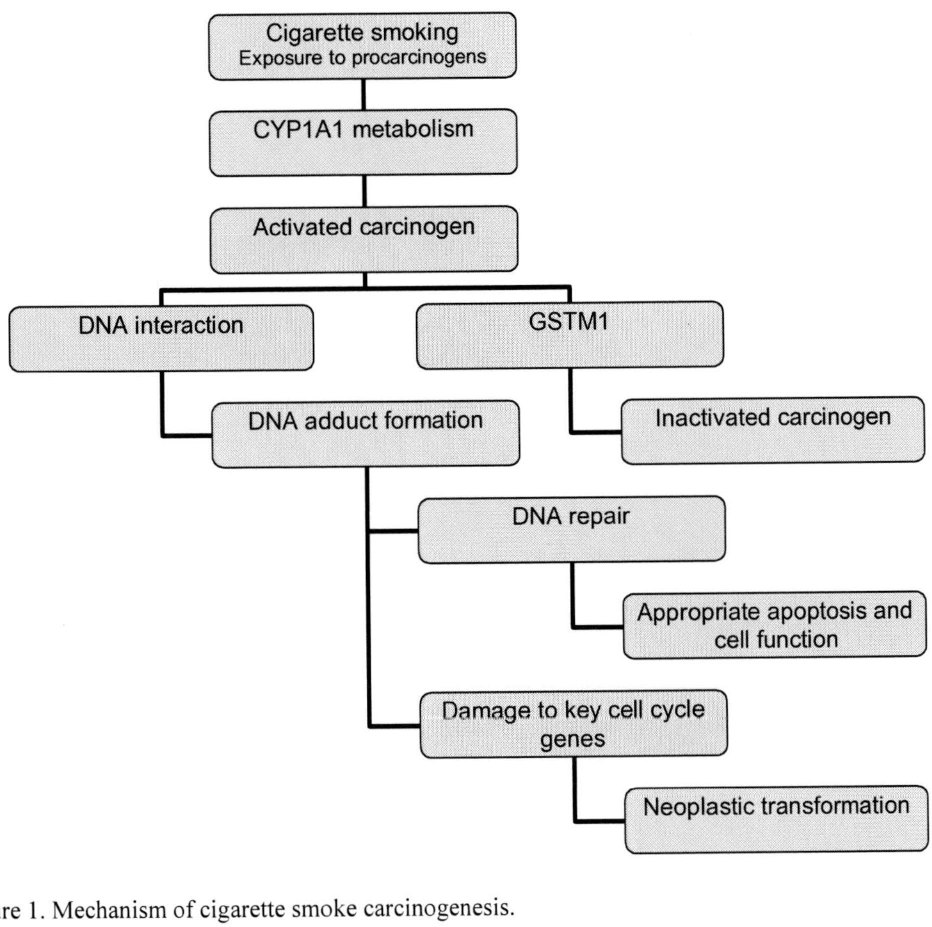

Figure 1. Mechanism of cigarette smoke carcinogenesis.

Glutathione-- Transferase M1 (GSTM1)

Reactive PAH species generated by cytochrome P450 enzymes can be neutralized by Phase II detoxification enzymes that include glutathione-S-transferase. These enzymes catalyze the conversion of the electrophilic metabolites to inactive conjugates, preventing adduct formation with DNA. In 40-50% of the general population, the GSTM1 gene is absent [23]. Molecular epidemiologic case-control studies have noted that the GSTM1 null genotype is significantly associated with lung cancer for women but not men [24]. In a study evaluating DNA extracted from peripheral mononuclear cells, the combined genotype of CYP1A1 exon 7 mutation and null GSTM1 in women has an odds ratio of 6.54 for the development of lung cancer as compared to 2.36 in men [25]. Polymorphisms in cytochrome P450 and GSTM1 may be a contributing factor to the increased risk of lung cancer in women.

DNA Repair Capacity

Observational studies have consistently shown higher levels of DNA adducts in women than men [22.26.27]. The impact of these adducts and their association with the development of malignancy is dependent on the ability of the cells to repair DNA damage. DNA repair capacity (DRC) has been evaluated in a case-control study of patients with lung cancer. The DRC of patients' cultured lymphocytes was determined by measuring the activity of a reporter gene exposed to a reactive intermediate of PAH metabolism, B(a)P diol epoxide [28]. In this study, women had a lower DNA repair capacity than men. A statistically significant trend of increased lung cancer risk with lower levels of DRC was observed, suggesting that women are at higher risk of disease development.

p53

The impact of DNA adduct formation depends on the location of damage and the disruption of key cell cycle genes. Specifically, p53 and K-ras have been examined as a target of PAH cigarette damage. Cigarette smoke and PAH exposure associated p53 mutations are typically G:C to T:A transversions and have been linked to several hotspots in the p53 gene [29]. An analysis of the 2002 International Agency for Research on Cancer mutational database demonstrated that 36% of smoking women had a G to T transversion mutation as compared to 13% of non-smoking women with lung cancer indicating the mutational impact of smoking [30]. In contrast, 31% of smoking and 27% of non-smoking men with lung cancer were observed to have this type of mutation. This suggests that susceptibility to DNA damage is increased in women exposed to tobacco smoke.

K-ras

Activation of K-ras causes downstream signaling via the MAP kinase cascade, amongst others, resulting in cell proliferation and tumor growth. Codon 12 of K-ras is frequently mutated in lung adenocarcinomas and is associated with cigarette smoke exposure and poor outcomes. A prospective study evaluating K-ras mutational status in 200 lung cancer patients found that mutations were only present in current or former smokers. In addition, a higher proportion of women (26.2%) had the mutation as compared to men (17.4%) [31]. Even after controlling for pack years of smoking, there was a statistically significant association between K-ras mutation and female sex. In contrast, a retrospective analysis of K-ras mutational status in patients treated on the TRIBUTE trial (carboplatin and paclitaxel with or without erlotinib, n=264) demonstrated that the mutation rate was the same in men and women (approximately 20%). However, similar to the previous study, K-ras mutations were only observed in smokers.

Overall, environmental exposure to cigarette smoke and its toxins appears to have a greater impact at the biological level in women than in men. This appears to be due to differences at multiple steps along the carcinogen pathway. Women have increased metabolism of PAH resulting in increased DNA adducts and have a lower capacity for DNA repair. In addition, essential proteins for regulated cell growth are targeted and altered by the PAH adducts resulting in an even higher propensity for cancer development. Dose for dose, these studies suggest the carcinogenic effects of cigarettes are greater for women.

Hormone Receptors in Lung Cancer

While the importance of hormones and their receptors have long been recognized in breast and prostate cancer, the potential role of a hormonal influence on lung cancer has not been as well studied. Estrogen receptors (ER α and ER β) regulate transcription processes by binding at the estrogen response element (ERE) and the AP1 response element (Figure 2). Interaction of estrogen-bound ER α and β with the ERE results in increased transcription of key proteins; in contrast, anti-estrogens causes transcription downregulation [32]. Responses differ at the AP1 site with ER α binding of estrogen and anti-estrogens increasing transcription and ER β binding of estrogens causing transcription inhibition, while anti-estrogen binding results in transcription activation. This suggests that ER α and β have different roles in transcription modification.

It has been hypothesized that the presence of ER β, the most common ER detected in lung tissue, is a negative prognostic indicator in women with lung cancer because of endogenous estrogen binding resulting in transcription activation. Retrospective studies examining pathological specimens, found that 45-67% of lung tumors were ER β positive [33,34,35]. In a retrospective, population-based, case-control study (n=278), for women with ER β positive tumors, there was a non-significant trend towards increased mortality compared to ER β negative tumors [35]. Approximately 40% of the women had used HRT; however, the analysis did not look at outcomes in this subset of women or specifically define HRT use. In contrast, men with ER β positive tumors had a reduction in mortality compared to their negative counterparts. Overall, women had better survival rates than men, regardless of ER β status. Expression of ER β may be related to histology, with one report indicating higher levels of ER β expression in adenocarcinoma (85%) compared to squamous cell carcinoma (30%) [33]. Wu et al did not find a correlation between histology and ER β status but noted increased ER β expression in females, non-smokers, smaller tumors ($\leq$ 3 cm), well-differentiated tumors and absence of lymph node metastasis [34]. The prognostic implications of ER β status are unclear, possibly due to the dual mechanism of transcription modification through the ERE and AP1 pathways.

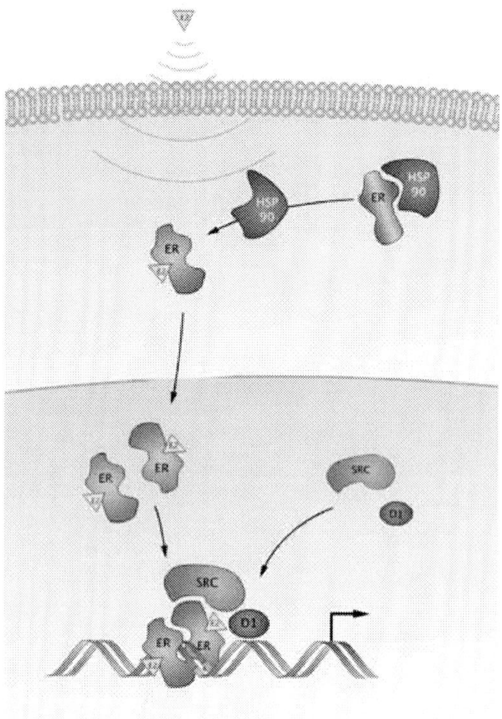

From: http://mekentosj.com/science/er/overview.html.

Figure 2. Estrogen receptor signaling and transcription activation (ER - estrogen receptor, E2 - estrogen, HSP 90 - heat shock protein 90, D1 – cyclin D1).

Progesterone receptors (PR) have been detected in NSCLC and have been identified as a positive prognostic indicator in both sexes. In a study by Ishibashi et al, 46% of tumors were PR positive, and PR were more commonly observed in females and adenocarcinoma histology [36]. Their pre-clinical models demonstrated that progesterone inhibited cell proliferation *in vitro* and in tumor xenografts. Tumor xenografts growth inhibition by progesterone was associated with increase p21 and p27 levels with decreased cyclin A, cyclin D1, cyclin E and Ki-67. Endogenous progesterone may have a role in suppressing progression of PR positive NSCLC tumors. The positive prognostic role of PR and the impact of progesterone needs validation in future studies as it may provide therapeutic options for patients with PR positive tumors.

In addition to the presence of ER and PR, immunohistochemistry of archival NSCLC tissue has demonstrated expression of aromatase, the enzyme that converts androgens (testosterone) into estrogens, in 86% of samples [37]. Higher levels of aromatase activity were found in tumor cells compared to adjacent normal lung tissue. Evidence to support a potential therapeutic intervention includes the *in vitro* application of an aromatase inhibitor, anastrazole, which reduces enzyme activity, cell growth and causes tumor growth inhibition in A549 tumor xenografts in ovariectomized nude mice [37].

The hormone mediated proliferation pathway may overlap with the epidermal growth factor receptor (EGFR) cascade, a well recognized pathway, important in the growth of lung cancer. In studies of lung tumor cell caveolae, ER and EGFR have been localized in close proximity [38] and *in vitro*, estrogen and epidermal growth factor are known to stimulate cell proliferation. Thus, both ER and EGFR pathways have been targeted together in lung cancer cell models. NIH N23 lung adenocarcinoma cells were treated with fulvestrant, an ER antagonist and gefitinib, an EGFR tyrosine kinase inhibitor *in vitro* [38,39]. Marked inhibition of cell growth was noted with this combination compared to the hormonal agent alone. Similarly, Stabile et al found that in A549 (bronchioloalveolar), 201T (adenocarcinoma) and 273T (squamous) cell lines and mouse 201T xenografts, there was improved anti-tumor effect with the combination therapy [39]. This correlated with evidence of increased apoptosis, decreased phospho-MAPK, a downstream proliferation-signaling molecule, and decreased Ki-67, a proliferation index, compared to single agent therapy. This pre-clinical work has been translated to the clinic, where a small trial (n=22) was conducted in post-menopausal women combining gefitinib and fulvestrant [40]. Thus far there is no apparent correlation between ER α, ER β, EGFR expression and response to treatment. The treatment was well tolerated with 6 patients experiencing stable disease and an additional 2 with confirmed partial responses.

The presence of hormone receptors and aromatase activity in lung cancer tissue raise interesting questions regarding the role of endogenous and exogenous estrogens in NSCLC growth and development. There are clearly complex interactions between hormones and hormone receptors that warrant further investigation to increase our understanding for potential therapeutic interventions in lung cancer.

Table 2. Summary of studies evaluating the association between hormone replacement therapy and lung cancer risk in women

Year published	Author	Source	Study design	n	Hormonal therapy and lung cancer risk
1988	Wu	Southern California database	Case-control	336	Same
1994	Taioli	American Health Foundation	Case-control	483	Increased
1996	Persson	Sweden	Cohort	22,597	Same
2002		Women's Health Initiative	Cohort	16,608	Same
2002	Blackman	Four centres United States	Case-control	662 cases	Same
2003	Kreuzer	Germany	Case-control	1,723	Decreased
2003	Olsson	Sweden	Cohort	29,508	Decreased
2004	Schabath	MD Anderson	Case-control	1018	Decreased
2005	Ganti	US community based teaching hospital	Case-control	498	Detrimental effect on overall survival

Hormone Replacement Therapy

The impact of hormone replacement therapy (HRT) on lung cancer risk has been examined in multiple studies. Data has been collected from case-control and cohort studies without reaching a consensus on risk (Table 2). Three studies have demonstrated a decreased risk of lung cancer with HRT, including a case-control study by Kreuzer et al performed in Germany [41]. After adjusting for the age, region, pack years, time since smoking cessation and education level, the odd ratio (OR) for lung cancer associated with the use of exogenous hormones was 0.69 for oral contraceptives and 0.83 for HRT. However, the study lacked information regarding the composition and dose of the hormone therapy. A second study, a population-based cohort study involving over 29,000 women, noted a protective benefit from HRT [42]. Long-term HRT users had a decreased incidence of all smoking related malignancies including lung cancer. This advantage was observed in progestin and non-progestin users, regardless of smoking dose. Similarly, in a study conducted at MD Anderson, HRT, estrogen alone and estrogen with progesterone, was associated with a reduction in the risk of lung cancer with an odds ratio of 0.66 [43]. Their model incorporated age, ethnicity, smoking status, education, body mass index and menopausal status.

Several studies have shown no change in lung cancer risk with the use of HRT. A population-based case-control series in the United States found, after accounting for other risk factors including HRT, that only personal smoking, personal and family history of lung disease were associated with increased risk [44]. A large cohort study in Sweden found no adverse or protective effects against lung cancer with the use of HRT after 13 years of follow-up [45]. In 662 female lung cancer patients in four American centers, comparing use $<$ 3 months of HRT to $\geq$ 3 months, the odds ratio was 1.0 [46]. The Women's Health Initiative, designed primarily to assess the impact of HRT on cardiovascular and breast cancer outcomes, found no HRT influence on the incidence of lung cancer (hazard ratio 1.04) [47]. According to these analyses, HRT is not associated with increased or decreased incidence of lung cancer.

One study suggests that the incidence of lung cancer is increased in women taking HRT. Taioli et al, in a case-control study, observed that the use of HRT was significantly associated with the incidence of adenocarcinoma (OR 1.7) [48]. The risk of adenocarcinoma was significant higher in women who smoked and used HRT compared to those who only smoked. Like other studies, there are limitations to this study with the absence of information regarding dose and composition of HRT.

Multiple studies have conflicting results regarding the use of HRT and risk of lung cancer; perhaps the more important question is not about the impact of HRT in incidence but rather outcomes of women on HRT with lung cancer. Ganti et al performed a hypothesis-generating retrospective chart review of almost 500 women with lung cancer [49]. The use of HRT was defined as 6 continuous weeks of estrogen and progestin or estrogen alone prior to the diagnosis of lung cancer, excluding oral contraceptive use. In comparing non-hormone and hormone user, the only statistically significant difference was the median age at diagnosis, with the non-hormone users being slightly older (68 versus 63 years); histologic and stage distribution was similar in both groups. The overall survival was significantly reduced in patients treated with HRT compared to those that were not (39 versus 79 months,

HR 1.97, 95% CI, 1.14-3.39). This raises the possibility of estrogen promoting tumor growth or contributing to more aggressive tumor behavior. Further evaluation of the potential detrimental effect of HRT on survival outcomes in women with lung cancer is required.

While multiple studies have attempted to evaluate biological differences between men and women in the development and progression of lung cancer it is difficult to draw solid conclusions based on the data to date. Recognizing the importance of this issue, the Southwest Oncology Group (SWOG) is conducting a molecular epidemiology case series study in smoking and non-smoking women and men diagnosed with lung cancer (S0424). This study will assess DNA adducts, alterations in specific genes, proteins and receptors (eg. ER, HER2, p53, k-ras), in tumor tissue and peripheral blood. Over 700 patients will be enrolled with the hope of gaining greater knowledge regarding the relationship between sex, smoking status and lung cancer.

Clinical Observations in Lung Cancer

Stage at Diagnosis

SEER data indicate that women and men have the same stage distribution at diagnosis [50]. From 1995-2001, 16% of individuals presented with localized lung cancer, 37% regional, 39% distant and 8% were unstaged. However, when diagnosed women are more likely to be younger, non-smokers, have better pulmonary function and less cardiovascular disease than men [51-55]. In keeping with this observation, women, stage for stage, appear to do better than men. The 5 year survival rates for men with localized, regional and distant disease are 44.8%, 14.2% and 1.7% compared to women, 53.5%, 17.1% and 2.2% respectively (Table 3).

Histology

Retrospective reviews of lung cancer patients have identified consistent trends in histological diagnoses [51-56]. The rates of squamous cell carcinoma are proportionally higher in men. In contrast, women proportionally had higher rates of adenocarcinoma and bronchioloalveolar carcinoma. Rates of small cell lung cancer, most closely associated with smoking, was also higher in women, approximately 25% compared to men, 20% [54].

Table 3. 5 year overall survival rates by stage and gender, SEER data

Stage	Male 5 year OS	Female 5 year OS
Localized	44.8%	53.5%
Regional	14.2%	17.1%
Distant	1.7%	2.2%

The reason for these differences is unknown, although it has been hypothesized that smoking behaviors and hormone receptors may play a role. This variation in histological distribution however, may contribute to the differences observed in survival between sexes.

Treatment

Surgery

The primary modality of treatment for early stage NSCLC is surgery. Several retrospective studies have examined prognostic factors in resected NSCLC and female sex consistently bodes for better survival [51,53-55]. Reviews that controlled for other factors including age, smoking status, pulmonary function, stage, histology and type of surgery continue to demonstrate a better outcome in women with surgically resected NSCLC.

Systemic Therapy

In advanced stage NSCLC, similar to early stage disease, female sex is a positive prognostic factor [56-59]. This may reflect a different underlying biology of advanced disease in women and may be related to likelihood of response to treatment. Studies utilizing chemotherapy and newer molecularly targeted therapies have examined the impact of sex on outcomes.

Chemotherapy (Further Subheading of Systemic Therapy)

Eastern Cooperative Oncology Group study, E1594, was a large Phase III trial comparing four platinum-based chemotherapy regimens in advanced NSCLC [60]. All treatment groups had similar outcomes with response rates of 17-22% and median survivals of 8 months. A retrospective analysis, including 437 women and 726 men, evaluated outcomes according to sex [61]. There was no statistically significant difference in performance status, weight loss > 10%, stage or incidence of brain metastasis. While response rates were similar (19%) median survival, accounting for known prognostic indicators, was prolonged in women compared to men (9.2 versus 7.3 months respectively, $p=0.004$). In addition, women had greater rates of toxicity with respect to nausea, vomiting, alopecia, neurosensory and neuropsychiatric symptoms.

Targeted Therapy (Further Subheading of Systemic Therapy)

The EGFR pathway plays a pivotal role in the development and progression of NSCLC and has become a key target in the treatment of advanced NSCLC. The epidermal growth factor receptor tyrosine kinase inhibitors (EGFR TKIs) block the signaling cascade initiated by activation of the EGFR, inhibiting cell proliferation, angiogenesis and metastasis. This pathway may be particularly important in the growth of NSCLC in women, and thus women may be more likely to benefit from EGFR-targeted therapies. Sensitivity to EGFR TKIs has been associated with activating EGFR mutations [64,65] and initially it was thought that these mutations were more common in women. However, larger series have demonstrated a similar incidence of these mutations in men and women [63,65,66]. Thus, presence of EGFR mutations does not explain the apparent increased benefit women obtain from treatment with these agents compared to men.

A recent phase II trial (Southwest Oncology Group study, S0126) evaluated gefitinib, an EGFR TKI, in advanced bronchioloalveolar carcinoma (a histological subtype of NSCLC) [62]. An unplanned subgroup analysis demonstrated that women (n=70) had a significantly longer median survival compared to men (n=67) (19 months versus 8 months, respectively, p=0.007). This benefit in survival was maintained in a multivariate model that incorporated rash (a common side effect of this class of drugs), smoking history and performance status. In a phase III National Cancer Institute of Canada (NCIC) led trial (BR 21) patients with advanced NSCLC that had progressed after front line therapy were randomized to erlotinib, another EGFR-TKI, or placebo. While women had higher response rates compared to men (14% vs 6%, p=0.007) [63], there was no difference in survival.

In contrast, a recent trial incorporating the novel antibody directed against vascular endothelial growth factor (VEGF), bevacizumab, did not show a survival benefit for women in an unplanned subgroup analysis. The ECOG 4599 trial compared carboplatin/paclitaxel -/+ bevacizumab (PC vs PCB) in 855 chemo-naïve advanced stage NSCLC patients [67]. The bevacizumab containing arm demonstrated an improved response rate (10% versus 27.2%, p<0.0001) and median survival (10.2 versus 12.5 months, p=0.007). In an unplanned subgroup analysis, the survival benefit with the addition of bevacizumab was only seen for men; hazard ratio for death PC vs PCB in men 0.69 (p=0.003) and women 0.96 (p=0.80). The reason for this lack of benefit in women is unclear; it may reflect differences in second and third line treatment, imbalances in unmeasured baseline prognostic factors or may in fact represent a true difference.

Outcomes

Despite the body of evidence that, at a biologic level, women may be more susceptible to the negative effects of cigarette smoke and estrogens may contribute to increase tumor proliferation, studies indicate that overall, women have a better prognosis once diagnosed with lung cancer than men. Women diagnosed with lung cancer are more likely to be younger, non-smokers, with better pulmonary function and less cardiovascular disease than their male counterparts [51-55]. When analyses have controlled for these potential confounding prognostic indicators, women still have a better survival. The 5 year survival rate from data compiled by the NIH from 1995-2001 was 13.6% for women compared to 5% for men, for all stages combined [68]. This observation may be the result of both different underlying disease biology and increase likelihood of response to current therapies.

Conclusion

Lung cancer in women is a significant health issue, responsible for more cancer related mortality than breast and colorectal cancer combined. There appear to be biological differences in lung cancer related to sex. Women seem to be more susceptible to the negative effects of smoke exposure possibly due to differences in carcinogen metabolism. The presence of hormone receptors may also impact the natural history of disease, playing a role in tumor proliferation and growth. Yet, despite this, once diagnosed with lung cancer women have a better overall prognosis than men. Clearly there are complex mechanisms involved and a better understanding of sex-related biology will enable us to more effectively direct research and apply treatments for both women and men.

References

[1] Society AC: *Cancer Facts and Figures* 2006, 2006.

[2] Giovino, GA. Epidemiology of tobacco use in the United States. *Oncogene*, 2002 21, 7326-40.

[3] Khuder, SA. Effect of cigarette smoking on major histological types of lung cancer: a meta-analysis. *Lung Cancer*, 2001 31, 139-48.

[4] Hackshaw, AK; Law, MR; Wald, NJ. The accumulated evidence on lung cancer and environmental tobacco smoke. *Bmj,* 1997 315, 980-8.

[5] Sasco, AJ; Secretan, MB; Straif, K. Tobacco smoking and cancer: a brief review of recent epidemiological evidence. *Lung Cancer 45 Suppl 2*, 2004, S3-9.

[6] Bolego, C; Poli, A; Paoletti, R. Smoking and gender. *Cardiovasc Res*, 2002 53, 568-76.

[7] WHO, 2006.

[8] Services USDoHaH: *National Survey on Drug Use and Health* 2004, 2006.

[9] Dalton, MA; Sargent, JD; Beach, ML; et al. Effect of viewing smoking in movies on adolescent smoking initiation: a cohort study. *Lance*t, 2003 362, 281-5.

[10] King, C, 3rd; Siegel, M. The Master Settlement Agreement with the tobacco industry and cigarette advertising in magazines. *N Engl. J. Med*, 2001 345, 504-11.

[11] Harris, RE; Zang, EA; Anderson, JI; et al. Race and sex differences in lung cancer risk associated with cigarette smoking. *Int. J. Epidemiol*, 1993 22, 592-9.

[12] Zang, EA; Wynder, EL. Differences in lung cancer risk between men and women: examination of the evidence. *J. Natl. Cancer Inst*, 1996 88, 183-92.

[13] Osann, KE; Anton-Culver, H; Kurosaki, T; et al. Sex differences in lung-cancer risk associated with cigarette smoking. *Int. J. Cancer*, 1993 54, 44-8.

[14] Risch, HA; Howe, GR; Jain, M; et al. Are female smokers at higher risk for lung cancer than male smokers? A case-control analysis by histologic type. *Am. J. Epidemiol*, 1993 138, 281-93.

[15] Henschke, CI; Miettinen, OS. Women's susceptibility to tobacco carcinogens. *Lung Cancer*, 2004 43, 1-5.

[16] Halpern, MT; Gillespie, BW; Warner, KE. Patterns of absolute risk of lung cancer mortality in former smokers. *J. Natl. Cancer Inst*, 1983 85, 457-64.

[17] Kreuzer, M; Boffetta, P; Whitley, E; et al. Gender differences in lung cancer risk by smoking: a multicentre case-control study in Germany and Italy. *Br. J. Cancer*, 2000 82, 227-33.

[18] Bach, PB; Kattan, MW; Thornquist, MD; et al. Variations in lung cancer risk among smokers. *J. Natl. Cancer Inst*, 2003 95, 470-8.

[19] Bain, C; Feskanich, D; Speizer, FE; et al. Lung cancer rates in men and women with comparable histories of smoking. *J. Natl. Cancer Inst*, 2004 96, 826-34.

[20] Kouri, RE; Rude, TH; Curren, RD; et al. Biological activity of tobacco smoke and tobacco smoke-related chemicals. *Environ. Health Perspect*, 1979 29, 63-69.

[21] McLemore, TL; Adelberg, S; Liu, MC; et al. Expression of CYP1A1 gene in patients with lung cancer: evidence for cigarette smoke-induced gene expression in normal lung tissue and for altered gene regulation in primary pulmonary carcinomas. *J. Natl. Cancer Inst*, 1990 82, 1333-9.

[22] Mollerup, S; Ryberg, D; Hewer, A; et al. Sex differences in lung CYP1A1 expression and DNA adduct levels among lung cancer patients. *Cancer Res*, 1999 59, 3317-20.

[23] Bell, DA; Taylor, JA; Paulson, DF; et al. Genetic risk and carcinogen exposure: a common inherited defect of the carcinogen-metabolism gene glutathione S-transferase M1 (GSTM1) that increases susceptibility to bladder cancer. *J. Natl. Cancer Inst*, 1993 85, 1159-64.

[24] Tang, DL; Rundle, A; Warburton, D; et al. Associations between both genetic and environmental biomarkers and lung cancer: evidence of a greater risk of lung cancer in women smokers. *Carcinogenesis*, 1998 19, 1949-53.

[25] Dresler, CM; Fratelli, C; Babb, J; et al. Gender differences in genetic susceptibility for lung cancer. *Lung Cancer*, 2000 30, 153-60.

[26] Ryberg, D; Hewer, A; Phillips, DH et al. Different susceptibility to smoking-induced DNA damage among male and female lung cancer patients. *Cancer Res*, 1994 54, 5801-3.

[27] Haugen, A. Women who smoke: are women more susceptible to tobacco-induced lung cancer? *Carcinogenesis*, 2002 23, 227-9.

[28] Wei, Q; Cheng, L; Amos, CI; et al. Repair of tobacco carcinogen-induced DNA adducts and lung cancer risk: a molecular epidemiologic study. *J. Natl. Cancer Inst*, 2000 92, 1764-72.

[29] Kure, EH; Ryberg, D; Hewer, A; et al. p53 mutations in lung tumours: relationship to gender and lung DNA adduct levels. *Carcinogenesis*, 1996 17, 2201-5.

[30] Toyooka, S; Tsuda, T; Gazdar, AF. The TP53 gene, tobacco exposure, and lung cancer. *Hum. Mutat*, 2003 21, 229-39.

[31] Nelson, HH; Christiani, DC; Mark, EJ; et al. Implications and prognostic value of K-ras mutation for early-stage lung cancer in women. *J. Natl. Cancer Inst*, 1999 91, 2032-8.

[32] Paech, K; Webb, P; Kuiper, GG; et al. Differential ligand activation of estrogen receptors ERalpha and ERbeta at AP1 sites. *Science*, 1997 277, 1508-10.

[33] Omoto, Y; Kobayashi, Y; Nishida, K; et al. Expression, function, and clinical implications of the estrogen receptor beta in human lung cancers. *Biochem. Biophys. Res. Commun*, 2001 285, 340-7.

[34] Wu, CT; Chang, YL; Shih, JY; et al. The significance of estrogen receptor beta in 301 surgically treated non-small cell lung cancers. *J. Thorac. Cardiovasc. Surg*, 2005 130, 979-86.

[35] Schwartz, AG; Prysak, GM; Murphy, V; et al. Nuclear estrogen receptor beta in lung cancer: expression and survival differences by sex. *Clin. Cancer Res*, 2005 11, 7280-7.

[36] Ishibashi, H; Suzuki, T; Suzuki, S; et al. Progesterone receptor in non-small cell lung cancer--a potent prognostic factor and possible target for endocrine therapy. *Cancer Res*, 2005 65, 6450-8.

[37] Weinberg, OK; Marquez-Garban, DC; Fishbein, MC; et al. Aromatase inhibitors in human lung cancer therapy. *Cancer Res*, 2005 65, 11287-91.

[38] Pietras, RJ; Marquez, DC; Chen, HW; et al. Estrogen and growth factor receptor interactions in human breast and non-small cell lung cancer cells. *Steroids*, 2005 70, 372-81.

[39] Stabile, LP; Lyker, JS; Gubish, CT; et al. Combined targeting of the estrogen receptor and the epidermal growth factor receptor in non-small cell lung cancer shows enhanced antiproliferative effects. *Cancer Res*, 2005 65, 1459-70.

[40] Traynor, AM; Schiller, JH; Stabile, LP; et al. Combination therapy with gefitinib and fulvestrant (G/F) for women with non-small cell lung cancer (NSCLC*). J. Clin. Oncol. (Meeting Abstracts)*, 2005 23, 7224-.

[41] Kreuzer, M; Gerken, M; Heinrich, J; et al. Hormonal factors and risk of lung cancer among women? *Int. J. Epidemiol*, 2003 32, 263-71.

[42] Olsson, H; Bladstrom, A; Ingvar, C. Are smoking-associated cancers prevented or postponed in women using hormone replacement therapy? *Obstet Gynecol*, 2003 102, 565-70.

[43] Schabath, MB; Wu, X; Vassilopoulou-Sellin, R; et al. Hormone replacement therapy and lung cancer risk: a case-control analysis. *Clin. Cancer Res*, 2004 10, 113-23.

[44] Wu, AH; Yu, MC; Thomas, DC; et al. Personal and family history of lung disease as risk factors for adenocarcinoma of the lung. *Cancer Res*, 1988 48, 7279-84.

[45] Persson, I; Yuen, J; Bergkvist, L; et al. Cancer incidence and mortality in women receiving estrogen and estrogen-progestin replacement therapy--long-term follow-up of a Swedish cohort. *Int. J. Cancer*, 1996 67, 327-32.

[46] Blackman, JA; Coogan, PF; Rosenberg, L; et al. Estrogen replacement therapy and risk of lung cancer. *Pharmacoepidemiol. Drug Saf*, 2002 11, 561-7.

[47] Rossouw, JE; Anderson, GL; Prentice, RL; et al. Risks and benefits of estrogen plus progestin in healthy postmenopausal women: principal results from the Women's Health Initiative randomized controlled trial. *Jama*, 2002 288, 321-33.

[48] Taioli, E; Wynder, EL. Re: Endocrine factors and adenocarcinoma of the lung in women. *J. Natl. Cancer Inst*, 1994 86, 869-70.

[49] Ganti, AK; Sahmoun, AE; Panwalkar, AW; et al. Hormone replacement therapy is associated with decreased survival in women with lung cancer. *J. Clin. Oncol*, 2006 24, 59-63.

[50] SEER: *SEER data for lung and bronchus cancer*, 2006.

[51] Ferguson, MK; Wang, J; Hoffman, PC; et al. Sex-associated differences in survival of patients undergoing resection for lung cancer. *Ann. Thorac. Surg*, 2000 69, 245-9, discussion 249-50.

[52] Radzikowska, E; Langfort, R; Giedronowicz, D; Estrogen and progesterone receptors in non small cell lung cancer patients. *Ann. Thorac. Cardiovasc. Surg*, 2002 8, 69-73.

[53] Alexiou, C; Onyeaka, CV; Beggs, D; et al. Do women live longer following lung resection for carcinoma? *Eur. J. Cardiothorac. Surg*, 2002 21, 319-25.

[54] Chatkin, JM; Abreu, CM; Fritscher, CC; et al. Is there a gender difference in non-small cell lung cancer survival? *Gend. Med*, 2004 1, 41-7.

[55] Batevik, R; Grong, K; Segadal, L; et al. The female gender has a positive effect on survival independent of background life expectancy following surgical resection of primary non-small cell lung cancer: a study of absolute and relative survival over 15 years. *Lung Cancer*, 2005 47, 173-81.

[56] Radzikowska, E; Glaz, P; Roszkowski, K. Lung cancer in women: age, smoking, histology, performance status, stage, initial treatment and survival. Population-based study of 20 561 cases. *Ann. Oncol*, 2002 13, 1087-93.

[57] Albain, KS; Crowley, JJ; LeBlanc, M; et al. Survival determinants in extensive-stage non-small-cell lung cancer: the Southwest Oncology Group experience. *Journal of Clinical Oncology*, 1991 9, 1618-26.

[58] Paesmans, M; Sculier, JP; Libert, P; et al. Prognostic factors for survival in advanced non-small-cell lung cancer: univariate and multivariate analyses including recursive partitioning and amalgamation algorithms in 1,052 patients. The European Lung Cancer Working Party. *Journal of Clinical Oncology*, 1995 13, 1221-30.

[59] Visbal, AL; Williams, BA; Nichols, FC, 3rd; et al. Gender differences in non-small-cell lung cancer survival: an analysis of 4,618 patients diagnosed between 1997 and 2002. *Ann. Thorac. Surg*, 2004 78, 209-15, discussion 215.

[60] Schiller, JH; Harrington, D; Belani, CP; et al. Comparison of four chemotherapy regimens for advanced non-small-cell lung cancer. *New England Journal of Medicine*, 2002 346, 92-8.

[61] Wakelee, H WW; Schiller, J; Langer, C; Sandler, A; Belani, C; Johnson, D. Survival differences by gender for patients with advanced non-small cell lung cancer in Eastern Cooperative Group trial 1594. *J. Thoracic Oncology In press*, 2006.

[62] West, H; Franklin, WA; Gumerlock, P; et al. *Gefitinib (ZD1839) therapy for advanced bronchioloalveolar lung cancer: Southwest Oncology Group Study S0126.*, ASCO. New Orleans, 2004.

[63] Tsao, MS; Sakurada, A; Cutz, JC; et al. Erlotinib in lung cancer - molecular and clinical predictors of outcome. *N Engl. J. Med*, 2005 353, 133-44.

[64] Pao, W; Miller, V; Zakowski, M; et al. EGF receptor gene mutations are common in lung cancers from "never smokers" and are associated with sensitivity of tumors to gefitinib and erlotinib. *PNAS* 101:13306-13311, 2004.

[65] Paez, JG; Janne, PA; Lee, JC; et al. EGFR Mutations in Lung Cancer: Correlation with Clinical Response to Gefitinib Therapy. *Science*, 2004 304, 1497-1500.

[66] Eberhard, DA; Johnson, BE; Amler, LC; et al. Mutations in the Epidermal Growth Factor Receptor and in KRAS Are Predictive and Prognostic Indicators in Patients With Non-Small-Cell Lung Cancer Treated With Chemotherapy Alone and in Combination With Erlotinib. *J. Clin. Oncol*, 2005 23, 5900-5909.

[67] Sandler, AB; Gray, R; Brahmer, J; et al. Randomized phase II/III trial of paclitaxel (P) plus carboplatin (C) with or without bevacizumab (NSC #704865) in patients with advanced non-squamous non-small cell lung cancer (NSCLC): An Eastern Cooperative Oncology Group (ECOG) Trial - E4599. *J. Clin. Oncol. (Meeting Abstracts)*, 2005 23, LBA4-.

[68] Health USNIo: *Surveillance Epidemiology and End Results (SEER)*, 2005.

In: Smoking and Lung Cancer
Editors: E. N. Powers and J. B. Cabbot
ISBN 978-1-60692-367-2

Chapter X

Perspectives on Smoking and Radon Related Lung Cancers

Anita Enflo*
Retired from the Swedish Radiation Protection Authority, SE 17116 Stockholm, Sweden

Abstract

The proportion between smoking and radon related lung cancer incidences is discussed with focus on the real situation in a region with high radon concentrations in dwellings. Special emphasis has been put on the exposition of children where there is a lack of data. The risks from domestic radon seem to be highly coupled with the risks from smoking. Smoking is by far the most leading risk factor for primary lung cancer, and the risks from radon seem to be overemphasised. The most effective method to reduce the number of primary lung cancer incidences seems to be to stop smoking, both what concerns smoking related as well as radon related lung cancers. Campaigns for testing all homes for radon should also include campaigns against smoking.

Introduction

Lung cancer is mainly a disease of elderly ages and is rare at young ages. There is no effective cure yet, but both diagnostic and therapeutic methods for early detection and cure are under development. The one-year survival after diagnosis has during the last decade risen from about 10% to about 30% of the incidences. The five-year survival is today still less than 10 %.

There seems to be a common opinion that smoking is the main cause of *primary* lung cancer. About 90 % of the cancer incidences occur among smokers. Residential radon has been considered the second leading cause. The proportion between these two risk factors is

* anita.enflo@swipnet.se.

unclear and there are reasons to believe that the risk from radon is overestimated. *Secondary* lung cancer, on the other hand, is a result of metastasis from cancers in other organs and can have many causes. In this paper only primary lung cancer is considered.

There are several studies about the risks for lung cancer from radon and several large evaluations by different international and national organisations, the most recent ones performed by the ICRP (International Commission on Radiological Protection) in 1994 [1], the NAS (National Academy of Sciences) in USA in 1999 [2], the Swedish Government Report in 2001 [3] and the EPA (U.S. Environmental Protection Agency) assessment of risks from radon in homes in June 2003 [4]. Whereas it seems fairly well established that lung cancer among miners is radon related with commonly accepted risk values, the risks from domestic radon seems still to be under debate. Due to the relatively low radon levels in homes, compared to mines, and many other factors, as for example, long exposure and latency periods and other environmental factors, it is difficult to find an accurate estimate of the radon risks. Still to day risk evaluations about residential radon is to a great extent based on extrapolations from data on miners. The present situation can be described as follows:

According to the U.S. Environmental Protection Agency (EPA) out of a total of 157,400 lung cancer deaths nationally in 1995, 21,100 (13.4%) were estimated to be radon related. Among non smokers an estimated 26% were radon related [4]. The absolute risk for non smokers was found to be lower than for smokers but the relative risk was found to be higher for non smokers than for smokers. As the baseline risk for lung cancer is low for non smokers, the number of radon related non smoking lung cancer incidences is still low.

In Sweden, which is a high radon country, the corresponding authorities, SSI (Swedish Radiation Protection Authority) estimate that in the Swedish population of about 9 million people, about 500 primary lung cancer incidences per year, i.e. 17%, are radon related (of a total of about 3000 incidences) [3]. The absolute risk for non smokers was lower than for smokers.

There are, however, weaknesses in these risk estimations that need further consideration and that may change the picture.

Methodology

The above referred risk values are based on several studies, mainly epidemiological, since the dosimetric estimations resulted in unrealistically high risk values exceeding the total number of lung cancer incidences. This made ICRP (International Commission of Radiological Protection) to recommend that the risk estimations should be based on epidemiological studies [1]. A comprehensive report of the state of the Art was elaborated from 1994 by the NAS (National Academy of Sciences) and published early 1999 (BEIR VI) [2]. The EPA assessment of risks [4] is a revision based on the findings and recommendations in BEIR VI.

Of the epidemiological studies, the ecological are the most simple. No individual data is required. Only the number of cases in one area with a certain property, as for example radon level, is compared with the number of cases in another area. The method has been extensively used by Cohen [5], who found a negative correlation between radon and lung cancer. This method has been fiercely critisised by many of the groups working with case-control studies as they find the method too simple [6-11]. It should be kept in mind that the case-control studies may also have their limitations, as shown below.

The first epidemiological studies about radon related lung cancer were performed among miners. There was little controversy about the precision of the risk estimations. Radon levels in mines were high and the miners were exposed to radon during well specified time periods. It was rather easy to follow the history of the miners and their living habits. Lately, however, some doubt has been raised concerning the effects of other factors as diesel gases, uranium and other dust particles as well as smoking habits, although most of the miners were also heavy smokers.

What concerns residential radon, the situation is different. Radon levels in dwellings are generally orders of magnitude lower than in mines. The inhabitants are exposed to low radon levels during long and often unspecified time periods. During these time periods the living habits may change considerably and it is not possible to completely control the exposure to other known or unknown risk factors, as for example passive smoking, other air contaminants, working environment or radon in work places, schools or other buildings. Mostly risk estimations about residential radon have thus been extrapolated from data about high radon levels among miners to the lower radon levels in dwellings. Such extrapolations are based on the LNT hypothesis, i.e. that there is a Linear Non Threshold relationship between the effects of high and low doses.

Lately, several case control studies concerning lung cancer and domestic radon have been performed, many of them pretty large what concerns the number of cases and number of controls. The larger the studies, the higher are their statistical power. Thus, there have been attempts to pool several studies together to get more statistical power, presuming that the studies are performed as similarly as possible. The risk estimations used today depend to a considerable extent on a meta-analysis of 8 different studies, taking into account their different designs [12].

Case-control studies are elaborate, as they handle each individual separately. Well performed case-control studies are considered reliable. For small risks large amounts of cases and controls are needed. It is a costly procedure to find cases and matching controls and follow up them all individually. It is not always possible to handle all parameters needed. If the input parameters are wrong, the final result will also be wrong, even though the mathematical data treatment is correct. Some examples of input variables that may affect the final result are:

- The number of cases is too small. This has been the case especially among the non-smoking lung cancer cases. They are so few so that it has been difficult to collect enough cases to perform good enough epidemiological studies.
- The controls do not match the cases to all parameters needed. This is the case for the smoking habits among cases and controls. Thus, for example in the Swedish nationwide case-control study [13] consisting of 1360 primary lung cancer cases and 2847 age matched controls, 87% of the cases were smokers but only 59% of the controls.

- The follow up time does not cover the whole exposure history. This can be the case in the studies about domestic radon, where the individuals are exposed to low doses during long time periods, as discussed below. This is not the case for radon in mines, where the miners are exposed to high doses under shorter time periods that can be followed from their working schemes.
- The period of latency is longer than the study period. This can be the case for long latency periods, as for example for lung cancer and radon, as discussed below.
- The exposure measurements are wrong or inaccurate. In all measurements there are always more or less severe measurement errors.
- The measured exposure is not the same as the individual exposure. This is the case especially for radon measurements hitherto performed. The radon measurements do not follow the individual, but are measured in the room where the individual is supposed to live. This is not necessary the case, and even if it is the case, the individual do not spend all its time there. An occupational factor of 0,8 is often used, but it can be much different. The individual can spend the rest of the time in places where the radon concentration can be much different, as for example on a working place with high radon levels.

In all studies, there are always some approximations and some limitations, which can more or less seriously affect the results. We will in this study mainly concentrate upon follow up times and latency periods. Epidemiological studies will always give us a number, which can be seriously in error if the input data is incorrect although the statistical treatment of the data is correct. There has to be some check that the final results are reasonable. These checks can be rather simple ones, as for example to check that the predicted numbers are realistic or in accordance with measured values.

Results

Data from Sweden

The situation in Sweden deserves special interest. Partly because Sweden is one of the countries where the radon levels are high and partly because there are good registers to be used in Sweden.

Register Studies

Due to the Swedish health care system, it is possible to register all diagnosed cancer incidences in Sweden. The Swedish cancer registry [14] has been working since 1958. Depending on the development of diagnostic methods, the register can be considered complete. For lung cancer, as long as most of the lung cancer incidences die within a year, the number of incidences is about the same as the number of deaths, but as the prognosis gets better and more patients are cured, the number of incidences gives a better measure of the risk than the number of deaths, which has been used in several of the epidemiologic studies. The problem with misclassification is also smaller in a register for incidences than in a register for deaths, because the cause of death can be another than the original illness.

Not only is the number of cases needed. The exposition history must also be known. The Swedish population is rather stationary, not moving around from place to place but often living in just a few places during their whole lifetime. Their living places are easy to follow through registers and people are also rather open for interviews. For smoking habits though, there is no register on the individual level.

Radon Levels in the Swedish Housing Stock

Sweden is a high radon country. The ground is rich in uranium, which during its decay process releases radon gas through the ground to the air. During a time period of economical growth, after World War II, when a large amount of the housing stock was built, a kind of blue concrete (unfortunately containing radium) was a popular building material. This building material was forbidden in 1975 but the houses still remain. The mean value of radon gas in Swedish dwellings has been estimated to be 108 Bq/m^3, only exceeded by Finland with a mean value of 128 Bq/m^3. These numbers can be compared with the corresponding numbers for some other countries as for example Norway 73 Bq/m^3, France 62 Bq/m^3, Denmark 53 Bq/m^3, Germany 50 Bq/m^3, USA 46 Bq/m^3, Canada 34 Bq/m^3, Great Britain 20 Bq/m^3 and Japan as low as 16 Bq/m^3 [15].

Although the mean values in the other countries are appreciably lower than the Swedish ones, there can be local regions with pretty high values. Such regions are for example the uranium mining areas in the Czech Republic and Eastern Germany (Saxony), and Cornwall in the UK. What is special for Sweden is that there are high radon houses as well as low radon houses spread rather smoothly all over the country without any big regional variations and thus there is no regional population especially much exposed or adjusted to radon. This makes Sweden especially suitable to study the radon issue as cases and matched controls should be rather easily found.

In the Swedish housing stock of about 4 million dwellings it is estimated [16] that about 4%, (i.e. 160 000 dwellings) has radon levels of more than 400 Bq/m^3 (10.8 pCi/l), which is the recommended action level for radon in existing buildings in Sweden and about 7% (i.e. 280 000 dwellings) has radon levels between 200 Bq/m^3 and 400 Bq/m^3. 200 Bq/m^3 (5.4 pCi/l) is the recommended upper level for radon in new buildings. Most of the buildings, 89% or about 3 million dwellings has radon levels well below 200 Bq/m^3, many as low as 20 Bq/m^3. The arithmetic average is 108 Bq/m^3 and the geometric average 56 Bq/m^3. The highest value measured in a Swedish dwelling was 86 000 Bq/m^3, but fortunately there does not seem to be so many buildings with so high levels. About 1% (i.e. 40 000 dwellings) has radon levels more than 800 Bq/m^3 [16].

Table 1. Total number of lung cancer incidences among men and women 1984-2002

Year	Men	Women	Men+women
1984	1982	726	2708
1985	1957	760	2717
1986	1932	781	2713
1987	1924	861	2785
1988	1882	828	2710
1989	1879	820	2699
1990	1904	865	2769
1991	1890	949	2839
1992	1841	952	2973
1993	1807	977	2784
1994	1909	1059	2968
1995	1732	1063	2795
1996	1713	1073	2785
1997	1724	1037	2761
1998	1771	1075	2846
1999	1727	1168	2895
2000	1727	1234	2961
2001	1785	1259	3044
2002	1713	1269	2982

Table 2. Age distribution of primary lung cancer incidences among men and women 1990-2002

Age at incidence	Men	Women	Men	Women	Men	Women	Men	Women
	1990	1990	1996	1996	2000	2000	2002	2002
0-19	0	0	0	1	0	0	1	0
20-39	12	9	7	6	13	7	9	7
40-59	327	201	281	293	287	336	298	316
60-79	1297	539	1214	666	1183	764	1136	775
80+	268	116	210	107	244	127	269	171

As these high radon values are supposed to cause several primary lung cancer incidences among the population living in the buildings, an epidemiologic case control study [13] consisting of 1360 primary lung cancer incidences and 2847 age matched controls was designed to determine the risk values from domestic radon. Based on the results from this study together with some other considerations it was estimated that there are about 500 radon related lung cancer incidences per year caused by the Swedish housing stock.

Annual Trends in Lung Cancer Incidences

Table 1 shows the total number of primary lung cancer incidences from year 1984 to year 2002 as well as the corresponding numbers for men and women [14]. The total number of primary lung cancer incidences shows a tendency to increase during the years, but is decreasing for men and increasing for women. These trends seem to follow the trends for the smoking habits among men and women: men stop smoking but women, especially young women, smoke more. The total number of incidences is higher for men than for women, which again can be explained by smoking habits as men smoke more than women. If there is any effect of varying radon levels, it is completely hidden by the much stronger effects of smoking habits.

Table 2 shows the age distribution of the primary lung cancer incidences among men and women from the years 1990 to 2002. Up to 40 years of age, no trends can be found and the numbers are small. There is clear trend in the age group between 60-79 years of increasing lung cancer incidences among women and decreasing among men from years 1990 to 2002. The same trends, but weaker, can be seen for the younger age groups of 40-59 years and also for the older age groups of more than 80 years. It could be of interest to point out that the number of incidences among men and women is of about the same in the age group between 40-59 years whereas the number of incidences among men is about the double than among women in the age groups from 60 years and older.

It could be suggested that women seem to be a little more sensitive to tobacco smoking and that lung cancer appears a little earlier among women then among men, but there could also be other reasons for these vague trends, as for example changes in smoking habits, different for men and women.

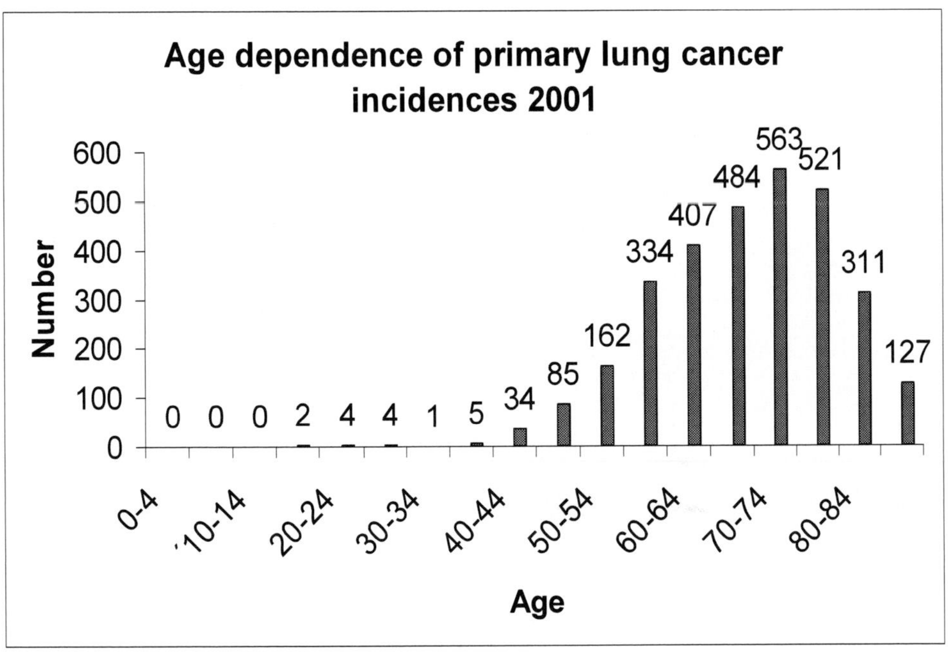

Figure 1. Showing the number of primary lung cancer incidence according to age.

Age Distribution of Primary Lung Cancer Incidences

Figure 1 shows the age distribution of the total number of primary lung cancer incidences in the year 2001 [14]. It should again be stressed that all cancer incidences are registered, there are no missing incidences other than misclassifications or mistaken diagnosis, which should be rather few with present diagnostic methods. Similar figures can be obtained for the other years [14, 17-19]. In table 3 the total number of primary lung cancer incidences among men and women, respectively, is given as a function of age. It is striking to see that there are so few primary lung cancer incidences at young ages. Below 15 years of age, there is no primary lung cancer incidence, and in the age group between 15-19 years there are 2 incidences and in the next age group (20-24 years of age) 4 incidences followed by 4 (25-29 years of age), 1 (30-34 years of age) and 5 (35-39) years of age. After the age of 40 years, the cancer incidences start to increase, first slowly, in the five year age period of 40 to 44 years with 34 more cases, then faster in the next 5-year of age period from 45 to 49 years of age with 85 more incidences, and so on up to the age group of 70-74 years for men and 65-69 years for women. Totally, in the 20 year period of age from 40 to 59 years, there were as many as 615 incidences. For elderly ages, the lung cancer incidences decrease, because elderly people die from other reasons too.

Table 3. Age distribution of primary lung cancer incidences among men and women. Year of incidence 2001

Age at incidence	Men	Women	Total
0-4	0	0	0
5-′9	0	0	0
10-′14	0	0	0
15-19	0	2	2
20-24	1	3	4
25-29	0	4	4
30-34	0	1	1
35-39	4	1	5
40-44	9	25	34
45-49	35	50	85
50-54	80	82	162
55-59	159	175	334
60-64	230	177	407
65-69	304	180	384
70-74	344	219	563
75-79	344	177	521
80-84	201	110	311
85+	74	53	127

The young age period from 0 to about 40 years of age is of special interest. Children generally do not smoke, at least not in their youngest ages, but are as much or even more exposed to domestic radon than adults. By studying the younger ages, the effects from radon should thus predominate, whereas the effects of smoking should predominate in the elderly age groups. In the age group from 0-39 years there was in 2001 totally 16 primary lung cancer incidences to be compared with a total of 2590 lung cancer incidences in the age group from 40-79 years.

There is no information about the individual smoking habits among the cancer incidences, but what could be said is that in the age group from 0-40 years, the effects of radon, smoking, passive smoking, genetic, statistic and other factors do not result in more than 16 primary lung cancer incidences before an age of 40 years. As Sweden belongs to one of the countries of highest domestic radon levels, these numbers could be taken as the upper limit for the number of radon related lung cancer incidences in this age group.

Exposition of radon or any other risk factor at young ages could very well cause lung cancer after the age of 40 years, which is even probable, at least for those who are exposed at elderly ages, but for those the effects of smoking may be considerable and it will be difficult to separate the effects from smoking from the effects from radon.

Discussion

Comparison with Predictions from Case Control Studies

According to the Swedish authorities, about 500 primary lung cancer incidences per year are radon related in the Swedish population of about 9 million people. Totally there are about 3 000 primary lung cancer incidences per year. About 90 % of the cases, i.e. about 2700 cases are smokers in a total population with about 59 % smokers. Few incidences occur at an age less than 40 years.

Age Distribution, Follow up Time and Latency

The risk estimations for domestic radon have mainly been extrapolated from the risk estimations for radon among miners. For the miners the latency period was about 20 years. The risk seemed to decrease as the time since exposure increased.

There are several pretty large case control studies concerning domestic radon and lung cancer today. By pooling different studies together it has been possible to get good statistical power [12]. Most of the studies have considered follow-up times of 20 years in retrospect. In one of the studies, the Swedish nationwide [13], a follow-up time of 35 years in retrospect has been considered. Radon measurements were performed in all dwellings where the study person, either a case or a control, had lived during the time of follow up, i.e. the last 20 (or 35) years. A period of 20 years was considered to safely cover the latency period obtained from the epidemiological studies on lung cancer and miners.

There are however several reasons to question if 20 years of follow up is enough. Later results from studies in Hiroshima and Nagasaki [20] have found that there is still an excess in cancer risk 50 years and more after the atomic bombs over Hiroshima and Nagasaki. If this is the case, there could be lung cancer incidences initiated earlier than the follow-up period covers, which means that a greater number of the lung cancer incidences than taken into account in the study is radon related. It could also mean that a higher dose is needed for the lung cancer to occur.

The other reason is seen from figure 1, namely that there are very few cancer incidences at young ages. The lung cancer incidences start increasing after the age of 40 years. The age periods up to 40 years of age are of special interest since they cover mostly non smoking cases and controls. Children are commonly not smokers at least not in their younger ages.

The case control studies performed until now do not include the youngest age groups, not at least to any statistical power, since the incidences are so few. There is little information about what is the cause of these young lung cancer incidences and more information is needed. To what extent exposition at young ages contributes to the risk is thus not answered by the case control studies.

There are always more or less severe approximations in the case control studies. It is not practically possible to take all variables and all data into account. It is of special importance to cover the whole exposure history, which can be impossible if the exposure history and the latency period is long. The more simple ecological studies take the exposure history implicitly into account as long as most of the population stays in the region. It can be of great value to check the results from case control studies with data from ecological studies or other well known or easily available facts. It is informative to use different methods and use different viewpoints.

Smoking Habits

According to Swedish statistics, about 90% of the lung cancer cases are smokers. This is in consistence with the countrywide case control study, where 87% of the cases were smokers. It is difficult to get any good statistics about the smoking habits in the whole population over the years, but a good approximation would be to compare with the age adjusted controls in the same study. 59% of the controls were smokers. Many of the case control studies performed until now suffer from the fact that the smoking habits are not matched between the cases and controls. It is obvious that there is a mixing between radon related lung cancer and smoking related lung cancer. It would be of great value to perform case control studies with only non smokers included. In a recent study [21] consisting of 436 never-smoking lung cancer cases and 1649 never-smoking controls (with a follow-up time of 35 years in retrospect) a small effect of radon was only seen among those exposed to environmental tobacco smoke.

It is gratifying to experience that the EPA assessment of risks from radon in homes now acknowledges that there is a synergistic effect between radon and smoking [4]. Smoking seems to be an important factor for the radon related lung cancer cases. Reducing smoking would also reduce the radon related lung cancer cases.

Other Risk Factors

It should in this context be pointed out that there are also other risk factors to take into account as a cause of lung cancer, such as passive smoking, air pollution, occupational chemicals as well as genetic and statistical factors. Little attention has been paid to these factors. Smoking seems to be the by far most leading cause of primary lung cancer.

Effective Methods to Reduce Radon Related Lung Cancer Cases

Smoking is by far the main risk factor for primary lung cancer. Smoking seems also to play an important role for radon related lung cancer. There are many indications that radon related lung cancer is rare among non smokers. Reducing smoking reduces also the radon related lung cancer incidences.

Reducing smoking seems to be the most effective and also cheapest way to reduce most of the lung cancer incidences. It is possible to stop smoking completely but it is not possible to completely reduce radon. Radon is always there, to higher or lower levels. Remediation is not always successful and remediation actions are not always long lasting. The radon levels tend to increase after some time, depending on for example that new cracks appear in the buildings or that ventilation fans stop working. Remediation actions are often expensive. If the radon levels can be reduced by simple means, there is no reason to keep high levels. High levels of radon can be an indication that the ventilation is bad and that the air quality is generally bad.

Table 4. Age distribution of causes of death. 2001

Age at incidence	lung cancer	traffic accidents	suicide
0-4	0	7	0
5-′9	0	5	0
10-′14	0	10	5
15-19	2	58	22
20-24	4	71	55
25-29	4	54	56
30-34	1	35	77
35-39	5	52	98
40-44	34	36	99
45-49	85	40	114
50-54	162	40	135
55-59	334	49	113
60-64	407	32	92
65-69	484	19	71
70-74	563	37	68
75-79	521	30	73
80-84	311	37	59
85+	127	25	59

Comparison with other Known Risks in the Society

When talking about risks, it can be useful to compare different risks with each other. In table 4 the age dependence of deaths caused by primary lung cancer, traffic accidents and suicides in Sweden during the year 2001 [21] are listed. At young ages deaths from traffic accidents as well as from suicides exceed by far the lung cancer deaths whereas the opposite is true at higher ages. There is certainly a need for reducing the lung cancer incidences and most effectively it can be done by reducing the smoking habits.

Summary

The risk for primary lung cancer from radon seems to be overestimated. Although radon is considered the second leading risk factor for primary lung cancer, the risk from smoking is by far predominant. There is a need for seeing the proportions between the risks from radon and the risks from smoking. To stop smoking reduces the risk from smoking as well as from radon. Radon levels can be reduced, but never eliminated completely. These findings have lately been supported by more elaborate nation wide case control studies performed both in Europe [22] and in the United States [23]

References

[1] ICRP 65, Protection against radon-222 at home and at work, Recommendations of the International Commission on Radiological Protection, *Pergamon*, Oxford, 1994.

[2] BEIR VI, Biological Effects of Ionization Radiation VI, National Research Council, Health Effects of Exposure to Radon, *National Academy Press*, Washington DC, ISBN 0-309-05645-4. 1999.

[3] SOU 2001:7, Radon, Betänkande från Radonutredningen 2000, ISBN 91-38-21392-3. Fritzes Offentliga Publikationer. Stockholm, Sweden (In Swedish), 2001. See also www.ssi.se and "*Naturally Occurring Radioactivity in the Nordic Countries – Recommendations*", 2000, ISBN 91-89230-00-0, available from the Swedish Radiation Protection Authority, SSI, S-171 16 Stockholm, Sweden.

[4] EPA ASSESSMENT OF RISKS FROM RADON IN HOMES. (June 2003). Office of Radiation and Indoor Air, *United states Environmental Protection Agency*, Washington, DC 20460.

[5] Cohen B L 2001 Radon exposure and the risk of lung cancer *J. Radiol.* Prot. 21 64-66 and references cited therein.

[6] Lubin J H 1998 On the discrepancy between epidemiologic studies in individuals of lung cancer and residential radon and Cohen´s ecologic regression. *Health Phys.* 75 4-10.

[7] Lagarde F and Pershagen G 1999 Parallel analyses of individual and ecologic data on residential radon, cofactors and lung cancer in Sweden *Am.. J. Epidemiol.* 149 268-74.

[8] Cohen B Lagarde F and Pershagen G 2000 RE: Parallel analysis of individual and ecologic data on residential radon, cofactors, and lung cancer in Sweden *Am. J. Epidemiol.* 152 194-5.

[9] Darby S and Doll R 2000 Reply to comment on "Explaining the lung cancer versus radon exposure data for USA counties" *J. Radiol. Prot.* 20 221-2.

[10] Darby S, Deo H, Doll R and Whitley E 2001 A parallel analysis of individual and ecological data on residential radon and lung cancer in south-west England *J. R. Stat. Soc.* A 164 193-203.

[11] Field R W and Becker K 2001 Does exposure to residential radon increase the risk of lung cancer? *Radiat. Prot. Dosim.* 95 75-81.

[12] Lubin J and Boice J Jr 1997 Lung cancer risk from residential radon: meta-analysis of eight epidemiologic studies *J. Natl. Cancer Inst.* 89 49-57.

[13] Pershagen G, Åkerblom G, Axelson O, Clavensjö B, Damber L, Desai G, Enflo A, Lagarde F, Mellander H, Svartengren M and Swedjemark G-A 1994 New England *J. of Medicine* 330 159-64

[14] Swedish National Board of Health and Welfare, Cancer Incidences in Sweden 1984-2002, *Socialstyrelsen*, S-106 30 Stockholm, Sweden, see also www.sos.se

[15] UNSCEAR 2000, United nations scientific committee on the effect of atomic radiation, *Report to the General Assembly*, with Scientific Annexes, United Nations, New York.

[16] Swedjemark G-A and Mäkitalo A 1991 Distribution of radon in houses as a basis for radiological protection, *Radiation Protection Dosimetry* 36 125-8.

[17] Enflo A 1998 Where are the radon induced lung cancer cases? In J. Inaba, Y. Nakamura (Eds.) Comparative Evaluation of Environmental Toxicants, Kodansha Scientific, Tokyo, 1998, ISBN 4-906464-06-8, pp 291-2. *Supplement* pp. 151-6, ISBN 4-938987-05-8.

[18] Enflo A 2002 Where are the radon-induced lung cancer cases? Is it time for a re-evaluation of the radon problem? *International Congress Series* 1236 23-5.

[19] Enflo A 2002 Lung cancer risks from residential radon among smokers and non-smokers *J. Radiol. Prot.* 22 A95-A99.

[20] Preston D L, Shimizu Y, Pierce D A, Suyama A and Mabuchi K 2003 Studies of mortality of atomic bomb survivors. Report 13: Solid cancer and non cancer disease mortality: 1950-1997. *Radiation Res.* 160 381-407

[21] Swedish National Board of Health and Welfare, Causes of Death 2001, Socialstyrelsen, S-106 30 Stockholm, Sweden, see also *www.sos.se*

[22] Darby S et. al. 2006 Residential radon and lung cancer – detailed results of a collaborative analysis of individual data on 7148 persons with lung cancer and 14 208 persons without lung cancer from 13 epidemiologic studies in Europe. In Scand. J. Work Environ. Health 32 suppl. 1:1-84.

[23] Krewski D et. al. 2006 A combined analysis on North American case-control studies of residential radon and lung cancer. In Journal of Toxicology and Environmental Health, Part A, 69:533-597.

Index

B

C

D

E

F

G

H

I

J

K

L

N

O

P

Q

R

S

T

U

V

W

X

Y

Z